We live life the way we want.

Don't tell me what to do.

OLO

DYNAMICS OF
HEALTH CARE
IN SOCIETY
REVISED EDITION

Roxann DeLaet, RN, MS

Professor of Nursing
Sinclair Community College
Dayton, Ohio

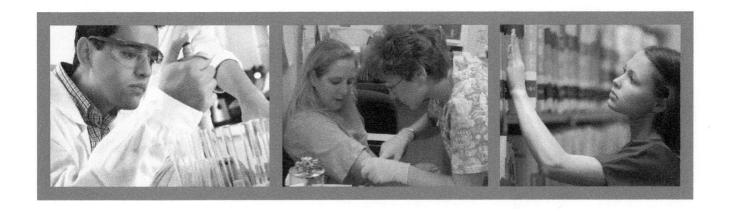

. Wolters Kluwer | Lippincott Williams & Wilkins
Health

Philadelphia · Baltimore · New York · London
Buenos Aires · Hong Kong · Sydney · Tokyo

Supervisor, Custom Solutions: Heather A. Rybacki
Executive Editor: David Troy
Creative Director: Doug Smock
Manufacturing Director: Phillip Lee
Prepress Vendor: S4Carlisle Publishing Services

Acknowledgments

Dynamics of Health Care in Society is an introductory textbook derived from key titles in the Lippincott Williams & Wilkins | Wolters Kluwer Health library. Chapters 1 through 20, the appendices, and the glossary are from the following textbook:

Introduction to Health Care and Careers
Roxann DeLaet, RN, MS
Professor of Nursing
Sinclair Community College
Dayton, OH
ISBN: 978-1-58255-900-1

Chapter 21 is from the following textbook:
The Ethical Component of Nursing Education:
Integrating Ethics Into Clinical Experience
Marcia Sue DeWolf Bosek, DNSc, RN
Associate Professor
Department of Adult Health Nursing
Rush University College of Nursing
Program of Ethics, Department of Religion, Health & Human Values
Rush University College of Health Sciences
Chicago, Illinois

Teresa A. Savage, PhD, RN
Assistant Professor-Research
Maternal-Child Nursing, College of Nursing
University of Illinois at Chicago
Associate Director
Donnelley Family Disability Ethics Program
Rehabilitation Institute of Chicago
Chicago, Illinois
ISBN: 978-0-7817-4877-3

Chapter 22 stems from the following textbook:
Nursing in Today's World:
Trends, Issues, & Management, Tenth Edition
Janice Rider Ellis, PhD, RN, ANEF
Professor Emeritus and Nursing Education Consultant
Shoreline Community College
Seattle, Washington

Celia Love Hartley, MN, RN, ANEF
Professor Emerita
College of the Desert
Palm Desert, California
Curriculum Consultant
Camano Island, Washington

Illustrations by Tomm Scalera
ISBN: 978-16054-7707-7

Contents

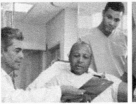
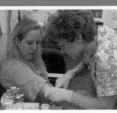
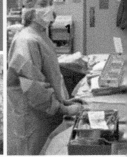

Today's Health Care System

CHAPTER OBJECTIVES

After careful study of this chapter, you should be able to:

* Recognize the importance of major health care events throughout the ages.

* Identify major health care facilities and the purpose of each.

* Describe five types of health care professionals and their roles.

* List four trends that influence health care.

KEY TERMS

acute care facility
assisted-living facility
complementary therapies
extended care facility
general practitioner
Hippocratic Oath
  (hip-ə-KRAT-ik ōth)

home health care
homeopathy
  (hō-mē-OP-ǎ-thē)
hospice (HOS-pis)
independent-living facility
inpatient

interdisciplinary team
microbiology
outpatient
pandemic (pan-DEM-ik)
prognosis (prog-NO-sis)
rehabilitation centers

sphygmomanometer
  (sfig-mō-ma-NOM-ə-
  ter)
stethoscope (STETH-ō-
  skōp)
subacute care facility

The practice of medicine and the health care system as we know them today are the result of the long evolution of human knowledge over the centuries. Health care facilities, as well as practitioner roles and responsibilities, have developed over time too. Health care will continue to evolve as research and other influences contribute to growth and development.

HEALTH CARE PAST AND PRESENT

Many forces have shaped our present health care. From the most primitive care of prehistoric times to space-age advances, many influences helped shape today's health care system. Many of those forces have had a significant impact on health care over the years. Understanding the past helps us understand the present.

Health Care Through the Ages

Health care is continually evolving. From medical research to technology, new developments in health care occur almost daily. In addition, institutions such as hospitals and the government have played major roles in the evolution of health care. As health care evolves, so do health concerns. For example, obesity, which was

Health Care Through the Centuries

0–3000 BC

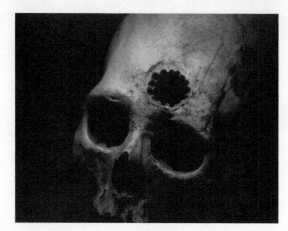

Procedure called trepanning is used to treat headaches, epilepsy, and insanity. Many believe these conditions are caused by evil spirits, so holes are drilled into a patient's skull in order to release the demons.

2600 BC

Egyptian physician Imhotep is credited with writing the Edwin Smith Papyrus. References to more than 90 anatomical terms and 48 injuries are found in this ancient medical text. The first reference to blood circulating around the body in a constant stream is recorded in *The Theory of the Body's Interior* by Chinese Emperor Huang-Ti.

1000 BC

First published work describing over 3,000 symptoms and their outcomes (*Treatise of Medical Diagnosis and Prognosis*) is published in Babylon.

600 BC

Indian doctor Sushruta, considered by many to be the father of Indian surgery, performs the first plastic surgery. He also provides a detailed description of rhinoplasty (nasal surgery).

460 BC–370 BC

Greek physician Hippocrates, widely considered to be the father of medicine, bases his medical beliefs on the theory of humorism. Humorism is the idea that the body is filled with four basic substances: yellow bile, black bile, blood, and phlegm. Hippocrates believes that illnesses are caused by an imbalance in these substances.

910

Persian physician Al-Razi details signs and symptoms of smallpox and measles.

1590

Zacharias Janssen, a spectacle maker from Holland, invents the microscope.

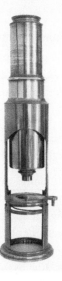

Health Care Through the Centuries

1628   English physician William Harvey publishes an explanation of how blood pumps from the heart, through the body, and then returns to the heart. This work, titled *An Anatomical Study of the Motion of the Heart and of the Blood in Animals*, forms the basis for future research on blood vessels, arteries, and the heart.

1800   British chemist and inventor Sir Humphry Davy recommends the use of nitrous oxide (laughing gas) as anesthesia in minor surgeries.

1816   French physician Rene Laënnec invents the stethoscope.

1853   French physician Charles Gabriel Pravaz and British physician Alexander Wood develop the syringe for drug administration.

1870   Robert Koch and Louis Pasteur establish the germ theory of disease.

1895   German-born physicist Wilhelm Conrad Roentgen produces the first x-ray image.

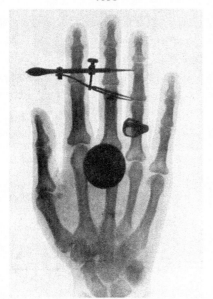

1941   Austrian physician Karl Dussik publishes a paper on the use of ultrasound as a diagnostic device.

1950   Canadian electrical engineer John Hopps develops the first cardiac pacemaker.

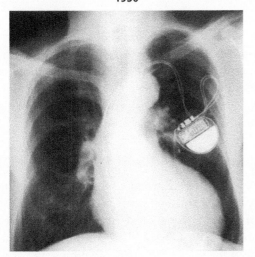

(continued)

1952

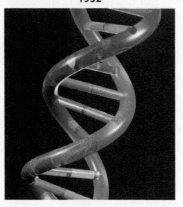

English molecular biologist Rosalind Franklin studies DNA (deoxyribonucleic acid) structure using x-ray diffraction.

1953   American molecular biologist James Watson and British graduate student/researcher Francis Crick uncover the code that identifies the structure of the DNA molecule.

1975   American physicist and radiologist Robert S. Ledley develops the first CT scanner.

1984   British geneticist Alec Jeffreys develops DNA fingerprinting.

1996   British embryologist and genetic engineer Ian Wilmut completes the first successful cloning experiment from a single mammary cell, producing Dolly the sheep.

2003   The Human Genome Project, a project coordinated by the U.S. Department of Energy and the National Institutes of Health, completes the mapping of the human genome.

once considered a sign of wealth and social status, is now regarded as a disease.

As the health care system has advanced in form and complexity, so has growth in personnel and tasks. While there are currently hundreds of health-associated careers to choose from, most health care professionals before the 1900s were in one of three categories: physician, dentist, or nurse. Health care career choices were more limited in the past.

Prehistoric Times (circa 8000 BC—3000 BC)

Although disease has always existed, early people were spared from many of the worst diseases, such as measles and smallpox. These diseases did not spread as easily through prehistoric tribes because of small communities and nomadic lifestyles. As civilizations advanced, so did their understanding of the human body and its functions. However, most medicine remained rooted in religious or spiritual beliefs throughout prehistoric times.

Ancient Times (circa 3000 BC—500 AD)

In ancient times, Egyptian medicine was considered highly advanced. Although religion prohibited the dissection of a body, Egyptians had some basic knowledge of the human anatomy. They also documented ideas that were advanced for their time, such as washing and shaving a

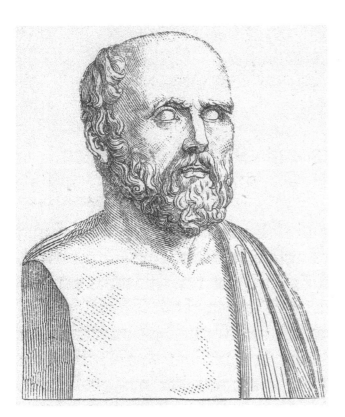

Figure 1-1 It's believed that Hippocrates wrote the Hippocratic Oath in the 4th or 5th century BC.

body before surgery. Their medical processes influenced Greek medical practices in this period.

An important figure in early Greek medicine was Hippocrates of Cos. Hippocrates rejected the idea that illnesses were caused by supernatural forces. Instead, he emphasized prognosis. Prognosis is a medical opinion about the likely outcome of a condition or disease. Hippocrates and some of his followers wrote a collection of early medical works known as the Hippocratic Corpus. Included in this collection are textbooks, lectures, research, notes, and essays on various medical subjects. One of the most famous works is the Hippocratic Oath, which serves as the moral basis for many medical regulations and guidelines still in use today. Figure 1-1 shows how Hippocrates may have looked when he was alive more than 2,000 years ago.

During this time period, Roman medicine used many Greek ideas. However, Roman medicine put more emphasis on preventive health care. Public health was encouraged by the Roman government. Structures were built to help pipe water in to cities, and sewage systems were constructed to remove waste from larger cities. Romans developed the first hospitals, which were used primarily for the military, as places where patients could stay until they had recovered fully. They also introduced the idea of medical specialists.

Medieval Times (circa 500 AD—1300 AD)

The fall of the Roman Empire suspended medical progress. Many religions taught that disease and illness were sent as punishments. Some believed that only God could heal, so they considered medicine an unsuitable profession for Christians. Many healers, such as nurses, midwives, and dentists, performed various medical tasks during this period. However, unlike physicians, most healers only practiced their trade part-time and weren't considered professionals.

A significant work produced during this period was the Canon of Medicine, written by Persian physician Avicenna. Influenced by a combination of sources, including Roman, Persian, Indian, and medieval Islamic medicine, Avicenna's Canon of Medicine explained the causes of many common diseases and set a new standard for medical practice throughout much of Europe and Asia.

The Renaissance (circa 1300 AD—1600 AD)

At the beginning of the Renaissance, many Western Europeans were living in unsanitary conditions that allowed the spread of plagues and other contagious diseases. These conditions led to one of the deadliest disease outbreaks in history—the spread of a highly contagious disease called the bubonic plague. Often referred to as Black Death, the bubonic plague became a pandemic—an infectious disease that affects entire continents or even the world. It caused the deaths of over half of the European population.

Following this tragedy, the 14th century had a renewed interest in the study of medicine. Greek and Roman medical texts were translated during this period, and many advances were made in science and research. For example, detailed studies were made of human anatomy. Andreas Vesalius was a physician who revealed detailed information on the human body through dissection. His writings and illustrations were published as the first comprehensive book of anatomy (Figure 1-2, following page). This information spread widely with the invention of the printing press.

This period also brought the establishment of the first medical universities. Some societies began requiring that a person have several years of training in order to qualify as a doctor of medicine. An unfortunate result of the stricter requirements was a smaller number of qualified physicians.

Modern Times (circa 1600 AD—present)

The last few centuries have produced significant medical developments. The 17th century brought improvements in surgical procedures and a better understanding of the circulatory system, digestive system, and respiratory system. The invention of the microscope allowed scientists

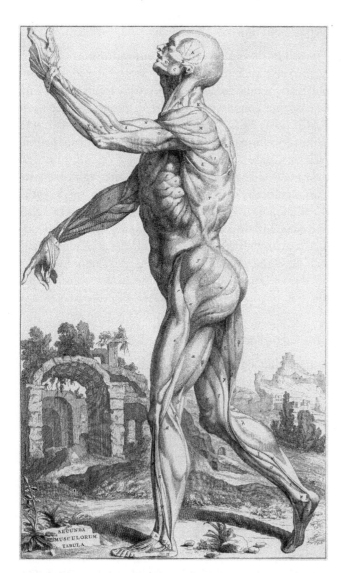

Figure 1-2 Anatomical drawings from Andreas Vesalius' book *On the Fabric of the Human Body* were shown in lifelike poses.

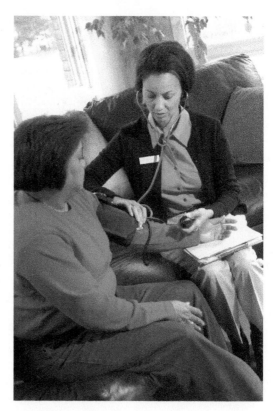

Figure 1-3 A sphygmomanometer is used in conjunction with a stethoscope to measure blood pressure.

to view previously unknown organisms. The development of the mercury thermometer allowed for the first accurate body temperature readings. The stethoscope let doctors listen to the internal sounds of a patient. Although several different methods were developed for measuring blood pressure during this period, the first sphygmomanometer (commonly referred to as a blood pressure cuff) didn't become a widely used diagnostic device until the early 1900s (Figure 1-3). These medical innovations remain important diagnostic tools today and are used by many different professionals.

Scientific and Technological Advances

Many scientific developments have occurred over the past few centuries. Advances ranging from improved medica-

tions to new diagnostic devices have brought significant improvements to all areas of health care.

Medication and Vaccinations

Infectious diseases were common killers as recently as 200 years ago. An English doctor named Edward Jenner found that a person who was inoculated, or treated, with a small amount of cowpox would be immune to smallpox. He called this material *vaccine* and gave the first successful smallpox inoculation in 1796. In 1798, Jenner coined the term *vaccination*. Despite early resistance, this process was eventually performed throughout the world. The World Health Organization (WHO) declared the smallpox virus eradicated, or completely eliminated, in 1972.

While studying microorganisms, a 19th century French chemist named Louis Pasteur developed the germ theory of disease—the theory that most infectious diseases are caused by germs. This theory laid the groundwork for large scale brewing of beer, wine-making, pasteurization, and antiseptic operations. It also led to a better understanding of the nature of contagious diseases. Through his research, Pasteur produced vaccinations to immunize against anthrax and rabies.

A German physician named Robert Koch also studied microorganisms in the late 19th century. Koch researched

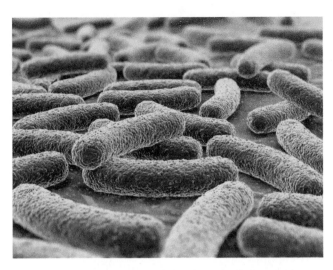

The work of 19th century scientists led to the study of microorganisms and our current understanding of bacteria and germs.

diseases such as anthrax and cholera. In 1905, he was awarded a Nobel Prize for his discoveries relating to tuberculosis. Pasteur and Koch are considered the founders of microbiology, the branch of biology that studies microorganisms and their effects on humans. Their studies led to the understanding that infectious diseases were caused by certain bacteria and germs.

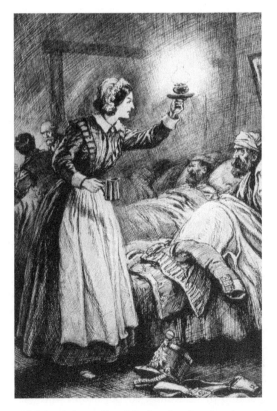

Florence Nightingale is considered the founder of modern day nursing.

Hygiene and Sanitation

Prior to the mid-1800s, few improvements were made in hygiene and sanitation in medicine. Florence Nightingale, an English woman, was a main force behind reform. Considered the founder of modern day nursing, Nightingale worked in a military hospital during the Crimean War. She improved standards of hygiene and sanitation, which dramatically reduced infections. After the war, she returned to England and began campaigning to improve the quality of nursing in military hospitals. Nightingale set the foundations of hospital design and nursing practice that are still in use today.

Military Actions

Military actions have always had a major effect on both innovation and delivery of health care. The first surgical procedures were undertaken during one of the French wars. The Mobile Army Surgical Hospital (MASH) was first used in combat during the Korean War. The use of helicopter ambulances in the Korean and Vietnam wars greatly reduced the time required to transport casualties to a hospital. Innovations in military medical procedures have significantly increased the number of lives saved in both war and peacetime.

Space Program

Research to support astronauts in the space program has led to important new medical technologies. A nonsurgical alternative to balloon angioplasty was derived from NASA-pioneered technology. The CT (computerized tomography) scan and the MRI (magnetic resonance imaging) are two of the most widely used body imaging techniques. The technology for both of these began with digital imaging developments for the Apollo moon landing program. The electron microscope, nuclear medicine, and life support techniques are just a few of the medical advances attributed to the space program. Researchers are currently using a process developed by NASA to analyze human chromosomes. Technology developed from this research could lead to disease prediction in infants.

Health Care Today

As a result of new technologies and medical advances, the U.S. has one of the most advanced health care systems in the world. Growth in the health care system has created new roles for health care professionals. The area of radiological technology is a perfect example. A single x-ray technician once performed all imaging procedures. Today a radiology department typically employs several highly trained professionals: a radiographer who takes the x-ray; a nuclear medicine technologist who uses radioactive materials to make an image; an ultrasound technologist who uses sounds waves to produce an image; a radiation therapist who uses radiation to treat cancer; and CT and MRI technologists who use computers to produce a sectional image of the patient.

This is a common theme in all areas of health care. From management to diagnostics, new careers have arisen to meet the needs of an evolving system. Several factors contribute to continuing growth in the industry. Innovative medical technology, an aging population, and longer life expectancies are some of the top reasons for our expanding system.

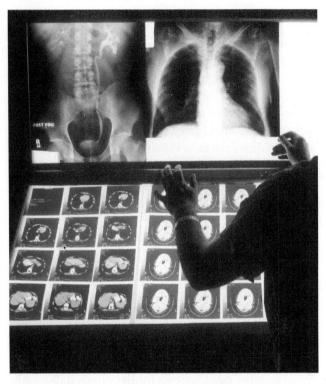

Though x-rays are still a major part of radiology, the field now also includes nuclear medicine technology, ultrasound technology, radiation therapy, and CT and MRI technology.

✔ CHECK POINT

1 How did Romans emphasize preventive health care in ancient times?

2 What are some significant medical innovations from the past few centuries that remain important diagnostic tools in today's health care system?

HEALTH CARE FACILITIES

Health care in the U.S. is available through a variety of facilities. Typically, only patients who require complex surgery or who are seriously injured need full hospital services. Most health care services are provided in settings other than a hospital.

As described below, subacute and extended care facilities offer care for patients who no longer require hospitalization, yet still need 24-hour care and supervision. Home health care agencies deliver medical care directly to patients who are either unable or unwilling to leave their homes. Many other health care facilities offer specialized care, such as rehabilitation, mental health evaluation and treatment, and hospice.

Patients in health care facilities are typically classified as either inpatients or outpatients. A person who remains in an acute care facility, such as a hospital, for more than 24-hours is considered an inpatient. Those who require health care but don't need to stay in a facility may receive outpatient care. An outpatient is one who is discharged within 23 hours, but may require ongoing treatment, care, and education.

Hospitals

Hospitals care for patients who have extremely serious, severe, or painful conditions that require immediate medical attention. This is known as *acute care*. Patients in hospitals are often people who are too ill to care for themselves at home, who are severely injured, or who require surgery or complicated treatments. In addition, many women deliver their babies in hospitals.

Traditionally, people who were admitted to a hospital weren't discharged until they either recovered fully or had used all of the hospital's available services. This policy has changed over the years with the rise of nontraditional care facilities, changing health care reimbursement practices, and federal regulations. The average length of stay in a hospital is now only 4.8 days. Because patients are discharged earlier, most hospitals focus on the most critical needs of the patient.

Hospitals are classified as public or private, and as for-profit or nonprofit. Public hospitals, which are nonprofit institutions, are financed and operated by local, state, or national agencies. Nonprofit institutions receive tax exemptions and must provide community benefit. One example of community benefit is uncompensated care, whereby services are provided at little or no cost to patients who do not have health insurance or the money to pay for services. Instead, tax revenue or public funds cover the cost. For-profit institutions, on the other hand, do not receive tax exemptions and are not required to provide community benefit. Private hospitals may be for-profit or nonprofit and are operated by churches, corporations, and charitable organizations.

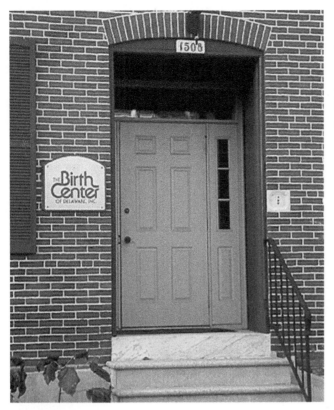

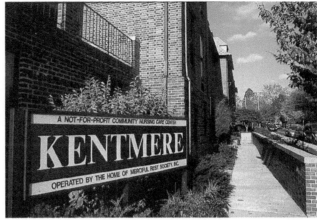

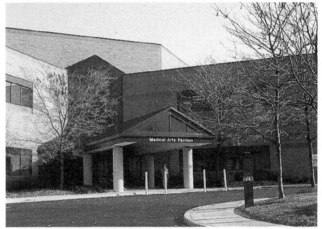

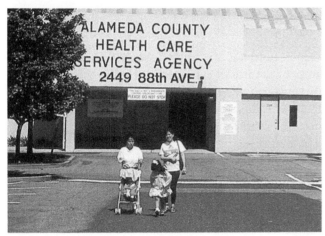

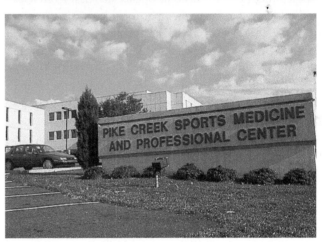

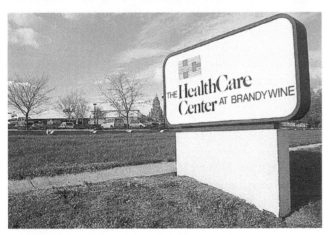

Several types of health care facilities.

Subacute Care Facilities

A relatively new and rapidly growing service in the U.S. is subacute care. A subacute care facility cares for a variety of patients with complex medical and rehabilitative needs. These facilities fill the gap between hospitalization and rehabilitation (therapy to restore patients to health or normal life). Subacute care patients are stable enough that they don't need acute care, yet they need more complex treatment than can be found in a nursing or rehabilitation facility. Extensive monitoring and intravenous therapy (giving fluids or medications through a needle or tube into a vein) often is required. Supervision is provided around the clock by personnel with acute care experience.

Many subacute centers are based in or near a nursing center or hospital. Technologically advanced equipment and specialized therapeutic treatments are available. Subacute care is typically 20 to 50 percent less expensive than similar care provided in a hospital.

Extended Care Facilities

Extended care facilities provide health care and help with the activities of daily living to people of any age. These people often are physically or mentally unable to care for themselves. This type of care may last from days to years. Extended care facilities include nursing homes and residential institutions for mentally or physically disabled patients. Independent-living and assisted-living facilities also offer extended care.

The number of extended care facilities has greatly increased in recent years. One reason for this is that many patients are discharged from the hospital earlier in their recovery period and require care that is beyond the scope of home care. Another reason is that many older adults cannot carry out the activities of daily living by themselves.

A new concept in extended care is called "aging in place." This type of care allows patients to remain in their own homes as long as they're able to care for themselves. Services such as home remodeling, communication and monitoring systems, and in-home care provide support for patients who want to preserve their independence.

An independent-living facility is often a group of apartments or houses for residents who can take care of themselves and are mobile, yet need some help with daily activities. Some independent-living facilities offer on-site amenities, such as a fitness club, banking center, and health care services, as well as local transportation. Meals and planned social activities also may be offered in a community setting.

An assisted-living facility generally provides housing, group meals, personal care, support services, and social activities in a community setting. Some health care also may be provided. Costs vary from around $1,000 up to $3,000 a month or more. Some states pay for personal care services for those with limited incomes.

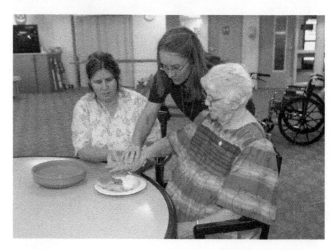

Extended care facilities included assisted-living facilities, which provide services and care for elderly patients who need help with activities of daily living.

Home Health Care Agencies

Home health care is one of the most rapidly growing areas of the health care system. Home health care, or care in a patient's home, may be provided through community health departments, visiting nurses' associations, hospital-based case managers, and home health agencies. These agencies provide many different health-related services, including assessment by nurses, teaching and support of patients and family members, and direct care for patients.

The growth of home health care is the result of several factors: (1) Health care reimbursement practices often encourage early discharge from the hospital, so patients may need skilled care at home. (2) Increasing numbers of older people are living longer with chronic illnesses (illnesses that last for a long time or often recur). (3) Sophisticated technology allows people to live and be relatively comfortable in their own homes.

Rehabilitation Centers

Rehabilitation centers specialize in services for patients needing physical or emotional rehabilitation or treatment of chemical dependency (addiction to a chemical substance, such as alcohol or drugs). These centers may be associated with a hospital or may provide services as an independent agency.

The goal of the rehabilitation centers is to return patients to the community as independent members of society who are in optimal health. They often use a team of physicians, nurses, physical therapists, occupational therapists, and counselors to meet the needs of patients.

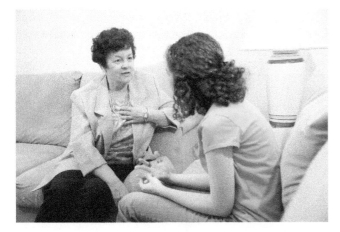

Rehabilitation may include emotional, as well as physical, therapy.

Mental Health Facilities

Mental health facilities may be either independent or associated with a hospital. They provide services for people in crisis or those needing long-term counseling. Patients receive outpatient care, including individual and group counseling, medications, and assistance with independent living.

Crisis intervention centers are also mental health centers. They typically provide 24-hour services and hotlines for people who are suicidal, abusing drugs or alcohol, or in abusive situations. These centers also provide information and services for victims of rape and abuse.

Hospice

Hospice is a care program focused on reducing pain, symptoms, and stress during the last stage of terminal illnesses. Physical, psychological, social, and spiritual care services are provided for dying persons, their families, and other loved ones. This care is provided most often in the home, but some hospitals also have hospice services. A hospice program is defined by the care it provides rather than its location.

Volunteer Agencies

Community agencies are often nonprofit voluntary agencies. These agencies are financed by private donations, grants, or fundraisers (although some may charge minimal fees).

Examples of volunteer agencies are the American Heart Association and the American Lung Association. Physicians and nurses are often active members of these organizations and provide health screenings and educational programs.

Another nonprofit voluntary community agency is Meals on Wheels. This agency and others like it provide meals and other nutritional services to older adults and homebound and disabled people who may go hungry otherwise. The purchase and delivery of meals is made possible through fundraising and community involvement.

✓ CHECK POINT

3 Why has home health care grown rapidly in recent years?

4 Describe some basic differences in extended care, independent-living, and assisted-living facilities.

HEALTH CARE PROFESSIONALS

In the modern health care system, care is provided by a diverse interdisciplinary team of professionals. This means that health care professionals with varied medical educations, backgrounds, and experiences work together to deliver the best possible care for each patient. Professionals in patient care, diagnostics, and health information fields are an integral part of this team. This section introduces health care professions. Specific health care professions will be described in more detail in Part IV.

Patient Care Professionals

For those who are interested in patient care, there are several career options. Different levels of care are provided by a variety of professionals in cooperation with traditional physicians and nurses. Medical assistants, physician assistants, surgical technologists, EMTs/paramedics, licensed practical nurses, and certified nursing assistants/ nurse assistants are all involved in direct patient care. Although the duties and educational requirements vary, professionals in this health care area share a common, and essential, interest in patient care.

Medical assistants (MA) and physician assistants (PA) are trained to assist physicians or other medical providers in clinical or administrative procedures. A licensed practical nurse (LPN) provides routine patient care under the direction of a registered nurse (RN) or physician. A certified nurse assistant (CNA) assists patients with daily health care needs and also may perform basic nursing procedures under the supervision of an RN.

Surgical technologists assist with surgical operations. An emergency medical technician (EMT) or paramedic is trained to perform emergency medical procedures.

Educational requirements for patient care professionals such as those previously mentioned range from 1 to 2 years of specialized training to an associate's or bachelor's degree. In addition to their initial training and education, many of these health care providers must be recertified annually.

Laboratory and Pharmacy Professionals

For those whose interests lean more toward the scientific side of health care, a laboratory or pharmacy career is worth looking into. Educational requirements in these fields range from 1 to 2 years of specialized training to a bachelor's, master's, or even a doctoral degree.

Laboratory and pharmacy professionals perform many duties. Laboratory jobs range from cleaning and maintaining laboratory equipment to conducting laboratory tests on tissues, fluids, and cells under the supervision of a pathologist. Some professionals may specialize in a particular laboratory field. For example, cardiovascular technicians perform diagnostic tests related to the heart, and phlebotomists collect blood samples for testing or transfusions. A pharmacy technician performs various pharmacy-related functions under the supervision of a licensed pharmacist.

Diagnostic and Imaging Professionals

Some diagnostic and imaging professionals work directly with patients. For example, diagnostic medical sonographers perform ultrasound tests on patients to help physicians detect and diagnose various conditions. Other diagnostic professionals work behind the scenes. For example, clinical laboratory technologists work in laboratories, performing tests on tissue, blood, and other body fluids that aid physicians in diagnosing and treating patients.

The level of education required for careers in this field ranges from 1 to 2 years of specialized training to a bachelor's or master's degree. With ongoing advances in the areas of diagnostics and imaging, careers in this field are continually evolving.

Therapy and Rehabilitation Professionals

Therapy and rehabilitation professionals assist patients with a variety of physical and work-related issues. In addition to restoring health, they also educate patients on practices that reduce the likelihood of future injuries.

Professionals in this area often specialize in a field, such as occupational, physical, rehabilitation, speech, or massage therapy. In many of these careers, therapy involves personal contact with a patient over weeks or even months, so good interpersonal skills are essential. Educational requirements vary by field, but range from accreditation to an associate's, bachelor's, master's, or doctoral degree.

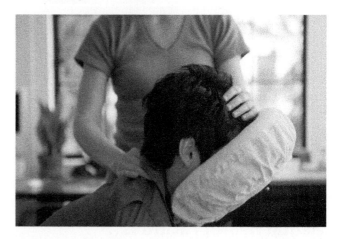

Massage therapy is one specialty within the field of rehabilitation.

Health Information and Administration Professionals

Professionals in the health information and administration area are responsible for managing medical, billing, insurance, legal, and governmental information. Medical records technicians, health information technicians, coding specialists, and medical transcriptionists are all part of this growing area.

Educational requirements in these fields range from 1 to 2 years of specialized training to an associate's or bachelor's degree. Computer skills are an essential requirement for anyone entering the health information field.

CHECK POINT

5 Briefly explain the idea behind the term "interdisciplinary team."

HEALTH CARE TRENDS

Health care has evolved to meet the needs of societies throughout the ages, and it continues to do so today. As our population ages, the need for medical advances becomes more urgent, and more and more attention is being focused on wellness and disease prevention. Holistic approaches to health care, which involve treating the whole person, not just the physical body, have become more popular. Therapies from a variety of cultures, including Indian and Chinese medicine, have become more mainstream and are being combined with Western medical practices. In addition, more and more health care professionals are specializing in the care of specific diseases or ailments. Trends like these are influencing and shaping today's health care.

Aging of the Population

Thanks in large part to scientific advances, people are living longer, more productive lives. This has led to a growing population of older adults, with many facing chronic health problems. This, in turn, has brought about a greater demand for health care providers—a trend that will only grow in the coming years.

According to U.S. Census Bureau projections, a substantial increase in the number of older people will occur when the Baby Boom generation (people born between 1946 and 1964) begins to turn 65 in 2011. The older population (people aged 65 and older) is projected to double from 36 million in 2003 to 72 million in 2030, and to increase from 12 percent to 20 percent of the population in the same time frame. By 2050, the older population is projected to number 86.7 million.

Wellness and Prevention

Today, more people are taking a proactive approach to their own health care, and more health care professionals are shifting their focus from treatment to wellness and prevention. Medical professionals know that simple changes in a person's behavior can bring about positive health benefits. A balanced diet, exercise, and stopping smoking are all changes that promote a person's health and prevent disease. Health care professionals also know that early detection is the key to fighting many diseases, such as heart disease and cancer. Routine examinations, like blood pressure and cholesterol screenings, Pap smears, and breast self-exams, save lives.

Complementary Therapies

Complementary therapies that use holistic methods also can improve a person's health. Sometimes referred to as alternative medicine, these therapies typically promote healing through nutrition, exercise, or relaxation. Many complementary therapies are culturally based, such as yoga and meditation. Others are more closely related to

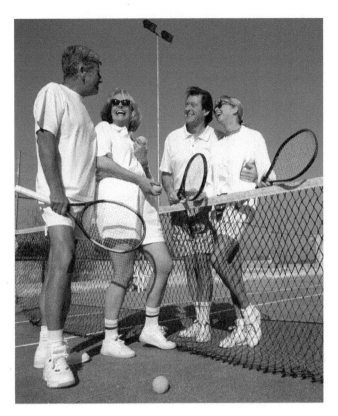

Getting enough exercise is one important way to maintain wellness and prevent disease.

conventional medical techniques, including chiropractic medicine and massage therapy.

Homeopathy is a holistic system of healing that focuses on stimulating the body's ability to heal itself by giving very small doses of highly diluted substances. Homeopathy is based on the *principle of similars* (or "like cures like"), which states that a disease can be cured by a substance that produces similar symptoms in healthy people. In other words, if a substance could cause disease symptoms in a healthy person, small amounts may cure a sick person who has similar symptoms. Homeopathic remedies are derived from diluted natural substances. Treatments are highly individualized, so patients with the same condition often receive different treatments.

Many Eastern-oriented therapies, such as acupuncture and aromatherapy, are designed to promote balance, peace, harmony, and relaxation. In *acupuncture*, needles are inserted through the skin at certain points to treat diseases or relieve pain. In *aromatherapy*, the face and body are massaged with oils made from herbs, flowers, and fruits. These treatments reduce anxiety and muscle tension, which helps relieve common aches and pains. More restful sleep, a boosted immune system, and an overall sense of well-being are just a few of the benefits from these treatments.

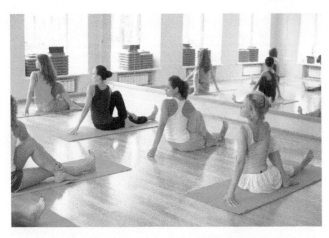

Yoga is a culturally-based therapy that has gained popularity in the U.S.

Chiropractic medicine uses adjustments of body structures (usually the spine) to promote healing. Chiropractic diagnosis typically is made by examining a person's health history, along with a physical exam and x-rays, if necessary. Treatment is administered by a licensed chiropractor, generally on an outpatient basis.

Health Care Specialization

Expanded health care research has led to much new technology and knowledge. Because many health care providers can no longer keep up with all the advances being made in all areas, specialization in smaller areas has become almost the rule rather than the exception.

Not too long ago, the only health care professional most people came in contact with was a general practitioner, a physician who diagnoses and treats a variety of common health problems. However, in today's world, a patient who needs diagnosis and treatment for a more complex problem usually is referred to a specialist. For example, a patient with a heart condition may be cared for by the family physician (general practitioner) or a cardiologist (a physician who specializes in heart problems).

Hospitalized patients come in contact with many different health care providers (such as registered nurses, physician assistants, respiratory therapists, pharmacists, dieticians, physical therapists, and students), and they also may be seen by other specialists who are called in for consultation or to do surgery. This fragmentation of care can cause patients to become confused about their care and treatments. It also can lead to a loss of continuity of care, resulting in conflicting plans of care, too much or too little medication, and higher health care costs. In today's expanding health care system, professionals need to make a concerted effort to remain focused on the needs of each individual patient. Part of your future role—especially if you will be engaged in direct patient care—is to help "humanize" each patient's health care experience by giving individualized care that focuses on the specific needs and circumstances of each patient.

✓ **CHECK POINT**

6 List a few of the health care trends discussed in this section and their effects on health care careers.

Don't forget to visit thePoint companion website for additional study resources!

CHAPTER HIGHLIGHTS

- Greek and Roman influences laid much of the foundation for modern health care.
- A better understanding of germs and disease made the discovery of several life-saving medications and vaccines possible.
- There are many different types of health care facilities. Hospitals provide acute care for patients suffering from conditions that require immediate medical attention. Subacute care facilities fill the gap between hospitals and rehabilitation facilities. Extended care facilities provide a variety of services to help with daily living and health care. Rehabilitation centers specialize in services for patients needing physical or emotional rehabilitation or treatment for chemical dependency. Mental health facilities provide services for people in crisis and those needing long-term counseling. Hospice programs focus on reducing pain, symptoms, and stress during the last stage of a terminal illness.
- Volunteer agencies are often financed through private donations, grants, or fundraisers and provide services such as health screenings, educational programs, meals, and local transportation.
- Professionals with varied medical educations, backgrounds, and experiences work together as an interdisciplinary team to deliver the best possible care for each patient.
- Complementary therapies, which are often culturally based, promote healing through nutrition, exercise, or relaxation.
- Increasing medical advances and information has led to a significant growth in health care specialization.

REVIEW QUESTIONS

Matching

1. _____ Most medicine was rooted in religious or spiritual beliefs during this period, and disease did not spread easily.
2. _____ Egyptian medicine was considered highly advanced during this period.
3. _____ The fall of the Roman Empire suspended medical progress during this period.
4. _____ The first medical universities were established during this period.
5. _____ The microscope was invented during this period, allowing scientists to view previously undetected organisms.

   a. Ancient times   **b.** Renaissance   **c.** Prehistoric times   **d.** Modern times
   e. Medieval times

Multiple Choice

6. This is the study of microorganisms.
   a. germ theory   **c.** microbiology
   b. dissection   **d.** anatomy

7. Patients who require health care but don't need to remain in a facility for more than 24 hours may receive this type of care.
   a. outpatient   **c.** subacute
   b. inpatient   **d.** independent-living

8. These health care professionals are trained to assist physicians or other medical providers in clinical or administrative procedures.
   a. medical assistants
   b. physician assistants
   c. surgical technologists
   d. both A and B

9. This health care professional provides direct patient care under the direction of a registered nurse (RN) or physician.
   a. emergency medical technician (EMT)
   b. phlebotomist
   c. coding specialist
   d. licensed practical nurse (LPN)

10. These therapies, sometimes referred to as alternative medicine, promote healing through nutrition, exercise, or relaxation.
    a. physical
    b. complementary
    c. occupational
    d. radiation

Completion

11. Obesity was once regarded as a sign of wealth and social status, but today is considered a/an _____.

12. _____ is a medical opinion about the likely outcome of a condition or disease.

13. A person who remains in an acute care facility, such as a hospital, for more than 24 hours is considered a/an _____.

14. _____ provides care for dying persons, their families, and other loved ones.

15. _____ skills are an essential requirement for anyone entering the health information field.

Short Answer

16. Hippocrates dismissed the idea that illnesses were caused by supernatural forces. Instead, what idea did he emphasize? Explain.

    _____

    _____

17. What important role did Florence Nightingale play in medical history?

    _____

    _____

18. What is the goal of a rehabilitation center?

    _____

    _____

19. Name at least three fields that therapy or rehabilitation specialists may specialize in.

    _____

    _____

20. Why is specialization becoming more prevalent in health care?

    _____

    _____

INVESTIGATE IT

1. Thanks to the efforts of medical professionals over the past few decades, many highly contagious diseases, such as smallpox and bubonic plague, have been eradicated through research, education, and immunization. Are medical researchers currently working toward the eradication of any other contagious diseases? Search the Internet and other available resources to find information about recent medical discoveries or advances that may wipe out other contagious diseases. Use the search term *medical discoveries contagious diseases* to begin your Internet search.

2. This chapter provided a brief look at just a few of the medical technologies made possible through the space program. Search the Internet and other available resources to find other medical advances made possible by this program. Use the search term *space program medical advances* to begin your Internet search.

RECOMMENDED READING

Association of the British Pharmaceutical Industry. *History of Medicine.* Available at http://www. abpischools.org.uk/res/coResourceImport/resources04/history/history2.cfm.

Bureau of Labor and Statistics. *Occupational Outlook Handbook, 2008–2009 Edition.* Available at http://www.bls.gov/oco/oco2003.htm.

Crystal, Ellie. *Ancient Egyptian Medicine—Smith Papyrus—Ebers Papyrus.* Available at http://www.crystalinks.com/egyptmedicine.html.

Luscombe, Stephen. *The History of Medicine: Pre-history.* Available at http://www.britishempire.co.uk/boniface/humanities/history/year10/prehistoric.html.

Newton, Giles. *Discovering DNA Fingerprinting.* Available at http://genome.wellcome.ac.uk/doc_wtd020877.html.

Rhee, Seung Yon. *Louis Pasteur (1822–1895).* Available at http://www.accessexcellence.org/RC/AB/BC/Louis_Pasteur.php.

Scott, Patrick. *Edward Jenner and the Discovery of Vaccination.* Available at http://www.sc.edu/library/spcoll/nathist/jenner.html.

The U.S. Army Medical Department Center and School. *Military Medicine During the Twentieth Century.* Available at http://www.au.af.mil/au/awc/awcgate/milmedhist/chapter3.htm.

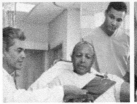
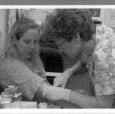
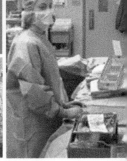

Overview of Health Care Careers

CHAPTER OBJECTIVES

After careful study of this chapter, you should be able to:

✳ List steps for planning a career in health care.

✳ Define and differentiate licensure, registration, and certification.

✳ Describe the typical work responsibilities; education, training, and legal requirements; employment; out-

look; and average earnings of selected occupations in therapeutic services, diagnostic services, health informatics, support services, and biotechnology research and development.

KEY TERMS

accreditation	certification	licensure	support services
biotechnology	diagnostic services	registration	therapeutic services
career ladder			

CAREER PLANNING IN HEALTH CARE

Health care has developed into a multibillion-dollar industry. It's the largest occupational field in the U.S. There are more than 300 occupations and career specialties within health care, with employment opportunities in many types of settings, from hospitals to homes.

Health Career Exploration

When thinking about a career in health care, it is important to explore thoroughly the many opportunities and resources available. They provide valuable information and experience that will help you choose and prepare for a satisfying career.

If you have not already chosen your career, a good way to learn more is to visit your school or public library. There

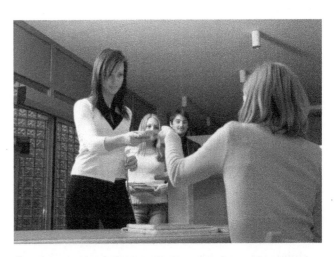

If you have not already chosen your career, a good way to learn more is to visit your school or public library.

you will find books that give a broad overview of many occupations; books written by nurses, paramedics, and other professionals about their experiences at work; databases; lists of web sites; and other references on health care careers. An entire section of the library is often devoted to careers. Librarians can assist in finding useful, up-to-date information about practically any health care occupation.

The Internet is a tremendously helpful resource as well. The first stop should be the *Occupational Outlook Handbook* at www.bls.gov/OCO/. This publication is produced by the U.S. Bureau of Labor Statistics (BLS) and is updated every two years. For any occupation, the *Occupational Outlook Handbook* provides:

- a detailed description of the work
- the training and education needed
- federal and state requirements
- professional certifications
- expected job prospects, backed by BLS research
- typical earnings
- opportunities for advancement
- links to employment projections and labor market resources, by state

On the Internet you can find almost any information about health care occupations, including schools that offer programs of study to prepare for the career, video interviews with workers in the occupation, and a wealth of other useful information.

A third useful resource is professional organizations, which represent most health care specialties. Visiting their web sites can yield helpful information. Contacting a local chapter is also a good way of gaining information. A local chapter can provide:

- details about the job market and employers in the area
- the chance to meet, talk with, and job-shadow people working in an occupation
- opportunities to network

A last important resource that shouldn't be forgotten is people. School career counselors can help set up interviews with health care workers, as well as job-shadowing appointments. You can also arrange these opportunities on your own. Physicians' offices, health clinics, and hospitals are often receptive to such requests. Spending a day on the job, and talking to people who work in that occupation, is often the best way to determine whether an occupation is right for you. The more information you gather, the better prepared you are to make a good choice.

Educational Requirements

Training for a health care occupation is very important. Educational requirements depend on the specific occupation, which often require graduation from an accredited school. **Accreditation** means that a school is recognized by an outside agency, such as a national board or commission, as having standards that qualify graduates for professional practice. Accredited programs must cover the skills determined by the accrediting agency.

Be sure to carefully check the requirements for any occupation that interests you. The *Occupational Outlook Handbook* and professional associations are good resources.

There are many different places to obtain training:

- four-year universities
- two-year community colleges
- technical institutions hospital-based schools
- trade schools
- private schools
- the military

If you are using this book, you have probably already enrolled in the type of educational institution that fits your situation and goals.

Credentials

For many health care occupations, workers must meet legal requirements in order to practice. In certain occupations, meeting standards may not be required but will confer professional distinction and, often, an advantage in the job market, including better pay and opportunities for advancement. Medical professionals can be licensed, registered, or certified.

Licensure

For many health care professions, state governments grant authority for individuals to work in that profession in a particular state. This act of granting authority by the state is known as **licensure.** As a licensed health care professional, you must practice your profession according to the guidelines and limitations set by the state in which you are licensed. A few examples of health care professions that are subject to licensure are practical nurses, registered nurses, physicians, dentists, and veterinarians.

Each state has agencies responsible for issuing and renewing licenses to health care professionals. If the health care profession you choose is a licensed one, you must obtain a license from the state in which you want to work. If you work in more than one state, you must obtain a license from each state.

Each state determines its own qualifications and requirements for licensure of a particular profession.

Generally, licensing requirements consist of graduating from a state-accredited school or training program and passing a state licensor exam. To find out about the licensing requirements in your state, ask the instructors at your school, or search online using the term *licensing*, followed by the specific occupation and the name of your state.

Registration

Registration means that you have graduated from an accredited school and have passed a standardized national exam administered by a nongovernmental agency. This examination is usually administered by a professional organization. Radiological technologist, respiratory therapist, physical therapist, and occupational therapist are a few of the professionals that can become registered. National registries are available to verify a potential employee's status.

Certification

A professional organization, rather than the government, controls certification. Certification demonstrates that a health care worker meets the requirements set by the certifying organization to demonstrate mastery of the job. Certification generally isn't required to work in health care professions, but many employers prefer to hire certified employees. Certification assures employers that the person meets a certain competency level. Workers with certification often have more and better job opportunities and earn higher pay.

In many occupations, health care workers can also be certified in areas in which they are specializing. For example, a registered nurse may be certified in intensive care nursing. Recertification and continuing education, through exams, courses, and other means, are required in certain occupations.

✓ **CHECK POINT**

1 Name four resources for information about health care careers.

2 Explain the differences among licensing, registration, and certification.

HEALTH CARE CAREERS

Not all of the more than 300 health care occupations and career specialties can be described here. The careers profiled in the following sections are representative examples, grouped according to the five National Consortium

Table 2-1 Employment Growth, 2008–2018

If the Statement Reads:	Employment is Projected to:
Much faster than average	Increase 20 percent or more
Faster than average	Increase 14 to 19 percent
About as fast as average	Increase 7 to 13 percent
More slowly than average	Increase 3 to 6 percent

Source: *Occupational Outlook Handbook*.

for Health Science Education (NCHSE) career clusters for health science. These five career clusters are:
- therapeutic services
- diagnostic services
- health informatics
- support services
- biotechnology research and development

Many allied health careers are described in more detail in the following chapters. The career profiles in Part IV draw heavily on information from the *Occupational Outlook Handbook*. Table 2-1 explains certain key phrases that the *Handbook* uses to describe employment growth.

Within some of the career fields discussed in this chapter, it is possible to move from one occupation to another. When that is the case, a table outlining the career ladder, or hierarchy of careers in that field, is provided. In nearly all cases, a person needs more education or training to move from a lower career on the ladder to a higher one.

Therapeutic Services

People in therapeutic services provide treatment for patients or animals. These services may include counseling, use of medications, surgery, radiation, physical therapy, occupational therapy, psychiatric treatment, or some combination of these. Those who provide therapeutic services also help clients to maintain or improve their health over time.

Physicians

The professionals with the greatest overall responsibility for medical care are physicians. They examine patients, diagnose medical problems, and treat illnesses and injuries.

Becoming a physician requires rigorous and time-consuming education and training. Typically, candidates must obtain their bachelor's degree, complete four years of medical school, and spend three to eight years in an internship or residency, depending on their specialty. In every state, the District of Columbia, and U.S. territories, physicians must be licensed.

In 2008, physicians held about 661,400 jobs. The BLS projects that employment will grow by 22 percent from 2008 to 2018.

According to a 2008 survey, primary care physicians had total median earnings of $186,044. For specialists, total median earnings were $339,738.

Physician Assistants

Physician assistants, or PAs, perform many of the same tasks as physicians. They provide primary care in places where physicians are sometimes in short supply. They also free up busy physicians by assuming responsibility for routine tasks. PAs work under the supervision of a physician, but they have much independence in their work.

In every state and the District of Columbia, practicing as a PA requires a license, obtained by completing an accredited program and passing a national exam. Applicants to these education programs must have completed at least two years of college and, for nearly all of these programs, must have some work experience in health care. According to the American Association of Physician Assistants (AAPA), applicants usually have a bachelor's degree and have worked in the field for about four years.

PAs must pass a recertification examination every six years. They must also complete 100 hours of continuing medical education every two years.

PA is a popular occupation. It accounted for about 74,800 jobs in 2008, and the BLS projects that the occupation will grow 39 percent between 2008 and 2018. Jobs will be available in both office settings and institutions like hospitals, public clinics, and academic medical centers.

The median annual salary for PAs was $81,230 as of May 2008, but salaries vary depending on specialty, location and experience. In a 2008 census report, AAPA cited salaries by specialty, ranging from $78,956 to $110,468. This occupation is profiled in more detail in Chapter 3, "Patient Care: Medical and Surgical."

Medical Assistants

Medical assistants work in physicians' offices and other health care facilities. They often perform both administrative and certain clinical tasks. They handle general office duties, such as greeting patients and answering phones, as well as work that's specific to a medical setting, such as scheduling procedures and filing insurance forms. Clinical duties vary. Examples include assisting in physical examinations, obtaining medical histories, and taking vital signs. A major goal of medical assistants is to keep the office running smoothly.

Some medical assistants are trained on the job, but many complete a one- to two-year medical assisting program.

ZOOM IN

Money Talk: Understanding Career Salaries

- **Wages.** Most health care workers are paid by the hour. For instance, a person who works 40 hours at $16 per hour earns $640.
- **Salary.** Some health care workers get a salary instead of an hourly wage. For instance, a receptionist might earn $27,000 a year, regardless of the number of hours worked. This sum may be paid out weekly, every two weeks, or monthly.
- **Median.** The median is a way of expressing a middle-range salary. It is the number in the middle when a set of number is put in numerical order. For example, if three workers earn salaries of $50,000, $65,000, and $80,000, the median salary is $65,000. Median salaries are often used to give a more realistic picture of typical salaries for a career.
- **Mean.** The mean, or average, salary in a career field is found by adding all of the salaries in that field together and then dividing this total by the number of individual salaries.

Medical assistants are not licensed. Although certification is not required, more than 90 percent of medical assistants become certified.

Medical assistants held more than 470,000 jobs in 2008, with the majority (about 62 percent) working in physicians' offices. The BLS projects job growth of 34 percent from 2008 to 2018, making medical assisting the 16th fastest-growing occupation.

A medical assistant's earnings depend on experience, skill level, and location. As of May 2008, median annual earnings were $28,300.

This occupation is profiled in more detail in Chapter 3, "Patient Care: Medical and Surgical."

Surgical Technologists

Surgical technologists are essential members of the operating room team. They perform many tasks before, during, and after an operation. For example, they set up the operating room and get the patient ready. They help count sponges, needles, and instruments to ensure that nothing is left inside the patient, and they make sure that the operating area stays germ-free. They may also pass instruments to the surgeon. After a procedure, the surgical technologist takes the patient to the recovery room and prepares the operating room for the next procedure.

Surgical technologists complete a nine-month to two-year training program leading to a certificate, diploma, or associate's degree. Programs are available at community and junior colleges, vocational schools, universities, hospitals, and in the military. Surgical technologists are not licensed, although state law may limit the scope of their work. Certification is also not required, but most employers prefer to hire certified technologists. Two organizations award credentials.

In 2008, surgical technologists held about 91,500 jobs. The BLS predicts an impressive job growth rate of 25 percent from 2008 to 2018. Hospitals will continue to be the main employers, but much faster job growth is expected in physicians' offices and outpatient care centers. Certified surgical technologists and those willing to relocate will have the best job opportunities.

The median annual salary for surgical technologists was $38,740 as of May 2008. In the settings employing the largest numbers of surgical technologists, salaries ranged from $36,380 to $40,880.

This occupation is profiled in more detail in Chapter 3, "Patient Care: Medical and Surgical."

Physical Therapists

Physical therapists help people who have suffered impairment due to injury, pain, or some other disabling condition. Physical therapists examine patients and develop a treatment plan that addresses one or more of these goals:
- restoring function
- improving mobility
- relieving pain
- preventing or limiting permanent physical disabilities

Physical therapists may work directly with the patient to carry out the plan, or that responsibility may be delegated to a physical therapist assistant. Physical therapists monitor the patient's progress and modify the plan when necessary. They also develop fitness and wellness programs and conditioning programs for athletes. Like many

other health care professionals, physical therapists often work in teams, with physical therapist assistants, physicians, nurses, occupational therapists, and others.

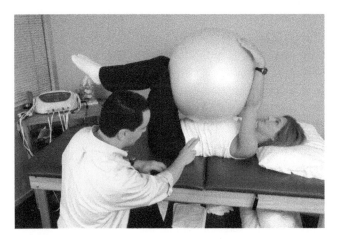

Physical therapists examine patients who have suffered impairment due to injury, pain, or some other disabling condition, then develop a treatment plan that addresses one the needs of the individual's needs.

Physical therapists must have a master's degree from an accredited physical therapy program, although a doctoral degree is fast becoming standard. Licensing, required in every state, typically requires a physical therapy degree, a national exam, and other criteria. Many physical therapy programs require volunteer work in the physical therapy department of a hospital or clinic prior to admission.

In 2008, physical therapists held about 185,500 jobs. Roughly 60 percent worked in hospitals or in the offices of other health care practitioners. From 2008 to 2018, the BLS anticipates job growth of 30 percent. Listing it as one of its best careers of 2010 (and 2009), *U.S. News & World Report* noted that in a recent survey, physical therapists ranked second only to members of the clergy in job satisfaction.

The median annual earnings of physical therapists were $72,790 as of May 2008. In the settings employing the largest numbers of physical therapists, median annual earnings ranged from $71,400 to $77,630.

This occupation is profiled in more detail in Chapter 8, "Therapy and Rehabilitation."

Physical Therapist Assistants

Once a physical therapist has developed a patient's treatment plan, a physical therapist assistant, or PTA, may implement it. PTAs work one-on-one with patients to rehabilitate them under the direction or supervision of the physical therapist. (*Rehabilitation* is the restoration, after a disease or injury, of the ability to function in a normal or near-normal manner.) For example, a PTA may put a patient with an injured leg through range of motion exercises, helping the patient regain the ability to move the leg. Once the patient

📷 ZOOM IN

Health Care Technician or Health Care Technologist?

The basic difference between a technician and a technologist is education. Generally, technicians hold an associate's degree, while technologists have a bachelor's degree.

Educational programs for technicians emphasize practical skills. Technologists have more advanced knowledge. They may have supervisory roles, make decisions and solve problems at a higher level, and perform more advanced procedures. In practice, the duties of technicians and technologists often overlap.

can do the exercises alone, the PTA monitors, corrects, and adds more challenging routines, according to the treatment plan. PTAs may massage injured tissues, apply heat or ice, or administer other therapies.

Most states regulate PTAs through licensure, registration, and certification, requiring an associate's degree from an accredited program and a national exam. In some states, PTAs must pass a state exam.

PTA ranks as the 17th fastest-growing occupation in the nation. Physical therapist assistants held about 64,000 jobs in 2008. The BLS projects that employment will increase by 33 percent from 2008 to 2018. As of May 2008, the median annual salary of PTAs was $46,140. In the settings employing the largest numbers of PTAs, median annual earnings ranged from $43,390 to $51,950.

This occupation is profiled in more detail in Chapter 8, "Therapy and Rehabilitation."

Occupational Therapists

Occupational therapists help people who are disabled in some way to work and to perform common tasks of everyday life. Clients who benefit from occupational therapy include people who have suffered strokes, have a mental illness, have disabilities like cerebral palsy, or use a wheelchair. The goals of occupational therapy are to help patients become independent and productive and to improve their quality of life.

Occupational therapists assess patients and prepare an intervention plan. This might include doing exercises or performing various activities, from dressing to grocery shopping to finding a job. Occupational therapists may perform therapy themselves or delegate it to an occupational therapy assistant.

Occupational therapists must have at least a master's degree. All educational programs include supervised fieldwork. Some institutions offer combined bachelor's and master's degree programs. Therapists may focus on a particular area of practice (such as mental health) or on an age group or disability. In every state, occupational therapists must be licensed, although the exact licensing requirements vary by state. Applicants must graduate from an accredited program and pass a national certification exam.

In 2008, occupational therapists held about 104,500 jobs. BLS predicts that, between 2008 and 2018, jobs for occupational therapists will increase by 26 percent. Those working with older patients and in specialized areas, such as evaluating and training older drivers, will enjoy especially good job prospects.

Median annual earnings of occupational therapists were $66,780 as of May 2008. In the settings employing the largest numbers of occupational therapists, median annual earnings ranged from $60,020 to $74,510.

This occupation is profiled in more detail in Chapter 8, "Therapy and Rehabilitation."

Occupational Therapy Assistants

Occupational therapy assistants work under the direction of an occupational therapist to provide occupational therapy services. Typically, their role is to carry out the intervention plan, working directly with clients, but they may also administer tests, contribute to the treatment plan, and participate in other ways at each stage of occupational therapy. Occupational therapy assistants can fill a wide variety of other roles. For instance, some serve as the directors of residential activities at nursing homes, and others lead exercise and stress reduction programs.

Employment typically requires an associate's degree from an accredited occupational therapy assistant program. Accredited programs include academic courses and at least 16 weeks of supervised fieldwork. Forty states and the District of Columbia regulate occupational therapy assistants. Requirements vary. A credential from the National Board for Certifying Occupational Therapy, awarded upon passing an exam, meets the requirements of some states.

In 2008, occupational therapy assistants held about 26,600 jobs. Job seekers should have very good prospects, as jobs are expected to grow by 30 percent from 2008 to 2018.

Median annual earnings of occupational therapy assistants were $48,230 as of May 2008. In the settings employing the most assistants, median annual earnings ranged from $41,850 to $53,090.

This occupation is profiled in more detail in Chapter 8, "Therapy and Rehabilitation."

Orthotists/Prosthetists

These health care professionals design, make, and custom-fit artificial limbs (prosthetists) and orthopedic devices such as leg braces (orthotists). Orthotists and prosthetists use computers and a wide array of traditional tools. For artificial limbs (which can be anything from a finger or toe to an entire arm or leg), they work with the patient to choose the parts that will make up the prosthesis. A patient might want a waterproof knee or feet designed for sprinting, for example. After making the device, the orthotist or prosthetist fits the device and makes any adjustments that are needed so that it works properly and is comfortable.

People who pursue one of these occupations must earn a bachelor's degree in the field and then complete a residency program with a licensed professional. To be certified, orthotists and prosthetists must pass an exam administered by the American Board for Certification in Orthotics, Prosthetics & Pedorthics. Some states require licensing, a trend that is likely to continue. Licensing requirements vary but generally include both education and testing.

As of 2008, BLS estimated that 5,900 people were employed as orthotists and prosthetists. In 2007, their mean hourly wage was estimated at $30.90, and their mean annual salary at about $64,300. Growth for these occupations from 2008 to 2018 is expected to be faster than average.

Respiratory Therapists

Respiratory therapists assess, treat, and care for patients with breathing and other cardiopulmonary disorders. For example, they run tests for lung capacity, as well as stress tests, and they do sleep studies to screen for disorders like sleep apnea. These workers administer oxygen, give aerosol medications, provide many other types of treatment, and monitor a patient's responses. Both tests and treatment are given under a physician's direction.

Respiratory therapists work in every area of a hospital and with patients of all ages. They are often among the first health care workers to assess a patient, and they play an essential role in emergency response teams. Respiratory therapists can specialize in a number of areas, such as diagnostics and disease management. They also provide other services, such as smoking cessation counseling.

Respiratory therapists need at least an associate's degree, but a bachelor's or master's degree may help them to advance. Colleges and universities, medical schools, vocational-technical institutes, and the armed forces offer training programs. Most programs award an associate's degree.

All states, except Alaska and Hawaii, require respiratory therapists to be licensed. Licensing generally follows the National Board for Respiratory Care's certification requirements, including an accredited program and one or two exams.

In 2008, respiratory therapists held nearly 106,000 jobs. Most—about 81 percent—worked in hospitals. According to the BLS, employment in this occupation will grow by 21 percent from 2008 to 2018. In addition to hospitals, jobs will be increasingly available in home health care services, offices of physicians and other health care practitioners, and companies that rent respiratory equipment for home use.

Respiratory therapists had median annual earnings of $52,200 as of May 2008.

This occupation is profiled in more detail in Chapter 8, "Therapy and Rehabilitation."

Paramedics

Paramedics give emergency medical care at the scene of accidents, in homes, and in other places and continue to care for patients on the way to a hospital or other medical facility. Paramedics are the most highly trained of emergency medical technicians (EMTs), with the greatest level of responsibility.

Becoming a paramedic requires a one- to two-year training program and, in all states, a certifying exam. Applicants need a high school diploma or GED and a driver's license. In addition to advanced skills, paramedics must be able to perform the skills taught at the basic EMT level.

Together with other EMTs, paramedics held about 210,700 jobs in 2008. From 2008 to 2018, the BLS projects job growth of 9 percent. Job prospects should be good, especially in cities and private ambulance services.

Earnings depend on where a paramedic works, as well as training and experience. The median hourly wage for paramedics and other EMTs was $14.10 as of May 2008.

This occupation is profiled in more detail in Chapter 3, "Patient Care: Medical and Surgical."

Emergency Medical Technicians

Emergency medical technicians (EMTs) care for people who are ill or injured away from a hospital or other medical facility. They treat victims at the scene and then transport them, continuing to care for them on the way. Starting an IV, performing CPR, and doing a rapid trauma assessment are examples of the many procedures an EMT may perform.

The services EMTs provide depend on their level of training and certification. All EMTs must complete a formal training program. Admission requires a high school diploma or GED and a driver's license. Training is offered at three levels, with certification required by all states at each level.

All levels of EMTs must be able to perform the skills taught at the EMT-Basic level. Each level includes both classroom instruction and work at a hospital or clinic and/or in the field. Depending on the state, certification may be by a national exam administered by the EMTs' professional organization, a state certifying exam, or the applicant's choice of either exam.

The employment and salary figures given for paramedics above apply to other EMTs as well, as the BLS classifies them together.

This occupation is profiled in more detail in Chapter 3, "Patient Care: Medical and Surgical."

Registered Nurses

Like physicians, nurses are very familiar to the public. Nursing is one of the oldest health care professions, and nurses work in nearly every health care setting and situation. They establish or contribute to a plan of treatment,

CAREER LADDER Paramedics and EMTs

Occupation	Requirements	Median Earning	Growth Rate
EMT-Paramedic	• 1- to 2-year training program • Hospital and field work; field internship • Written and practical (certifying state) exam	$14.10	9%

EMT-Intermediate	• Training requirements vary by state. Typically:
	  • 30 to 350 hours of training based on scope of practice
	    • Hospital and field work
	• Written and practical (certifying state) exam
		$14.10	9%

EMT-Basic	• About 110 hours of classroom instruction Practical work with experienced EMTs in the field or in emergency rooms or clinics • Written and practical (certifying state) exam	$14.10	9%

help perform diagnostic tests and analyze the results, give treatments and medications, and help care for patients who cannot care for themselves. Nurses work with patients and their families, providing advice and emotional support and assisting with rehabilitation and home care. They also educate patients and the public about medical problems and good health.

Registered nurses (RNs) can specialize in one or more areas of patient care. The BLS identifies four ways for RNs to specialize:

• focusing on a particular setting or type of treatment (like emergency or cardiac catheter laboratory nursing)
• concentrating on specific health conditions (like HIV/AIDS nursing)
• specializing in one or more organs or body system types (like pulmonary nursing)
• serving a well-defined population (like pediatric nursing)

Most RNs work as staff nurses, as part of a health care team. RNs can also become advanced practice nurses, who work independently or collaborate with a physician. Advance practice nurses specialize in one of four areas: clinical nurse specialist, nurse anesthetist, nurse-midwife, or nurse practitioner.

People who want to become registered nurses can choose from three main educational paths:

• a bachelor of science degree in nursing (colleges and universities—four years)
• an associate's degree in nursing (community and junior colleges—two to three years)
• a diploma (hospitals—three years)

Many RNs with an associate's degree or diploma later return to school for their bachelor's degree, often making use of tuition reimbursement programs offered by employers. A variety of options, including accelerated options, are available to earn a master's degree in nursing, and there are doctoral programs as well. The BLS recommends a bachelor's degree or higher because of the enhanced career opportunities.

All states, the District of Columbia, and U.S. territories require registered nurses to be licensed. They must complete an approved nursing program and pass a national exam, the National Council Licensure Examination for Registered Nurses (NCLEX-RN). Other requirements vary by state.

Registered nursing is the largest health care occupation. In 2008, registered nurses held about 2.6 million jobs. The BLS projects job growth of 22 percent for this occupation from 2008 to 2018, resulting in the largest number of new jobs for any occupation (581,500). Good sources of jobs from 2008 to 2018 will be physicians' offices, home health care services, nursing care facilities, employment services, and hospitals.

As of May 2008, the median annual salary for registered nurses was $62,450. In those settings employing the largest numbers of registered nurses, the highest median annual salary was in employment services ($68,160) and general medical and surgical hospitals ($63,880).

This occupation is profiled in more detail in Chapter 4, "Patient Care: Nursing."

Licensed Practical Nurses

Licensed practical nurses (LPNs) work under the direction of a physician or registered nurse to care for patients. LPNs perform many different kinds of nursing tasks. They provide basic bedside care, including taking vital signs, giving injections, dressing wounds, and helping with personal hygiene. LPNs monitor patients and talk with them about their medical history and condition, sharing the information with physicians and RNs when it may help in a patient's treatment. Most LPNs work in all areas of health care.

LPNs are licensed in every state and the District of Columbia. To obtain a license, a person must complete a state-approved practical nursing program and pass a national exam, the National Council Licensure Examination for Practical Nurses (NCLEX-PN). Programs are typically offered at technical and vocational schools and community and junior colleges. Most programs last about a year and require a high school diploma or the equivalent for admission.

In 2008, licensed practical nurses held more than 750,000 jobs. The BLS projects that employment of LPNs will grow by 21 percent from 2008 to 2018. Nursing care facilities and home health care services will offer the best job growth.

LPNs had a median annual salary of $39,030 as of May 2008. Among settings employing the largest numbers of LPNs, the highest median annual earnings were in employment services ($44,690), nursing care facilities ($40,580), and home health care services ($39,510).

This occupation is profiled in more detail in Chapter 4, "Patient Care: Nursing."

Nursing Assistants

Nursing assistants, also known as certified nursing assistants (CNAs) and nursing aides, help care for patients by performing simple, basic nursing functions. Some typical tasks that nursing assistants perform are bathing patients, transferring them safely (from a bed to a chair, for example), serving meals, answering patients' call lights, taking vital signs, and helping nurses with equipment.

For many jobs, nursing assistants need a high school diploma or the equivalent. Federal law requires all nursing assistants who work in nursing care facilities to complete a state-approved training program of at least 75 hours and to pass a competency test, including both a written component and an assessment of practical skills. Nursing assistants who pass the exam are certified, and the state places their names on a registry. State requirements vary. Training is available at high schools, vocational schools, community colleges, and health care facilities.

The BLS places nursing assistants in a category called *nursing aides, orderlies, and attendants.* In 2008, this group of employees held more than 1.5 million jobs, 70 percent of them in nursing facilities and hospitals. From 2008 to 2018, the BLS projects job growth of 19 percent for these occupations, with more jobs available in nursing and residential care facilities than in hospitals. Nursing aides, orderlies, and attendants had a median hourly wage of $11.46 as of May 2008.

This occupation is profiled in more detail in Chapter 4, "Patient Care: Nursing."

Home Health Aides

When older or disabled individuals need more care than family members can provide, they often turn to home health aides. Home health aides help people with basic health care needs so that they can stay in their own homes instead of a health care facility. Older adults, people with disabilities, and those recovering from illnesses and injuries receive their services.

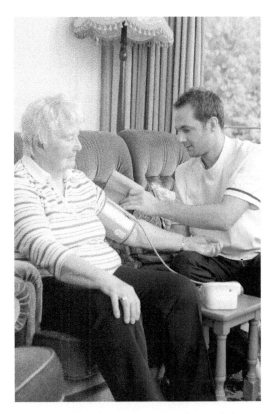

Some common tasks that home health aides perform include giving medicines, taking vital signs, helping clients in and out of bed, helping them with grooming and getting dressed, and assisting them with exercises and other therapies.

Many home health aides work for certified home health or hospice agencies that receive government funding. According to the regulations that are a condition of that funding, they must work under the direction of a nurse or other medical professional. Some common tasks that home health aides perform include giving medicines, taking vital signs, helping clients in and out of bed, helping them with grooming and getting dressed, and assisting them with exercises and other therapies. With experience and training, home health aides may also use, or help patients use, certain kinds of medical equipment.

Home health aides are usually trained on the job by RNs, LPNs, experienced aides, or their supervisor. Requirements vary widely from state to state, but a high school diploma usually isn't necessary.

Federal law requires aides whose employers are reimbursed by Medicare or Medicaid to complete a training program of at least 75 hours and a competency evaluation or state certification program. It also requires at least 16 hours of supervised practical training before having direct contact with a client. Some states require additional training. An aide may be certified without training by passing a competency exam. Professional certification is available from the National Association for Home Care and Hospice (NAHC).

Home health aides held about 921,700 jobs in 2008. The BLS predicts that 460,900 new jobs will be created from 2008 to 2018, a job growth rate of 50 percent. This places home health care aides third among all occupations in rate of expected job growth and second in numerical job growth.

As of May 2008, home health aides had a median hourly wage of $9.84.

Audiologists

When patients have hearing, balance, or related problems, they're often referred to an audiologist. Audiologists assess these problems and then develop and carry out treatment programs. They fit patients for hearing aids and other devices and teach people to use them. They also help patients adjust to hearing loss in other ways. Some audiologists measure noise levels in workplaces and lead hearing-protection programs. Others specialize in the care of certain groups, such as older adults, children, or hearing-impaired individuals requiring special treatment.

In all states, audiologists must be licensed, which requires at least a master's degree in audiology. In 18 states, a doctoral degree or the equivalent is necessary. The professional doctorate in audiology (Au.D.) requires four years of graduate university training. Audiologists can earn professional credentials from the American

CAREER LADDER Nursing Occupations

Occupation	Requirements	Median Earnings	Growth Rate
Registered nurse	Main educational paths: • Bachelor of science degree in nursing (4 years) • Associate's degree in nursing (2 to 3 years) • Diploma (hospital—3 years) Licensing required in all states, D.C., U.S. territories 1. Approved nursing program 2. National exam (NCLEX-RN). 3. Other state requirements vary.	$62,450	22%

Licensed practical nurse	• Training program (about 1 year)
	• Licensing required in all states and D.C.
	  1. State-approved practical nursing program
	  2. National exam (NCLEX-PN).
		$39,030	21%

Nursing assistant (CNA, nursing aide)	• High school diploma or equivalent (most jobs)
	• State requirements vary.
	• Federal requirements for work in nursing care facilities:
	  1. State-approved training program (minimum 75 hours)
	  2. Competency test.
		$11.46/hour	19%

Home health aide	• High school diploma usually not necessary.
	• Usually trained on the job.
	• State requirements vary widely.
	• Federal requirements if employers are reimbursed by Medicare or Medicaid:
	  1. Training program (minimum 75 hours)
	  2. Competency evaluation
	  3. 16 hours of supervised practical training
	Or Competency exam (Replaces 1–3.)
		$9.84/hour	50%

Speech-Language-Hearing Association (ASHA) or the American Board of Audiology. These certifications may satisfy some or all of a state's licensing requirements. Some states license separately for fitting hearing aids.

Audiologists held about 12,800 jobs in 2008. The BLS predicts this occupation will grow by 25 percent from 2008 to 2018.

As of May 2008, the median annual salary of audiologists was $62,030.

Audiometric Technician

When people need their hearing tested, the person doing the testing may be an audiometric technician. Audiometric technicians use audiometry equipment, which emits sounds at different pitches and volumes. The patient, wearing headphones, signals upon hearing a sound, and the technician records and reports the results. Other titles for this occupation include audiologist's (or audiology) assistant and oto-tech.

Audiometric technicians may perform a variety of routine tasks under the direction of an audiologist. Examples include cleaning, fitting, checking, and making minor repairs to hearing aids; teaching people to use them; and making ear mold impressions.

Employment may require a high school diploma or GED and a brief (several-day) training course conducted by a state board of health or another organization. Several institutions, as well as the American Academy of Otolaryngology, offer training programs leading to a certificate. Practicing audiologists also conduct programs. Another avenue for training is the military. The Department of Veterans Affairs and the armed forces use audiometric technicians in their clinics, and they provide training.

According to ASHA, 32 states regulated audiometric technicians, as of 2009. Standards vary widely. People interested in this occupation should check the requirements for their state. The strong job growth that the BLS projects for audiologists (due in large part to the needs of an aging population) should create a demand for more audiometric technicians as well.

Speech-Language Pathologist

Speech-language pathologists help people who have speech or language disorders. Their clients include people who stutter, children with developmental disabilities that retard their speech, people who've suffered strokes or other trauma, people with cerebral palsy or other diseases that impair their ability to speak, and people with swallowing disorders. Speech-language pathologists evaluate these patients, make a diagnosis, and develop and implement a treatment plan.

Forty-seven states regulate speech-language pathologists. Typically, candidates must have a master's degree from an accredited college or university, pass a national exam, and complete 300–375 hours of supervised clinical experience and nine months of postgraduate professional clinical experience. In some states, a professional credential offered by ASHA meets some or all licensing requirements. Some states impose different regulations for working in public schools.

In 2008, speech-language pathologists held about 119,300 jobs. Roughly half were employed in educational institutions. Others worked in hospitals and other health care settings. The BLS projects that employment will grow by 19 percent from 2008 to 2018.

Speech-language pathologists had a median annual salary of $62,930 as of May 2008. In the settings employing the largest numbers, median annual earnings ranged from $58,140 to $79,120.

Speech-Language Pathology Assistants

Speech-language pathology assistants work with clients individually or in groups, implementing treatment plans designed by speech-language pathologists. They use a wide variety of tools and techniques to help people speak or improve their speech. Examples include sign language, multimedia computer programs, sound analyzers, pictures, and toys.

Some speech-language pathology assistants specialize in particular age groups or disorders. They also perform a variety of support services, always under a speech-language pathologist's supervision. Speech-language pathology assistants work in schools, hospitals, rehabilitation centers, and other places. Some are in private practice.

ASHA reports that 32 states regulated speech-language pathology assistants as of 2009. The tasks that states allow assistants to do vary, as do state requirements. Educational requirements range from a high school diploma to a bachelor's degree with graduate credit hours. ASHA recommends an associate's degree program for speech-language pathology assistants. As of 2009, it listed 22 such programs. Speech-language pathology assistants cannot practice in some states.

According to ASHA, speech-language pathology assistants typically receive 60 to 75 percent of the salaries of speech-language pathologists and professionals in similar occupations.

Ophthalmologists

Ophthalmologists are physicians who specialize in vision and eye care. They perform routine eye exams, prescribe glasses and contact lenses, diagnose and treat eye diseases like

CAREER LADDER Audiology and Speech-Language Pathology Occupations

Occupation	Requirements	Median Earnings	Growth Rate
Speech-language pathologist	Licensed or registered in 47 states. • Master's degree from accredited college or university • 300–375 hours of supervised clinical experience and nine months of postgraduate professional work • National exam	$62,930	19%
Audiologist	Licensed in all states • Master's degree in audiology (doctoral degree or equivalent in 18 states)	$62,030	25%
Audiometric technician	Regulated in 32 states. Standards vary widely. • High school diploma or GED and, often, a brief training course • Certificate or training program • Training through military	Not available	Not available
Speech-language pathology assistant	• Regulated in 32 states. Requirements vary. • ASHA recommends associate's degree program.	60%–75% that of a speech-language pathologist	Not available

cataracts or glaucoma, and diagnose other diseases that affect the eyes, such as diabetes or hypertension. Ophthalmologists also prescribe medications and perform eye surgery.

Ophthalmologists have the same medical education as other physicians. After medical school, they typically complete a three-year ophthalmology residency that focuses on medical and surgical eye training. Ophthalmologists are licensed like other physicians.

Optometrists

Optometrists are primary eye care providers, supplying most of the eye care services that people need. Optometrists offer many of the same services that ophthalmologists do. They are not medical doctors, however, and they cannot prescribe some medications, treat some diseases, or perform eye surgery, except for certain procedures. States differ in the scope of practice for optometrists.

In all states and the District of Columbia, optometrists must be licensed. To get a license, an applicant must have a doctor of optometry degree from an accredited optometry school and must pass a written and a clinical exam. Many states require an additional exam on state laws that affect optometry practice.

Optometry school is a four-year program. To be admitted, candidates must complete at least three years of pre-optometric study at an accredited college or university, and most optometry school applicants have a bachelor's degree.

In 2008, optometrists held about 34,800 jobs. The BLS projects that employment for optometrists will grow by 24 percent from 2008 to 2018. Salaried optometrists had a median annual salary of $96,320 as of May 2008.

Ophthalmic Medical Technicians

Ophthalmic medical technicians help ophthalmologists in their work. They assist in procedures, and they perform some procedures and tests on their own. Ophthalmic medical technicians teach patients to use medications properly and to perform tasks like inserting and caring for contact lenses. They also record patients' medical histories. These technicians may have office duties, such as scheduling appointments, as well.

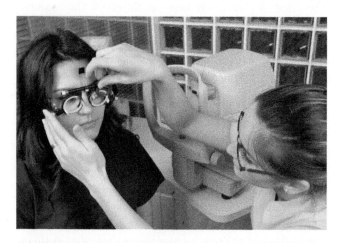

Ophthalmic medical technicians help ophthalmologists in their work by assisting in procedures, and sometimes performing some procedures and tests on their own.

Those considering this occupation need a high school diploma or GED. Skills can be learned on the job (usually in conjunction with independent study courses or online training), in an accredited program lasting three months to four years, or through independent study and online learning.

The Joint Commission on Allied Health Personnel in Ophthalmology (JCAHPO) certifies ophthalmic medical technicians at three core levels. The commission also offers certification for a subspecialty and three specialties. According to JCAHPO, studies show that technicians with certification earn higher salaries and have more opportunities for advancement.

Most states do not regulate ophthalmic medical technicians. People interested in this occupation should check with their state's regulatory agency.

In the 2010–2011 *Occupational Outlook Handbook*, ophthalmic medical technicians were classified as medical assistants, a field projected to grow 35 percent from 2008 to 2018. According to the Association of Technical Personnel in Ophthalmology, typical salaries for ophthalmic medical technicians range from $30,000 to $70,000, depending on their level of training and experience.

Athletic Trainers

Athletic trainers teach people to condition themselves so that they may participate in sports and other physical activities without injury. They also help treat injuries and help people who have been injured to recover. Athletic trainers work in physicians' offices, sports medicine clinics, schools, and hospitals. They work with dancers, industrial workers, high school and professional athletes, coaches, military recruits, and injured service people.

Most jobs as athletic trainers require a bachelor's degree from an accredited college or university. According to the National Athletic Trainers' Association, nearly 70 percent of athletic trainers have at least a master's degree.

In 2009, 47 states required athletic trainers to be licensed or registered. This requires certification from the Board of Certification, Inc. To be certified, athletic trainers must earn a bachelor's degree from an accredited athletic training program and pass an exam. For high school positions that involve teaching, athletic trainers may also need a teaching certificate or license.

In 2008, athletic trainers held roughly 16,300 jobs. Between 2008 and 2018, employment is expected to grow 37 percent. The best job prospects will be in health care and high schools.

Salaries of athletic trainers vary with job setting, experience, and responsibilities. As of May 2008, the median annual salary was $39,640.

Pharmacists

Pharmacists are health care professionals authorized by law to dispense prescription medicines. Pharmacists must carefully read prescriptions from physicians and fill them correctly. They counsel patients on side effects, drug interactions, and over-the-counter medications, and they confer with physicians about the medicines patients are using. Pharmacists also prepare medicines, but it's a small part of their work, because today most medicines are already in prepared form.

All states, the District of Columbia, Guam, Puerto Rico, and the U.S. Virgin Islands require pharmacists to be licensed. Candidates generally must earn a doctor of pharmacy degree from an accredited school or college of pharmacy and pass several exams, most of which vary by state. Admission requirements for pharmacy programs include at least two years of undergraduate work. Most applicants have completed three or more.

In 2008, pharmacists held about 268,900 jobs. The BLS projects that employment will grow by 17 percent from 2008 to 2018. As of May 2008, the median annual salary of pharmacists was $106,410.

This occupation is profiled in more detail in Chapter 6, "Laboratory and Pharmacy Services."

Pharmacy Technicians

Pharmacy technicians help pharmacists fill prescriptions by performing many routine tasks. For instance, they count pills, weigh and measure materials, prepare prescription labels, review prescription information for accuracy, and prepare insurance forms. Their work with prescriptions is checked by a pharmacist for accuracy. Pharmacy technicians must refer questions about prescriptions, drug information, or health matters to pharmacists.

Most pharmacy technicians are trained on the job. Formal training, however, is an advantage in getting a job, as are certification and relevant previous experience. Community colleges, vocational schools, hospitals, and the military all offer technician education programs. Programs range in length from six months to two years and lead to a diploma, certificate, or associate's degree.

Some states require pharmacy technicians to have a high school diploma or the equivalent. There is no national training standard. Students interested in this occupation should contact their state board of pharmacy for information. Certification, required by some states and employers, is available from several organizations, including the Pharmacy Technician Certification Board and the Institute for the Certification of Pharmacy Technicians.

In 2008, pharmacy technicians held about 381,200 jobs, roughly three-quarters of them in retail settings.

The BLS projects that employment for pharmacy technicians will increase by 25 percent from 2008 to 2018.

Pharmacy technicians had median hourly wages of $13.32 as of May 2008.

This occupation is profiled in more detail in Chapter 6, "Laboratory and Pharmacy Services."

Dentists

Dentists are doctors who care for people's teeth and gums. They check that teeth are healthy and advise patients on how to keep them that way with proper brushing, flossing, and other care. Dentists identify problems such as cavities, gum disease, and teeth that should be removed. They fill, extract, and straighten teeth; do surgery to correct gum disease; put protective sealants on children's teeth; make molds; and fit crowns.

To become a dentist, a person must graduate from an accredited dental school. Most are four-year schools. Admission requires a minimum of two years of undergraduate study (many schools require three or more years), including pre-dental education classes. Each dental school has its own list of such classes. Most applicants have at least a bachelor's degree. All schools require applicants to take the Dental Admission Test (DAT). Admission is quite competitive.

In all states and the District of Columbia, dentists must be licensed. In most states, obtaining a license requires graduation from an accredited dental school and a written and a practical exam.

In 2008, dentists held about 141,900 jobs. From 2008 to 2018, employment will grow by 16 percent according to the BLS.

Salaried dentists had a median annual salary of $142,870 as of May 2008. Salaries are affected by years in practice, location, hours worked, and specialty. Generally, self-employed dentists in private practice earn more than salaried dentists.

This occupation is profiled in greater detail in Chapter 5, "Patient Care: Dental."

Dental Hygienists

Dental hygienists clean people's teeth. They remove plaque and other materials, and they polish teeth, removing stains. They also teach patients about good dental hygiene. Dental hygienists take x-rays and apply fluoride treatments. They may perform a variety of additional tasks, depending on the state in which they practice.

Dental hygienists are licensed by each state. Almost every state requires graduation from an accredited dental hygiene program and a written and a clinical exam. In most states, candidates must also pass an exam on state law as it affects their work. Dental hygiene admission requirements typically include a high school diploma or GED and college entrance tests. Most programs grant an associate's degree.

Dental hygienists held about 174,100 jobs in 2008. Among all occupations requiring an associate's degree, dental hygiene ranks 12th in projected job growth for 2008–2018, at 36 percent.

As of May 2008, the median annual salary of dental hygienists was $66,570. They may be paid by the hour, daily, by salary, or on a commission basis. Pay is affected by location, employment setting, and years of experience.

This occupation is profiled in greater detail in Chapter 5, "Patient Care: Dental."

Dental Assistants

Dental assistants perform a wide variety of tasks, working closely with dentists and under their supervision. For example, dental assistants sterilize equipment and instruments, and they teach patients to brush and floss correctly. They assist during dental procedures, handing instruments and materials to the dentist and using compressed air and suction to keep the patient's mouth clean and dry. Dental assistants may also take and develop x-rays.

Dental assistants are often trained on the job. A growing number, however, attend dental assisting programs offered by community and junior colleges, trade schools, technical institutes, or the military. Most programs take a year to complete and lead to a certificate or diploma. To be admitted, a candidate must have a high school diploma or the equivalent. Some programs require applicants to have taken computer and science courses.

In some states, dental assistants must have a license or be registered. This may require an accredited dental assisting program and an exam. In addition, most states regulate the duties that dental assistants may perform. Advanced tasks, like taking x-rays, may require a national exam or additional training. Dental assistants can seek certification from the Dental Assisting National Board (DANB). As of 2009, 37 states and the District of Columbia recognized or required successful completion of a DANB exam to meet state regulations or to perform advanced tasks.

Dental assisting is a rapidly growing occupation. In fact, at 36 percent, it ranked 14th among all occupations in projected job growth for the period 2008–2018. Dental assistants held about 295,300 jobs in 2008. As of May of that year, the median annual salary was $32,380. This occupation is profiled in greater detail in Chapter 5, "Patient Care: Dental."

Dental Lab Technicians

Dental lab technicians make crowns, bridges, dentures, and other dental prostheses. They custom-design each

CAREER LADDER Dental Support Occupations

Occupation	Requirements	Median Earnings	Growth Rate
Dental hygienist	• Associate's degree in dental hygiene • Licensed by states. Requirements of most: 　1. Accredited dental hygiene program 　2. Written and clinical exam 　3. Exam on relevant state law	$66,570	36%
Dental assistant	• Most trained on the job • A growing number attend dental assisting programs (mostly one-year programs) • Licensed or registered in some states 　• Accredited dental assisting program 　• Exam	$32,380	36%

item, working from molds and x-rays that dentists provide. There are several steps in this process. These include making a model of the patient's mouth, hand-carving a wax model of the tooth or teeth, casting the metal framework, forming the metal, and bonding layers of porcelain to it. A single technician may perform some or all of these tasks, depending on the lab. Technicians may specialize in orthodontic appliances, crowns and bridges, complete or partial dentures, or ceramics.

Most technicians learn their skills on the job. However, formal training is a strong advantage in getting hired. In 2009, there were five dental orthotic and prosthetic technician programs accredited by the National Commission on Orthotic and Prosthetic Education. These programs offer either an associate's degree or a one-year certificate. There were also 20 programs in dental laboratory technology accredited by the Commission on Dental Accreditation in conjunction with the American Dental Association. Most of these programs take two years to complete and lead to an associate's degree.

In 2008, dental lab technicians held about 46,000 jobs. Employment growth for this occupation is projected to be 14 percent between 2008 and 2018. The BLS predicts that job opportunities will be favorable, particularly for those with formal training.

As of May 2008, the median annual salary of dental lab technicians was $34,170. In the settings that employed the most technicians, medical equipment and supplies manufacturing and dentists' offices, median annual earnings were $33,700 and $35,000, respectively.

Chiropractors

Chiropractors work mostly with people suffering from pain—pain in the back, neck, or wrists, headaches, or pain in other places. The main principle of chiropractic is that there is a close relationship between the body's structure, particularly the spine, and its function. When part of the body is out of adjustment, or misaligned, pain and other health problems can result. Chiropractic techniques include *manipulation*, or loosening joints and stretching tight muscles, and *mobilization*, putting joints through a full range of motion. Chiropractors emphasize overall health and do not use drugs in treatment.

In all states and the District of Columbia, chiropractors must be licensed. They must complete two to four years of undergraduate education (depending on the state), followed by a four-year program at an accredited chiropractic college. Candidates must then pass national and state examinations.

In 2008, chiropractors held about 49,100 jobs. The BLS projects that employment of chiropractors will increase by 20 percent from 2008 to 2018. Chiropractors earned a median annual salary of $66,490 as of May 2008.

Massage Therapists

Massage therapy helps reduce stress and promotes general health. People may also seek the services of a massage therapist when they have a painful ailment, a sports injury, or tired and overworked muscles. Massage therapists can specialize in more than 80 types of massage. Most have several specialties. This is a good occupation for people who want to work part-time or to be self-employed.

As of May 2009, 44 states and the District of Columbia had laws regulating massage therapy, and four additional states had introduced or were drafting legislation. (Idaho and Wyoming were the exceptions.) Most states require a formal, state-approved education program and an exam. Program applicants generally need a high school diploma or the equivalent. People interested in this occupation should check information on licensing, certification, and accreditation for the state where they would practice.

After training, many massage therapists choose to take one of two national certification exams administered by the National Certification Board for Therapeutic Massage and Bodywork. Many states require this test. The Federation of State Massage Therapy Boards offers a licensure program accepted by many states.

Massage therapists held about 122,400 jobs in 2008. The BLS predicts that employment will increase by 19 percent from 2008 to 2018. Median hourly wages, including tips, as of May 2008 were $16.78.

This occupation is profiled in greater detail in Chapter 8, "Therapy and Rehabilitation."

Dieticians

Dietitians apply the principles of nutrition to food choice and meal preparation. They educate people about eating well and work with individuals to manage illnesses. Many dieticians manage food services for large institutions, like schools, where they are in charge of everything from budgeting, purchasing, and hiring to planning meals and overseeing their preparation.

A dietician usually must have at least a bachelor's degree in dietetics, food and nutrition, food service systems management, or a related area, and many also hold master's degrees. The American Dietetic Association (ADA) awards the registered dietician (RD) credential to those who have completed approved coursework and an internship and have passed an exam.

Thirty-five states require dieticians to be licensed. In those states, only licensed individuals can work as dieticians. Twelve require certification. In those states, people who aren't certified can practice, but they cannot use certain titles, such as *dietician* or *nutritionist*. California requires registration.

The BLS reports that dieticians and nutritionists held about 60,300 jobs in 2008. The Bureau expects employment to increase by nine percent from 2008 to 2018. As of May 2008, the median annual salary of dieticians and nutritionists was $50,590.

Dietetic Technicians

Dietetic technicians help dieticians do their work. They plan meals and menus for individuals and groups, develop food selections for cafeterias, advise people on what to eat to stay healthy or to manage a medical problem, and gather information from patients for analysis by dieticians or physicians. Dietetic technicians analyze menus and recipes, order food, supervise its preparation, and help develop new products. They perform a variety of other tasks as well, under a dietician's supervision.

To become a dietetic technician, a person should complete an accredited dietary technician associate's degree program. The ADA awards the Dietetic Technician, Registered (DTR) credential to candidates who complete such a program, including a minimum of 450 hours of supervised practical experience, and pass a national exam. Some states require dietetic technicians to be licensed, certified, or registered.

In 2008, dietetic technicians held about 25,200 jobs. The BLS predicts that this occupation will add 11,000 new jobs from 2008 to 2018. According to an ADA compensation survey, the median hourly wage of registered dietetic technicians was $18.75 as of April 1, 2009.

Psychologists

Psychologists deal with human behavior and how it is affected by brain function and the environment. They usually specialize in a particular area, with the largest specialty being clinical psychology. Clinical psychologists help people in mental or emotional distress cope with life in general, as well as with illnesses and injuries and major events like the death of a parent. They interview patients, give tests, and counsel individuals, families, and groups.

CAREER LADDER Dietetic Technicians and Dieticians

Occupation	Requirements	Median Earnings	Growth Rate
Dietician	• Usually at least a bachelor's degree • For the RD credential, approved coursework, an internship, and an exam • Regulated by 48 states	$50,590	9%
Dietetic technician	• Accredited dietary technician associate's degree Regulated in some states	$18.75/hour	Faster than average

Clinical psychologists may work with physicians, nurses, social workers, and other health care professionals in caring for a patient.

Most psychologists need a doctoral degree, which usually requires five years of study. Candidates for admission to graduate psychology programs face strong competition. Some schools require a bachelor's degree in psychology. Others accept a bachelor's degree that included classes in basic psychology; biological, physical, and social sciences; statistics; and math.

All states and the District of Columbia have certification or licensing requirements for psychologists who work with patients. In addition to a doctorate in psychology, clinical psychologists usually need an approved internship and one to two years of professional experience. In every state, psychologists must also pass an exam. The American Board of Professional Psychology certifies psychologists in 13 specialties, including clinical psychology.

In 2008, psychologists held about 178,200 jobs. The BLS projects that employment will grow by 12 percent from 2008 to 2018. As of May 2008, the median annual salary of clinical, counseling, and school psychologists was $64,140.

Social Workers

Social workers help people with a variety of special problems and challenges in everyday life. For instance, they counsel couples with marital problems, assist with adoptions, and find foster homes for children. They arrange services for clients who are mentally ill or in poor health, connect older adults with community resources, give classes on managing stress, and assess and help treat people with substance abuse problems. Social workers are found in many different settings, from social agencies to schools to veterans' hospitals, and they provide or arrange a wide range of services and types of care.

To become a social worker, a person needs at least a bachelor's degree. Usually, it must be in social work, but for some jobs, a major in psychology, sociology, or a related field is acceptable. For many positions, a master's degree is required.

In all states and the District of Columbia, social workers must be licensed, registered, or certified. State requirements vary. The National Association of Social Workers offers three credentials and a dozen specialty certifications.

In 2008, social workers held about 642,000 jobs. From 2008 to 2018, the BLS projects job growth for social workers of about 12 percent. As of May 2008, median annual salaries of social workers ranged from the low $30s to nearly $70,000, depending on specialty.

Veterinarians

Veterinarians care for animals. Many care for pets, but veterinarians also work with livestock and animals at zoos, racetracks, and research facilities. They diagnose and treat illnesses and injuries, give advice on pet care, perform surgery, vaccinate against diseases, provide other preventive treatments, and euthanize animals when necessary. Some veterinarians take part in research to prevent and treat human medical problems. Others work in food safety and inspection.

In every state and the District of Columbia, nearly all veterinarians must be licensed. To get a license, a veterinarian must earn a doctor of veterinary medicine degree from an accredited college of veterinary medicine and pass a national exam. In most states, candidates must also pass an exam on state laws and regulations. Some states administer an additional test on clinical skills.

Students applying to veterinary schools face strong competition. A bachelor's degree is not required, but most applicants have one. All schools require 45 to 90 semester hours of college work. Experience working with animals is an advantage.

In 2008, veterinarians held about 59,700 jobs. From 2008 to 2018, employment is projected to increase by 34 percent. According to the BLS, veterinarians earned a median annual salary of $79,050 as of May 2008.

Veterinary Technicians

Veterinary technicians work for veterinarians, performing many routine tasks in veterinary care. For example, they weigh pets, take histories, do laboratory tests, give vaccinations, and assist in surgery. Most technicians work in private clinics and animal hospitals.

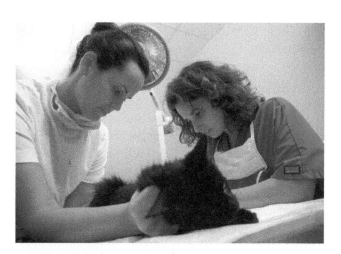

Veterinary technicians work for veterinarians, performing many routine tasks in veterinary care such as weighing pets, taking histories, performing laboratory tests, giving vaccinations, and assisting in surgery.

Most entry-level veterinary technicians have a two-year associate's degree from an accredited veterinary technology program at a community college. Some colleges offer a bachelor's degree. All states require veterinary technicians to be licensed, registered, or certified. State regulations vary, but they all include coursework and an exam.

Veterinary technology is projected to be the 13th fastest-growing occupation from 2008 to 2018. The BLS predicts that employment will grow by 36 percent, adding 29,000 new jobs.

As of May 2008, veterinary technicians had median annual earnings of $28,900.

CHECK POINT

3 What is the difference between a physical therapist and an occupational therapist?

4 What is the difference between a dental hygienist and a dental assistant?

Diagnostic Services

Diagnosis is the determination of the nature and cause of an illness. Professionals in diagnostic services careers determine the presence, absence, or extent of disease and provide data on the effectiveness of treatment.

Cardiovascular Technologists

Cardiovascular technologists perform diagnostic tests on the heart and blood vessels and help treat patients with cardiovascular illnesses. Their work is done at a physician's request or under a physician's supervision. Cardiovascular technologists may specialize in one or more of three areas: invasive cardiology (procedures that involve entering the body with a tube, needle, or other device), noninvasive cardiology (procedures that don't involve entering the body or breaking the skin), and peripheral vascular study (ultrasound scans of the blood vessels). Technologists can perform noninvasive procedures on their own. During invasive procedures, the technologist assists the physician. Tasks may include positioning and preparing the patient and monitoring blood pressure and heart rate.

Cardiovascular technologists have a variety of other tasks. They schedule appointments, review physicians' interpretations and patient files, and compare findings to a standard to identify problems. They operate and care for testing equipment and explain test procedures.

The majority of cardiovascular technologists complete a two-year training program at a junior or community college. Some opt for four-year programs, which are increasingly available. People who are already qualified in another allied health profession may take just one year of specialized instruction.

Two organizations certify cardiovascular technologists: Cardiovascular Credentialing International (CCI) and the American Registry of Diagnostic Medical Sonographers (ARDMS). Most employers require certification.

Cardiovascular technologists and technicians held about 49,500 jobs in 2008. About 77 percent were in hospitals. The rest were in physicians' offices and medical or diagnostic labs, including diagnostic imaging centers. Cardiovascular technologists and technicians had a median annual salary of $47,010 as of May 2008.

Cardiovascular technology is a rapidly growing occupation. The BLS predicts that employment will grow by 24 percent from 2008 through 2018. Technologists who hold multiple credentials and can perform a variety of procedures will have the best job prospects.

This occupation is profiled in more detail in Chapter 7, "Diagnostic and Imaging Services."

Cardiographic Technicians

Cardiographic technicians perform basic *electrocardiograms (ECGs or EKGs)*, which are studies of the heart's electrical activity. People in this occupation are also known as *electrocardiograph technicians* or *EKG or ECG technicians*. With additional training, they may perform these other types of tests:

- Specialized EKG tests
- Stress tests (EKG monitoring while walking on a treadmill)
- Holter monitor tests (using portable EKG devices worn by the patient)

For all tests, cardiographic technicians set up the equipment, explain the procedure to the patient, conduct the test, and communicate the results to the physician. They also may schedule appointments, review patients' files, and perform other tasks required by their employers.

Cardiographic technicians are usually trained on the job. There are one-year certificate programs for basic EKGs, stress tests, and Holter monitor tests. Other training programs, including training for specialized EKG testing, can take 18 months to two years to complete.

Most employers require technicians to be certified. CCI awards the Certified Cardiographic Technician credential to technicians who pass an exam.

The BLS groups cardiographic technicians with cardiovascular technologists, so the information about the number of jobs and the job outlook for cardiovascular technologists applies to cardiographic technicians as well. The BLS predicts that there will be less demand for technicians who can perform only basic EKGs, because hospitals are training nurses and nursing aides to perform EKGs. Cardiographic technicians who can also perform

CAREER LADDER Cardiology Diagnostic Occupations

Occupation	Requirements	Median Earnings	Growth Rate
Cardiovascular technologist	• 2-year training program (most) • Professional certification (required by most employers)	$47,010	24%
Cardiographic technician	• Usually trained on the job. • 1-year certificate for basic EKG, stress, and Holter monitor tests • 18 months to 2 years required for other training programs, including specialized EKG testing • Professional certification (required by most employers)	$22,760 (EKGs) $27,060 (other tests)	24%

stress tests, Holter monitor tests, and specialized EKGs will have better job prospects.

According to a survey by the Alliance of Cardiovascular Professionals, the average salary for technicians performing EKGs was $22,760. For technicians performing Holter and stress tests, it was $27,060. This occupation is profiled in more detail in Chapter 7, "Diagnostic and Imaging Services."

Electroneurodiagnostic (END) Technologists

Electroneurodiagnostic (END) technologists perform a variety of diagnostic tests for brain-related illnesses and injuries. The most common is the *electroencephalogram*, or *EEG*. For this test, the technician uses a paste to attach electrodes to the patient's scalp. The electrodes are wired to a computer, which records the brain's electrical activity. END technologists may also:

• monitor the nervous system during surgery for any warning signs of damage
• conduct scans while patients sleep to screen for sleep disorders
• do long-term monitoring of hospitalized patients to analyze seizures

Some END technologists are trained on the job. However, most employers prefer to hire graduates of accredited END programs. The CAAHEP is the accrediting agency. In 2009, there were 18 accredited programs leading to a diploma, certificate, or, most often, an associate's degree.

For most types of scans, states do not require technologists to be licensed, although efforts toward licensing are being made in some states. Many states do require a professional credential (and Louisiana and New Jersey require licensure) for technologists performing sleep studies. Three organizations offer professional credentials in scan specialties: the American Board of Registration of EEG & EP Technologists, the American Association of Electrodiagnostic Technologists, and the Board of Registered Polysomnographic Technologists.

According to a survey by the American Society of Electroneurodiagnostic Technologists, END technologists earned an average salary of $48,173 in 2006.

Clinical Laboratory Technologists

When blood needs to be typed and cross-matched for a transfusion or when a physician needs to assess a patient's response to drug treatment, the person performing the tests is often a clinical laboratory technologist. Sometimes called medical technologists or clinical laboratory scientists, clinical laboratory technologists perform a wide array of tests on tissues, blood, and other body fluids. These tests provide essential information for diagnosing and treating diseases and improving health.

Clinical laboratory technologists prepare specimens, perform tests, and interpret the results. Some tests are done manually, while others use sophisticated instruments and equipment. Clinical laboratory technologists may develop new tests under supervision. They sometimes set up procedures to help ensure that test results are accurate. They may also supervise technicians. In larger labs, like those in hospitals, clinical laboratory technologists often specialize in particular types of tests.

Entry-level jobs typically require a bachelor's degree with a major in medical technology or a life science. For some jobs, a combination of education, on-the-job training, and specialized training is acceptable. Medical technology programs are available at universities and hospitals.

In some states, laboratory personnel must be licensed or registered. A state's department of health or board of occupational licensing can provide information about requirements. Technologists who perform very complex tests are required by federal law to have at least an associate's degree. Three organizations offer certification. This is optional, but it confers a strong advantage in the job market.

Clinical laboratory technologists held about 172,400 jobs in 2008. The BLS projects employment growth of 12 percent and excellent job opportunities from 2008 to 2018. As of May 2008, the median annual salary of clinical laboratory technologists was $53,500.

This occupation is profiled in more detail in Chapter 6, "Laboratory and Pharmacy Services."

Clinical Laboratory Technicians

Clinical laboratory technicians, also known as medical laboratory technicians, perform tests on tissues, blood, and other body fluids, working under the supervision of a clinical laboratory technologist, a laboratory manager, or another health care professional. Their work typically involves a variety of tests that are routine or less complex than those performed by clinical laboratory technologists. Some are done manually, and some require the use of sophisticated instruments and equipment.

Clinical laboratory technicians collect specimens for testing, prepare them, and perform the tests. They must understand the different procedures required for each test and the instruments used. They check that tests are conducted under the appropriate conditions to ensure accurate results. Caring for laboratory instruments and equipment is another common responsibility.

Clinical laboratory technicians may specialize. For example, they may become phlebotomists (profiled later in this chapter) or histotechnicians, who cut and stain tissue specimens.

A few clinical laboratory technicians learn their skills on the job. However, most have an associate's degree from a community or junior college or a certificate from a hospital, a vocational or technical school, or the armed forces.

Laboratory personnel must be licensed or registered in some states. People interested in this occupation should check with their state department of health or board of occupational licensing. Federal law requires technicians who perform very complex tests to have at least an associate's degree. Clinical laboratory technicians, like clinical laboratory technologists, don't have to be certified, but certification is an advantage in getting jobs. Four organizations offer certification.

Clinical laboratory technicians held about 155,600 jobs in 2008. The BLS projects that this occupation will add 25,000 jobs from 2008 to 2018, an increase of 16 percent. As of May 2008, the median annual salary of clinical laboratory technicians was $35,380.

This occupation is profiled in more detail in Chapter 6, "Laboratory and Pharmacy Services."

Laboratory Assistants

Laboratory assistants, also known as clinical assistants or medical laboratory assistants, provide a variety of clinical and administrative support services. They work under the supervision of laboratory technologists, pathologists, or other lab personnel.

Laboratory assistants collect samples, label them, and prepare them for analysis. They set up routine tests, preparing materials according to established procedures, and record data. They may also perform certain tests. An important part of a laboratory assistant's work is maintaining the laboratory's storage system for specimens. They also maintain supplies and care for equipment, and they may be responsible for cleaning and sanitizing equipment and work areas.

Administrative responsibilities include entering patient data into computer systems, answering phones, assisting callers with inquiries, and referring calls to other personnel when necessary. Laboratory assistants are often the first level of assistance for people requiring services from the laboratory.

Laboratory assistants must have a high school diploma or the equivalent. Many are trained on the job, but some complete a formal training program. Programs typically last nine to 18 months and lead to a certificate. Some programs combine laboratory assistant training with phlebotomist and EKG technician training.

In some states, laboratory personnel must be licensed or registered. As with other laboratory occupations, people interested in becoming laboratory assistants should check with their state department of health or board of occupational licensing for requirements. In addition, federal law regulates the tests they can perform. Laboratory assistants can obtain the Certified Medical Laboratory Assistant (CMLA) credential from American Medical Technologists (AMT) or the National Healthcare Association (NHA). Certification isn't required, but it can help in getting jobs.

A 2009 survey by the American Society for Clinical Pathology (ASCP) found a serious shortage of personnel in the laboratory workforce, including laboratory assistants. According to the same survey, laboratory assistants earned a median salary of $28,080 in 2008.

CAREER LADDER Laboratory Occupations

Occupation	Requirements	Median Earnings	Growth Rate
Clinical laboratory technologist	• Bachelor's degree (typically) • Licensed or registered in some states	$53,500	12%
Clinical laboratory technician	• Associate's degree or certificate (generally) • Licensed or registered in some states	$35,380	16%
Laboratory assistant	• High school diploma or the equivalent • Often trained on the job, or may complete formal training program • Licensed or registered in some states	$28,080	

This occupation is profiled in more detail in Chapter 6, "Laboratory and Pharmacy Services."

Pathologists

When a blood sample or biopsy is rushed to the lab or a body must be examined to determine the cause of death, the person responsible for accurate answers is a pathologist. *Pathology* is the study of diseases, specifically their nature and effects. Pathologists examine blood and tissue samples, check lab tests, and interpret the results. Their work is often essential in diagnosing and treating diseases. Pathologists also make sure that the blood supply is safe. Forensic pathologists (as featured in the popular *CSI* television series) examine bodies to determine the cause of death.

Pathologists are physicians and have the same medical education as other physicians. After medical school, they complete a four-year residency in pathology and then take a certification exam. For many, the next step is training in one of the more than 20 subspecialties of pathology. Pathologists are licensed as other physicians are.

In a survey conducted annually by the ASCP, 47 percent of pathology residents who accepted jobs in 2008 had a starting salary of more than $150,000.

Pathologists' Assistants

Pathologists' assistants examine, dissect, and process tissue specimens and also assist pathologists in performing autopsies.

When biopsied tissue, removed during surgery, arrives in the lab for processing, the pathologists' assistant describes its features, photographs it, dissects it, sends samples for testing, and gives the resulting information to the pathologist. Pathologists' assistants do not make diagnoses.

For an autopsy, a pathologists' assistant has many tasks. These include reviewing the patient's medical history, coordinating information and requests, assisting in the autopsy, selecting and preparing specimens for testing, taking photographs, and helping prepare the autopsy report.

A pathologists' assistant may be placed in charge of billing, budget, supplies, recordkeeping, supervision, or other functions to help keep the lab running smoothly.

The minimum educational requirement for a pathologists' assistant is a bachelor's degree from a regionally accredited university and completion of an accredited pathologists' assistant program. Programs are accredited by the National Accrediting Agency for Clinical Laboratory Sciences (NAACLS), and they are typically master's degree programs. Once the training program has been completed, a pathologists' assistant can take the ASCP national certification exam and assume the title of pathologists' assistant.

Nevada and New York regulate the practice of pathologists' assistants. California requires them to have different levels of supervision depending on whether or not they are certified. The federal government requires pathologists' assistants to hold the equivalent of an associate's degree in a laboratory science and to be appropriately supervised by a pathologist.

The ASCP predicts growth in this occupation in the coming years. According to the society, during 2008, pathologists' assistants earned a median wage of $35 per hour and a median salary of $72,008.

Phlebotomists

A phlebotomist is a clinical laboratory technician who draws blood samples for testing. Phlebotomists must be able to draw blood from patients of all ages, and they must be skilled at different techniques, such as *venipuncture* (drawing blood from a vein), capillary puncture, and finger stick. Phlebotomists are responsible for labeling blood samples, preserving them, and sometimes transporting them. They must apply safety precautions to guard themselves and patients from blood-borne diseases.

Phlebotomists work in hospitals, commercial laboratories, physicians' offices, blood banks, public health clinics, and other places. They even visit patients in their homes.

Phlebotomists need a high school diploma, or the equivalent, and training. Some learn their skills on the job, while others complete formal education programs. These are either independent, stand-alone programs or combination programs (combining, for example, phlebotomist training with laboratory assistant and EKG technician training). Many two-year programs offer phlebotomy certification. Programs are available at hospitals, junior and community colleges, vocational schools, and medical laboratories.

A number of organizations certify phlebotomists. Examples are the National Phlebotomy Association and the American Phlebotomy Association. Certification may fulfill or partially fulfill state requirements, and it confers an advantage in securing jobs. As of 2010, only a handful of states regulated phlebotomists.

The BLS predicts that job opportunities for clinical laboratory technicians, including phlebotomists, will be excellent, with employment growing faster than average. According to the ASCP, the median earnings of phlebotomists in 2008 were $13 per hour and $27,040 per year.

This occupation is profiled in more detail in Chapter 7, "Diagnostic and Imaging Services."

Radiologists

A radiologist is a physician who specializes in interpreting medical images and treating injuries and diseases with medical imaging techniques. The four main techniques are x-ray, computerized tomography (CT), ultrasound, and magnetic resonance imaging (MRI).

Radiologists examine medical images, sometimes still images and sometimes a scan in progress. They may compare what they see to previous scans and to the results of other tests. Then they make recommendations for additional scans or treatment. Radiologists also treat diseases through radiation, *nuclear medicine* (the use of radioactive substances to create diagnostic images or to treat disease), and image-guided surgery.

Radiologists have the same medical education as other physicians. After medical school, they complete a four- to five-year residency in radiology. Following their residency, they often spend one to two years in a fellowship program learning a specialty.

Radiologists are licensed as other physicians are. Typically, they also seek to become board-certified in diagnostic radiology and/or a specialty by the American Board of Radiology or the American Osteopathic Board of Radiology.

Radiologists command high salaries. According to a 2009 survey by the American Medical Group Association, the median salary of diagnostic radiologists in 2007 was $438,115.

Radiologic Technologists/Radiographers

Radiologic technologists perform diagnostic medical imaging tests and give radiation therapy treatments. They work in one of four practice areas: radiography, sonography (ultrasound), nuclear medicine (profiled later in the chapter), and radiation therapy. This profile focuses on the first of those four practice areas.

Radiographers take x-rays for the purpose of diagnosing an injury or illness. In the process, they take precautions to avoid exposing themselves or coworkers to radiation or exposing the patient to more radiation than necessary. They develop the x-rays and determine whether they're satisfactory for diagnosis or need to be retaken. Radiographers do not make diagnoses. They have a variety of other duties, which include keeping patient records, adjusting and maintaining equipment, educating patients, and conducting quality assurance programs.

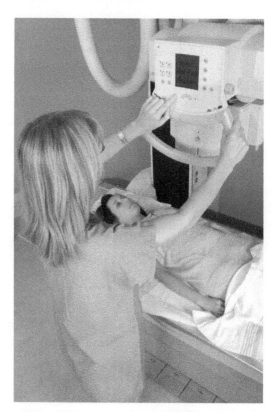

Radiographers take x-rays for the purpose of diagnosing an injury or illness.

Most people wishing to become radiographers complete a two-year associate's degree program. Other options are a certificate program typically lasting 21 to 24 months or a four-year bachelor's degree program. Radiographers can specialize in CT scans, MRIs, mammography, or other imaging procedures. As of 2010, 38 states had licensure or certification laws for radiographers. Students interested in becoming radiographers should check with their state's board of health.

Radiographers can seek certification from the American Registry of Radiologic Technologists (ARRT). As of 2010, 35 states used ARRT exams in licensing. Certification also gives an advantage in the job market.

In 2008, radiographers, together with other radiologic technologists, held about 214,700 jobs. More than 60 percent were in hospitals. Most of the rest were in physicians' offices, medical and diagnostic laboratories, and outpatient care centers. From 2008 to 2018, the BLS projects a 17 percent increase in jobs for these occupations. Because demand is regional, radiographers who are willing to relocate will enjoy better job prospects, as will those who can perform multiple diagnostic imaging procedures (for example, radiography *and* computerized tomography).

As of May 2008, the median annual salary of radiologic technologists was $52,210.

This occupation is profiled in more detail in Chapter 7, "Diagnostic and Imaging Services."

Computed Tomography (CT) Technologists

A computed tomography technologist is a radiographer who specializes in computerized tomography (CT) scans. This type of scan uses x-rays. The x-ray apparatus moves around the patient, taking images from many different angles. The result is a three-dimensional image, revealing body parts that might be hidden in a conventional x-ray.

CT technologists have the same basic education as other radiologic technologists. That is, many complete a two-year associate's degree program, while others choose to earn a one-year certificate or complete a four-year bachelor's degree program. Accredited programs include courses in computerized tomography. In some four-year programs, students can specialize in computerized tomography during their final year.

Practicing radiologic technologists can be trained to do CT scans on the job. However, many return to school for additional formal training, often in programs leading to a one-year certificate. The ARRT offers a certification in computerized tomography based on documented clinical experience and an exam.

The BLS reports that CT scans are replacing x-rays as a first choice for certain kinds of imaging because of their accuracy, giving CT technologists excellent job prospects. Being skilled in multiple imaging procedures and being willing to relocate will further increase a technologist's marketability.

According to a 2007 survey by the American Society of Radiologic Technologists (ASRT), the median salary for CT technologists in 2006 was $56,180.

Magnetic Resonance (MR) Technologists

A magnetic resonance technologist is a radiographer who specializes in magnetic resonance, or MR. MRI (magnetic resonance imaging) uses a magnetic field and radio waves. MRIs are used to detect tumors, aneurysms, and blockages in blood vessels, as well as many other uses.

MR technologists have the same basic education as other radiologic technologists. Many earn a two-year associate's degree. Others opt for a one-year certificate or a four-year bachelor's degree program. Radiologic technologists who want to do MRIs are often trained on the job. A second option is to return to school for a certificate or degree.

ARRT offers certification in magnetic resonance imaging to graduates of accredited schools who pass a certifying exam. For practicing technologists, a second path to certification requires documented clinical experience and an exam. The American Registry of MRI Technologists also offers certification based on completion of an approved program, employment in a related field, or work experience, in addition to passing an exam. As of 2009, three states regulated MR technologists.

The BLS notes that MRI scans are used increasingly for diagnosis, giving MR technologists an advantage in the job market. According to the ASRT's 2007 survey, the median salary for MR technologists in 2006 was $59,677.

Diagnostic Medical Sonographers

Ultrasound is used to diagnose and treat certain medical conditions. Health care workers who perform this type of imaging procedure are known as diagnostic medical sonographers. As they conduct a scan, sonographers decide which images should be shown to the physician. They analyze the results of the scan, prepare preliminary ndings, and make a record of the procedure. Diagnostic medical sonographers may specialize in different systems or parts of the body.

People can prepare for this occupation in several different ways. Training programs are available in hospitals, vocational-technical schools, and the armed forces.

Colleges and universities offer two- and four-year programs leading to an associate's or bachelor's degree. Two-year programs are the most common. The Commission on Accreditation of Allied Health Education Programs (CAAHEP) accredits programs. There are also a few one-year programs that typically lead to a certificate, which are used by practicing health care professionals who want to add sonography to their skills.

New Mexico and Oregon recently became the first two states to require diagnostic medical sonographers to be licensed. Policies and procedures were yet to be established, however. Generally, employers prefer to hire sonographers who have completed accredited programs and who have professional certification. Several organizations, including the ARDMS, offer credentialing.

In 2008, diagnostic medical sonographers held about 50,300 jobs. Roughly 59 percent were in hospitals. Most of the rest were in physicians' offices, medical and diagnostic laboratories, and mobile imaging services. From 2008 to 2018, the BLS projects employment in this occupation to grow by 18 percent. Diagnostic medical sonographers with several specialties or credentials will have the best job opportunities.

Diagnostic medical sonographers had a median annual salary of $61,980 as of May 2008. This occupation is profiled in more detail in Chapter 7, "Diagnostic and Imaging Services."

Positron Emission Tomography (PET) Technologists

A positron emission tomography (PET) technologist is a radiologic technologist who specializes in positron emission tomography, or PET. PET scans use a small amount of radioactive material that is designed to concentrate in a particular area of the body. These scans show changes in cells that occur when serious diseases like cancer are in their early stages and often more treatable. Another common use of PET scans is to reveal the extent of damage after a heart attack.

There are several paths to becoming a PET technologist. One is to complete a two- or four-year nuclear medicine technology program leading to an associate's or a bachelor's degree. (PET scanning is a specialty in nuclear medicine technology.) The Joint Review Committee on Education Programs in Nuclear Medicine Technology (JRCNMT) accredits these programs. Another path is to pursue a bachelor's degree with courses that provide a scientific grounding for nuclear medicine and then to

obtain a certificate in nuclear medicine. Radiologic technologists who already have an associate's degree and wish to specialize, or other health care professionals who want to change professions, can complete a one-year certificate program.

Licensing requirements for PET technologists vary. People interested in this occupation should check the requirements of the state in which they plan to work. The Nuclear Medicine Technology Certification Board (NMTCB) offers a specialty exam in positron emission tomography.

The BLS reports that while the use of nuclear medicine imaging technologies, such as PET scans, is increasing, only moderate job growth can be expected, due to costs and other factors. Technologists who can also perform other types of scans will have the best job prospects. Salaries of PET technologists are comparable to those of other nuclear medicine technologists (see "Nuclear medicine technologists," below). In a survey by NMTCB, salaries of PET technologists were slightly higher than those of nuclear medicine technologists.

Nuclear Medicine Technologists

A nuclear medicine technologist is a radiologic technologist who specializes in *nuclear medicine*, the use of radioactive materials to create diagnostic images or treat diseases. For diagnostic scanning, the nuclear medicine technologist prepares and administers the radioactive material. The material is attracted to a particular part of the body and concentrates there for a brief time. The technologist looks for lower or higher concentrations of the material than expected, which can indicate disease. The technologist then selects images to show the physician and does some preliminary analysis. Examples of nuclear medicine scans are PET scans, single photon emission computerized tomography (SPECT) scans, bone scans, and cardiovascular imaging.

Nuclear medicine technologists also assist in therapy. They ensure that the correct dosage is prepared and perform other tasks such as verifying the patient's identity and observing radiation safety procedures.

A person can become a nuclear medicine technologist by completing an associate's degree, bachelor's degree, or certificate program in nuclear medicine technology. Two-year programs are typically offered at community colleges, bachelor's degree programs at four-year colleges and universities, and certificate programs at hospitals. Certificate programs are intended for health care professionals who already hold an associate's or bachelor's degree but wish to specialize in nuclear medicine or change careers.

More than half of all states have licensure or certification laws for nuclear medicine technologists. Requirements differ, so people interested in this occupation should investigate the rules for the state where they plan to work. Certification, while voluntary, is a professional standard that employers typically expect. The ARRT and the NMTCB offer certification.

In 2008, nuclear medicine technologists held about 21,800 jobs. The BLS projects that this occupation will add 3,600 jobs from 2008 to 2018, for a growth rate of about 16 percent. Technologists who can do different types of diagnostic scans will have the best job prospects. The median annual salary of nuclear medicine technologists in 2008 was $66,660.

This occupation is profiled in more detail in Chapter 7, "Diagnostic and Imaging Services."

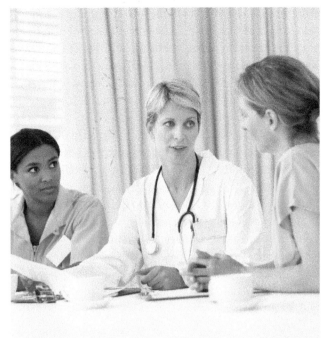

Health services administrators, also known as health care administrators and medical and health services managers, plan, direct, coordinate, and supervise the delivery of health care.

> ### CHECK POINT
>
> **5** Laboratory scientist is another name for which health care occupation?
>
> **6** If a laboratory assistant wanted to advance, what would be the most logical position to seek next, and what would that person have to do to prepare for it?

Health Informatics

Most of the careers in the health informatics career cluster involve managing medical information, using computers and other means. Some health informatics workers document client care. Others provide medical information to health care professionals, insurers, patients, and the public. Still others serve as managers.

Health Services Administrators

Health services administrators help keep departments, facilities, and systems running smoothly. Also known as health care administrators and medical and health services managers, they plan, direct, coordinate, and supervise the delivery of health care.

The responsibilities of health services administrators vary depending on the size and type of facility they manage. In smaller facilities, such as nursing homes, top administrators handle many details of daily operations. In larger facilities, administrators may have one or more assistants to whom they delegate responsibility for some areas. In clinical departments, the administrator often has relevant clinical experience. For example, a clinical laboratory technologist might serve as the laboratory manager. Health services administrators also work for small groups of physicians, for large practices, and in managed care settings.

A master's degree is the standard level of education for this occupation. The degree may be in health services administration, long-term care administration, health sciences, public health, public administration, or business administration. For some jobs, a bachelor's degree or on-the-job experience is acceptable.

Many areas of medical and health services management are not licensed. All states and the District of Columbia require nursing care facility administrators to have a bachelor's degree, pass an exam, and complete a state-approved training program. Some states also license administrators of assisted living facilities. Health services administrators can seek the Registered Health Information Administrator credential from the American Health Information Management Association.

Health services administrators held about 283,500 jobs in 2008. The BLS projects that employment of health services administrators will grow 16 percent from 2008 to 2018. As of May 2008, the median annual salary of health services administrators was $80,240. Earnings vary depending on the type and size of the facility and the level of responsibility.

Medical Librarians

Medical librarians provide information about new medical treatments, clinical trials, and standard procedures to physicians, other health care professionals, and researchers. They train medical students and others to find and use medical resources, and they give patients and consumers authoritative information about health topics. Medical librarians work at medical colleges and universities, corporations, hospitals, government agencies, research centers, and public libraries. They manage distance education programs, digital libraries, and web sites.

Medical librarians need a master's degree in library science (M.L.S.) and a strong background in the sciences. Admission to a library science graduate program requires a bachelor's degree in any undergraduate major. Medical librarians can apply for membership in the Academy of Health Information Professionals, a credentialing program of the Medical Library Association.

According to a 2008 survey commissioned by the Medical Library Association, the average (mean) salary for medical librarians was $65,796, and the median salary was $60,000.

Health Educators

Health educators teach people how to stay healthy, improve their health, and manage diseases. They may talk to high school students about the health effects of smoking, counsel a patient on how to manage high cholesterol, conduct a class for caregivers on coping with Alzheimer's disease, develop a brochure for pregnant women on good prenatal nutrition, or produce a video on HIV and STDs.

To secure an entry-level job as a health educator, a person generally needs a bachelor's degree in health education. Most higher-level jobs and jobs in public health require a master's degree. Many students earn a master's degree after majoring or working in a related field, like nursing.

Working health educators and those within three months of completing their degree can be certified by the National Commission of Health Education Credentialing by passing an exam on a health educator's basic areas of responsibility. Certification can provide an advantage in the job market and is required to work in a public health department in some states.

In 2008, health educators held about 66,200 jobs. The BLS projects employment will grow by 18 percent from 2008 to 2018. In most settings, demand will increase, but schools may see a decrease because of budget cuts.

Health educators had a median annual salary of $44,000 as of May 2008. In the settings employing the greatest numbers of health educators, annual earnings ranged from $36,050 to $56,390.

Health Information Coders

Health information coders assign codes to describe a patient's diagnosis and treatment. These codes determine what the patient's health insurance plan will pay. In assigning codes, accuracy, medical knowledge, and careful attention to detail are important. If a code is incorrect or incomplete, payment may be reduced, delayed, or denied. *U.S. News & World Report* named health information coder as a "Hot Healthcare Job" in 2009.

Most coders learn their skills on the job. A number of schools offer certificate programs in coding, and it is part of a health information technician associate's degree program.

Coders can seek certification from a number of professional organizations. The American Health Information Management Association (AHIMA), for example, offers 5 general credentials and 19 specialty credentials in areas such as general surgery and obstetrics and gynecology.

The BLS puts coders in the category of medical records and health information technicians. These workers held 172,500 jobs in 2008. The Bureau projects job growth of 20 percent for this group from 2008 to 2018.

A 2009 survey by the AAPC reports that certified coders earn an average annual salary of $44,750. Most employers prefer to hire credentialed coders.

This occupation is profiled in more detail in Chapter 9, "Health Information and Administration."

Medical Billers

Medical billers collect payment for services provided by a physician or other health care practitioner. They accept copayments, submit claims to insurance companies, and invoice patients. Depending on the office setup, they may also code. Medical billers answer patients' questions about health insurance and office billing procedures. Another important part of their job is negotiating with insurance companies and collection agencies, usually by phone.

People interested in this occupation need a thorough understanding of insurance and HIPAA regulations. They must be able to use medical billing software and submit claims both by mail and electronically. They must also have excellent organizational and communication skills. Medical billers work in physicians' offices, hospitals, clinics, and other settings. A growing number work at home.

Medical billers can learn their skills on the job. Several vocational schools and community colleges offer certificate programs, and medical billers can earn a certificate or an associate's degree in medical billing and coding. The American Medical Billing Association certifies members who pass an exam. Medical billers can also earn coding certifications as described in the profile of health information coders.

The BLS groups medical billers with billing and postal clerks and machine operators. Together, this group held nearly 529,000 jobs in 2008. The BLS predicts about 15 percent growth for these occupations from 2008 to 2018.

The median annual salary of billing and postal clerks and machine operators as of May 2008 was $30,950. Medical billers who do coding may expect earnings more consistent with those of health information coders. Certification may help in securing higher-paying jobs.

Health Information Technicians

Health information technicians work with patient information. People in this occupation are responsible for assembling and organizing medical charts and ensuring that all documentation—patient notes, treatment plans, test results, and so on—is properly recorded, entered in the computer, and added to the patient's file. Health information technicians must maintain the confidentiality of patient information and ensure that the people and agencies requesting it are authorized to have it.

Health information technicians may have a variety of additional duties. They may process business and government forms and prepare admission and discharge documents. They may also assemble data for research projects for medical staff and administrators and do some analysis of it. Health information technicians can specialize in two areas: coding (see "Health information Coders," above) and cancer registry (maintaining databases of cancer patients).

Health information technicians usually have an associate's degree. The Registered Health Information Technician (RHIT) credential, offered by the AHIMA, provides a strong employment advantage. Candidates must complete a two-year associate's degree program accredited by the Commission on Accreditation for Health Informatics and Information Management Education and pass a written exam.

In 2008, health information technicians held about 172,500 jobs, roughly 39 percent of which were in hospitals. Other employers included physicians' offices, nursing care facilities, outpatient care centers, and home health care services. The BLS projects that employment in this occupation will increase by 20 percent from 2008 to 2018. As of May 2008, the median annual salary of health information technicians was $30,610.

This occupation is profiled in more detail in Chapter 9, "Health Information and Administration."

Medical Transcriptionists

Medical transcriptionists listen to recordings dictated by physicians and other health care professionals and transcribe them into medical reports, letters, and other documents. Typically, they listen with a headset, using a foot pedal to pause the recording when necessary. Increasingly, streamed transcription is sent over the Internet. Medical transcriptionists key the transcription in word processing software and then edit for grammar and clarity. For this occupation, accuracy, attention to detail, and knowledge of medical terms, jargon, and abbreviations are essential.

CAREER LADDER Health Informatics Occupations

Occupation	Requirements	Median Earnings	Growth Rate
Health information coder	Education/training options: • Most learn on the job • As part of an associate's degree for health information technicians • Licensing not required	$44,750	20%
Health information technician	• Usually a two-year associate's degree • Licensing not required	$30,610	20%
Medical biller *May advance to health information coder*	Education/training options: • Learn on the job • Certificate or associate's degree in medical billing and coding • Licensing not required	$30,950	15%
Medical transcriptionist *May advance to health information technician or coder*	Education/training options: • Learn on the job • Two-year associate's degree • One-year certificate program Licensing not required	$15.41/hour	11%

Two trends in medical transcription are the outsourcing of transcription to foreign countries and the use of speech recognition technology. Both trends have generated jobs for medical transcriptionists in editing, proofreading, and formatting documents.

Employers prefer to hire transcriptionists with postsecondary training in medical transcription. Two-year associate's degrees and one-year certificate programs are available through vocational schools, community colleges, and distance learning programs. Some transcriptionists, especially those already familiar with medical terminology from other health care occupations, need only refresher courses and training.

As in many other fields, certification is recognized as a sign of competence. The Association for Healthcare Documentation Integrity awards two voluntary credentials, Registered Medical Transcriptionist (RMT) and Certified Medical Transcriptionist (CMT).

Medical transcriptionists held about 105,200 jobs in 2008. Nearly 60 percent worked in hospitals and physicians' offices. The BLS projects that employment will grow by 11 percent from 2008 to 2018. Job opportunities will be good, especially for transcriptionists who are certified.

As of May 2008, the median hourly wage of medical transcriptionists was $15.41.

This occupation is profiled in more detail in Chapter 9, "Health Information and Administration."

✓ CHECK POINT

7 For a person who enjoys learning about many different health topics, likes working with people, and wants a high-growth occupation, which health informatics occupation would be a good choice?

8 If a medical biller wanted to advance, what would be the most logical position to seek next, and what would that person have to do to prepare for it?

Support Services

Health care workers in support services provide care for patients, directly or indirectly. Or they create a therapeutic environment for providing health care.

Biomedical Engineers

Biomedical engineering is an engineering specialty. Engineers use technology to solve problems. They take ideas and transform them into reality. Biomedical engineers create devices and procedures that improve health care by solving medical and health-related problems. For example, biomedical engineers took a portable 3-D laser scanner, used in factories to check parts, and morphed it into a device that scans body parts to produce prosthetics.

For a woman who has lost a breast to cancer, the other breast can be scanned to produce a "twin." Products of biomedical engineering include instruments for medical procedures, artificial organs, prostheses and orthotic devices, and devices that deliver automatic insulin injections or control body functions.

Nearly all entry-level engineering jobs require a bachelor's degree in engineering. For biomedical engineers, many employers require or prefer a graduate degree. Most biomedical engineers need to combine their biomedical training with another engineering specialty, like mechanical or electronics engineering.

Biomedical engineers held about 16,000 jobs in 2008. This is the fastest-growing occupation in the country. The BLS projects 72 percent job growth for this occupation from 2008 to 2018. The median annual salary of biomedical engineers as of May 2008 was $77,400.

Biomedical/Clinical Technicians

Few workplaces have as many different kinds of equipment as a hospital. When something breaks down, the results can be more than inconvenient—they can be life-threatening. Who cares for equipment in hospitals and other health care facilities? That person is a biomedical/clinical technician.

Biomedical/clinical technicians, also known as biomedical or medical equipment technicians, install, calibrate, maintain, repair, and overhaul all kinds of medical equipment. They sometimes operate equipment or help acquire it, and they train people to use it. This occupation was rated as one of the best careers of 2009 (and of 2008) by *U.S. News & World Report*. To become a biomedical/clinical technician, a person can complete a two-year associate's degree program in biomedical equipment technology, electronics, or an engineering-related field at an accredited institution. Four-year programs are also available. Technicians who have an educational background in electronics may be trained on the job. The military also trains biomedical/clinical technicians.

Technicians typically spend their first three to six months on the job working closely with an experienced technician. Then, still under close observation, they begin to work more independently.

Technicians sometimes specialize in a particular type of equipment. The International Certification Commission for Clinical Engineering and Biomedical Technology offers certification for three specialties: biomedical, laboratory, and radiology equipment. Certification isn't required but can be helpful in getting a job and advancing. Criteria generally include an accredited educational program, work in the field, and an exam. If a candidate has worked for four years in the field, a degree isn't necessary.

CAREER LADDER Biomedical Occupations

Occupation	Requirements	Median Earnings	Growth Rate
Biomedical engineer	• Bachelor's or master's degree in engineering	$77,400	72%
Biomedical/clinical technician	Education/training options: • 2-year associate's degree in biomedical equipment technology, electronics, or engineering-related field • 4-year bachelor's degree • On-the-job training (technicians with education in electronics) • Military	$41,520	27%

The BLS predicts that employment growth for this occupation will be 27 percent from 2008 to 2018. As of May 2008, the median annual salary of biomedical/clinical technicians was $41,520.

Industrial Hygienists

Industrial hygienists examine workplaces to ensure that they present no dangers to employees or the surrounding community. Examples of the many threats they check for are poor indoor air quality, lead or asbestos, unsafe noise and radiation levels, and hazardous waste. Industrial hygienists take samples of potentially hazardous materials, analyze them, and make recommendations to remove or control the materials. They investigate incidents, and they do audits to ensure that companies and employees are following health and safety laws and procedures. They also make sure a workable emergency response plan is in place. Another responsibility of industrial hygienists is to educate employees and the public about potential risks to safety and health.

Industrial hygienists receive both classroom and on-the-job training. Typically, they hold a bachelor's degree in industrial hygiene, safety, a science or engineering area, or another related discipline. Many also have a master's degree in industrial hygiene or a related field.

In some states, industrial hygienists must be licensed. Licensing requirements vary but often include certification by the American Board of Industrial Hygiene. To sit for the certifying exam, applicants must have a B.A. or B.S. with 60 hours of undergraduate or graduate work in specific subjects, four years of professional experience, and college or continuing education courses in additional specified subjects.

The BLS predicts that employment for industrial hygienists and other occupational health and safety specialists will increase by 11 percent from 2008 to 2018. In a 2008 survey by the American Industrial Hygiene Association, the average salary was $94,947.

CHECK POINT

9 What do industrial hygienists do?

10 Of the occupations profiled in this section, which one was rated as one of the "Best Careers 2009" (and 2008) by *U.S. News & World Report*?

Biotechnology Research and Development

Biotechnology is the manipulation of genetic material in living organisms, or parts of living organisms, to make products and services. Biotechnology has produced pest-resistant crops, biofuels, and techniques for cleaning up the environment. In the field of health care, biotechnology workers create vaccines, drugs, medical treatments, diagnostic tests, and other products and services that improve diagnosis and treatment.

Microbiologists

If you open a newspaper or a magazine like *Discover* or *Popular Science*, there's often a fascinating story about the work of microbiologists. Can genetically engineered bacteria make antibodies in the human body? Will bacteriophages—bacteria-killing viruses—become the next superbug? Where did an outbreak of *E. coli* start, and how did it spread?

Microbiologists study microorganisms—their structure, how they behave, their dangers and benefits, and how they interact with people. Many microbiologists use biotechnology in their work.

A bachelor's degree in biology or microbiology opens the door to many jobs. Microbiologists at this level, for example, identify disease-causing microorganisms in water and food. They also check vaccines, antibiotics, and other products for safety. Those with a master's degree can be supervisors, laboratory managers, or research managers or associates. For higher-level positions, a Ph.D., M.D., or combined degree is almost always required. Scientists, research directors, consultants, and science advisors or administrators work at this level.

Microbiologists held 16,900 jobs in 2008. The BLS predicts that 2,100 new jobs will be added between then and 2018. As of May 2008, microbiologists had a median annual salary of $64,350.

Medical Scientists

Medical scientists research human diseases with the goal of improving people's health. Those working in biotechnology study viruses and bacteria and help develop vaccines, drugs, and other treatments. Many work with human genes, determining their functions and how they're linked to diseases. Others produce drugs based on substances in the human body, such as insulin.

People who want to become medical scientists should begin with a bachelor's degree in a biological science. After that, they can follow one of two main paths. The first is a university Ph.D. program in the biological sciences, which generally takes about six years. The second path is an M.D.-Ph.D. program at a medical college, which generally takes seven to eight years. After completing their studies, medical scientists typically do postdoctoral research. Medical scientists who perform invasive procedures on patients or give them drug or gene therapy must be licensed like other physicians.

In 2008, medical scientists held about 109,400 jobs. The BLS projects that employment of medical scientists will increase by 40 percent from 2008 to 2018, making medical science the sixth fastest-growing occupation. The median annual salary of medical scientists as of May 2008 was $72,590.

Research Scientists

Biological scientists study living organisms and their relationship to the environment. Biotechnology research scientists are biological scientists who apply that understanding to develop and improve products and services. Because biotechnology has such widespread applications, biological scientists in many different specialties work as biotechnology research scientists.

Biotechnology research scientists usually need a Ph.D. A master's degree is accepted for some jobs in applied research or product development. After obtaining a Ph.D., it is common for research scientists to take a temporary postdoctoral job. Here, a scientist can gain specialized research experience and have the opportunity to publish, which is often key to obtaining permanent research positions.

MONEY magazine rated biotechnology research scientist as one of its best jobs in 2006, based on salary and job prospects. That year, biological scientists held about 87,000 jobs. The BLS projects that employment will grow by 21 percent from 2008 to 2018. As of May 2008, the median annual salary of biochemists (including biological scientists) and biophysicists (which the BLS classifies together) was $82,840.

Research Assistants

The work of research assistants supports the efforts of microbiologists, medical scientists, research scientists, and an entire research and development team. Research assistants set up, run, and care for instruments. They monitor experiments, make detailed observations, analyze data, and interpret results. In addition, research assistants may prepare technical reports and plans for experiments or studies.

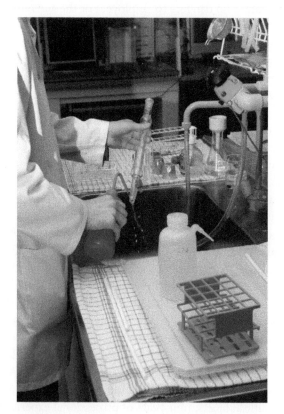

Research assistants set up, run, and care for instruments, as well as monitor experiments, make detailed observations, analyze data, and interpret results.

To become a research assistant, a person needs an associate's degree in applied science from a community college or technical school. Many research assistants earn a bachelor's degree and advance to the position of research associate. Research associates usually specialize and contribute their particular expertise to a project. They may develop methods of advancing projects, discover new ideas, do their own experiments, identify discoveries that could be patented, contribute to articles for professional journals, and attend conferences.

Biological technicians, including biotechnology research assistants, held 79,500 jobs in 2008. The BLS projects a growth rate for these occupations during 2008–2018 of 18 percent. As of May 2008, the median hourly wage of biological technicians was $18.46. The average salary for those working for the federal government was $39,538.

These are just a few of the many occupations within health care. The next few chapters will explore certain health care professions in greater detail.

CHECK POINT

11 What is biotechnology, and how is it used in the field of health care?

12 What would a research assistant need to do to advance to the position of research associate? What would be the professional advantages?

Chapter Wrap-Up

Don't forget to visit thePoint companion website for additional study resources!

CHAPTER HIGHLIGHTS

- When thinking about a career in health care, it is important to thoroughly explore the many opportunities and resources that are available. Libraries, the Internet, professional organizations, and people working in health care careers are good resources.
- Many health care professions are subject to licensure from the states. Licensed health care professionals must practice their profession according to the guidelines and limitations set by the state in which they are licensed.
- Registration means that a health care professional has graduated from an accredited school and has passed a standardized national exam administered by a nongovernmental agency, usually a professional organization.
- Certification, which is awarded by professional organizations, is generally optional but often leads to more and better job opportunities and higher pay.
- More than 300 occupations and career specialties are available in health care. This chapter has briefly profiled 67 careers in therapeutic services, diagnostic services, health informatics, support services, and biotechnology research and development.

REVIEW QUESTIONS

Matching

1. _____ Pathologists' assistant
2. _____ Phlebotomist
3. _____ Prosthetist
4. _____ Diagnostic medical sonographer
5. _____ Audiometric technician

   a. Might design an artificial knee **b.** Tests people's hearing **c.** Might help with autopsies
   d. Draws blood samples for testing **e.** Might do an ultrasound scan of the abdomen

Multiple Choice

6. Which of the following requires the most education?
   - **a.** certified nursing assistant
   - **b.** dental assistant
   - **c.** physician assistant
   - **d.** medical assistant

7. Which of the following takes x-rays?
   - **a.** MR technologist
   - **b.** END technologist
   - **c.** cardiographic technician
   - **d.** radiographer

8. Which of the following works with medical insurance payments?
   - **a.** health information coder
   - **b.** biomedical technician
   - **c.** medical transcriptionist
   - **d.** health educator

9. Which of the following checks workplaces for poor air quality, noise and radiation levels, and other hazards?
   - **a.** clinical technician
   - **b.** industrial hygienist
   - **c.** biomedical engineer
   - **d.** radiographer

10. Which of the following use radioactive materials in their work?
    a. radiologists
    c. nuclear medicine technologists
    b. PET technologists
    d. all of the above

Completion

11. In many health care professions, a/an _____ from the state is mandatory and shows that a health care professional has met the fundamental standards for performing the job.

12. Careers in the _____ career cluster are concerned with managing medical information.

13. A professional organization, rather than the government, controls _____, which isn't required to work but assures employers that a person has met a certain competency level.

14. _____ means that a school is recognized by an outside agency, such as a national board or commission, as having standards that qualify graduates for professional practice.

15. _____ are the most highly trained of emergency medical technicians (EMTs), with the greatest level of responsibility.

Short Answer

16. What is the difference between a registered nurse and a licensed practical nurse?

_____

_____

17. Name at least five specialties for radiologic technologists.

_____

_____

18. Explain some typical work responsibilities of a health information technician.

_____

_____

19. Describe what biomedical/clinical technicians do in their jobs.

_____

_____

20. What are the typical work responsibilities of a research assistant?

_____

_____

INVESTIGATE IT

1. Choose one of the occupations described in this chapter that interests you and that isn't profiled later in the text (Chapters 3–9). Investigate this occupation in depth. Use resources in the "Recommended Reading" and other resources as needed. Find details about what people in this occupation typically do, where they work, what their working conditions are like, and the job outlook and salaries for this occupation in your state. If possible, interview a person in this occupation.

2. Choose a health care occupation that isn't described in this chapter and profile it, including the kinds of information provided for occupations in this chapter. The web site of the Bureau of Labor Statistics (http://www.bls.gov) is a good resource for salary information and job growth prospects.

3. Research a legal or ethical topic that affects one or more of the health care professionals profiled in this chapter. Use Chapter 18, "Law, Ethics, and Professionalism in Health Care," as a resource. Be ready to explain the topic and what the health care professional should know or do about the topic. Here are some examples of topics (and search terms):
    - malpractice
    - implied and informed consent
    - the Controlled Substances Act
    - HIPAA
    - patient confidentiality
    - scope of practice
    - codes of ethics

RECOMMENDED READING

American Medical Association. Careers in Health Care. Available at: http://www.ama-assn.org/ama/pub/education-careers/careers-health-care.shtml.

Health Workforce Information Center. Professions. Available at: http://www.hwic.org/topics/professions.php.

Mayo Clinic. Career Exploration. Available at: http://www.mayoclinic.org/careerawareness/careerexploration.html.

National Institutes of Health. Office of Science Education. LifeWorks. Available at: http://science.education.nih.gov/LifeWorks.nsf/feature/index.htm.

U.S. Department of Labor. Bureau of Labor Statistics. *Occupational Outlook Handbook.* St. Paul: Jist Publishing. Updated every two years. Available at: http://www.bls.gov/OCO.

U.S. National Library of Medicine. Health Occupations. Available at: http://www.nlm.nih.gov/medlineplus/healthoccupations.html.

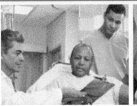
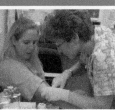
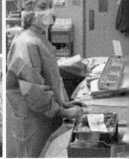

Patient Care: Medical and Surgical

CHAPTER OBJECTIVES

After careful study of this chapter, you should be able to:

* Explain the education, training, and legal requirements for becoming a medical assistant, surgical technologist, physician assistant, and EMT/paramedic.

* Describe the typical work responsibilities in each of these professions.

* List desirable personal characteristics of medical assistants, surgical technologists, physician assistants, and EMTs/paramedics.

* Identify employment opportunities and key trends for these occupations.

* List and explain the benefits of membership in a professional organization.

KEY TERMS

administrative tasks
clinical tasks
direct patient care

manual dexterity
medication administration
    record (MAR)

pathology
sharps container

sterile field
suture (SŪ-chŭr)

The health care occupations described in this chapter are different in many ways, but they all have one thing in common—they all involve direct patient care. Medical assistants, surgical technologists, physician assistants, and EMTs/paramedics are all part of health care teams that provide medical care to ill or injured people.

MEDICAL ASSISTANTS

Medical assistants often handle both the administrative tasks in a medical office and certain clinical tasks. Administrative tasks usually involve carrying out office proce-

dures. Clinical tasks are activities that involve examining patients and helping treat them. Medical assistants work in doctors' offices, hospitals, clinics, nursing homes, physical therapy facilities, imaging centers, laboratories, research facilities, and many other health care settings.

Medical assistants shouldn't be confused with physician assistants, profiled later in this chapter. Medical assistants may perform specific clinical procedures, but these tasks are more limited than those performed by physician assistants, and medical assistants do not have the authority to diagnose or treat patients.

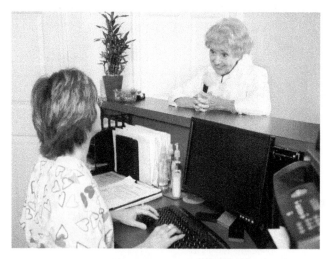

In addition to clinical tasks, medical assistants may perform administrative duties.

History of the Profession

The history of medical assisting can be traced to the early twentieth century. In the early years, office assistants were trained on the job to perform clinical procedures, or nurses were taught to do administrative work. In 1924, a biology teacher named M. M. Mandl opened the first school to train assistants to work in physicians' offices. That school still operates today.

In 1956, the American Association of Medical Assistants (AAMA) was founded. Its certification exam, first administered in 1963, set the standards for medical assistant education. Working with the American Medical Association (AMA), the AAMA developed a curriculum for accredited medical assisting programs, and AMA/AAMA became an accrediting agency. In 1977, the responsibility for accrediting programs passed to a committee sponsored by the AMA but independently operated. In the early 1990s, that committee was replaced by the Commission on Accreditation of Allied Health Education Programs (CAAHEP). The Accrediting Bureau of Health Education Schools also accredits medical assisting programs.

Education, Training, and Legal Requirements

Some medical assistants are trained on the job, but many complete a one- or two-year medical assisting program.

Such institutions as vocational-technical high schools, post-secondary vocational schools, and community and junior colleges offer these programs. Most one-year programs lead to a certificate or diploma; most two-year programs award an associate's degree. Two-year programs usually include general studies, such as English and math, in addition to professional courses. Medical assisting classes generally cover these areas:

- anatomy and physiology
- medical terminology
- typing and transcription
- computer applications
- office practices
- insurance processing
- recordkeeping and accounting
- patient relations
- clinical and diagnostic procedures
- laboratory techniques
- administration of medications
- pharmacology
- first aid
- medical law and ethics

As of 2010, nearly 600 accredited programs were available. Programs usually include an internship in which students work at a physician's office, hospital, or other health care facility, where they apply what they learn in class and gain practical experience.

For medical assistants who learn their skills on the job, a high school diploma or the equivalent is usually required. Volunteer experience in health care is also helpful. These medical assistants usually spend their first few months attending training sessions and working closely with experienced workers.

In some states, medical assistants can perform more advanced procedures, such as taking x-rays or giving injections, after passing a test or completing a course.

Professional certification is optional, but it offers advantages. Many employers prefer to hire medical assistants who are certified, and certified medical assistants often earn better salaries. Two nationally recognized credentials are

- CMA (AAMA): certified medical assistant, offered by the AAMA
- RMA (AMT): registered medical assistant, offered by American Medical Technologists (AMT)

Certification requirements vary but generally include graduating from an accredited medical assisting program and passing an exam. Medical assistants also may be certified in specialty areas, such as ophthalmology, optometry, or podiatry.

While working, many medical assistants continue to take courses for professional growth and development—

for example, in new computer programs, new clinical procedures, changes in medications, and new laws and regulations. Many certified medical assistants complete approved courses, workshops, and programs so that they can be recertified. Beyond that, continuing education is essential for them to keep current in the field and competitive in the job market.

Work Responsibilities

The duties of medical assistants vary depending on the type and size of the setting in which they work. In family practices, for example, medical assistants may do mostly clinical work. In psychiatric practices, they may perform mostly administrative duties. Administrative tasks include both work performed in any type of office and work that's specific to a health care setting. In large practices, medical assistants may specialize in a specific area.

Clinical responsibilities vary among employers. Laws regarding the clinical duties a medical assistant may perform differ from state to state, but most states leave it up to physicians to determine what the medical assistants they employ can and cannot do.

The following is a partial list of clinical duties:

measuring and recording a patient's height and weight

obtaining medical histories

assisting with physical examinations

preparing and administering medications

drawing blood samples

assisting with or performing diagnostic or basic laboratory tests

assisting with minor office surgery

preparing and sterilizing instruments

collecting and preparing laboratory specimens

recognizing and treating medical emergencies

educating patients about tests, procedures, medications, special diets, health maintenance, and disease prevention

Medical assistants may perform many different types of clinical procedures. Some specific examples are listed below:

measuring blood pressure

collecting a throat specimen

administering eye medications

performing blood glucose testing

assisting with therapeutic soaks

completing an EKG

changing dressings

removing sutures (materials used to close wounds)

disposing of biohazardous materials

measuring a patient for crutches

Personal Characteristics of Medical Assistants

Medical assistants need good communication skills. Since they are often the first staff members that patients meet in the office, their attitude and ability to communicate set the tone for future interactions. Medical assistants have to share information clearly and accurately with patients, physicians, and other health care workers. As a result, they must be good at verbal communication and be careful listeners. In addition, they must be able to write clearly and accurately.

Effective medical assistants are good organizers and good at managing time. They must keep schedules, medical records, financial data, supplies, and many other items

---

Typical Tasks of a Medical Assistant
Administrative

- Greet patients
- Answer telephones
- Manage appointments and schedules
- Arrange hospital admissions and laboratory services
- Organize, update, and file patients' medical records
- Complete medical reports from dictation
- Handle correspondence
- Manage office expenses and payroll
- Perform billing and collection procedures
- Manage supplies and equipment
- Fill out insurance forms and file claims

Clinical

- Measure and record a patient's height, weight, and blood pressure
- Obtain medical histories
- Assist with physical examinations
- Measure a patient for crutches
- Prepare and administer medications
- Draw blood samples and collect throat specimens
- Assist with or perform diagnostic or basic laboratory tests
- Prepare and sterilize instruments
- Assist with minor office surgery
- Change dressings
- Remove sutures (materials used to close wounds)
- Assist with therapeutic soaks
- Dispose of biohazardous materials
- Recognize and treat medical emergencies
- Educate patients about tests, procedures, medications, special diets, health maintenance, and disease prevention

SPOTLIGHT ON SKILLS Typical Task: Administer an Intradermal Injection

Position: Medical Assistant

When a patient needs medication, the most efficient way of administering it, other than orally, is by injection. *Intradermal injections* are administered into the *dermis*, the layer beneath the skin's surface. They are used to administer different kinds of skin tests for allergy testing and tuberculosis (TB) screening.

To prepare for an injection, a medical assistant washes his or her hands and gathers supplies. The medical assistant chooses the proper needle and syringe, reviews the physician's order, and selects the correct medication. The medical assistant must check the label three times—when taking the medication from the shelf, when drawing it up into the syringe, and when returning it to the shelf. The medical assistant then calculates the dosage, if necessary, and assembles or prepares the syringe.

When providing direct care to patients, the medical assistant should greet and identify the patient and explain what is about to happen. For an injection, the medical assistant must ask about any known medication allergies. Then he or she selects an appropriate site to administer the injection. Intradermal injections are usually given in the anterior forearm or the upper back. After cleaning the site, the medical assistant puts on gloves, pulls the patient's skin taut to allow the needle to enter the skin with less resistance and to secure the patient against movement, and inserts the needle at a 10- to 15-degree angle. This low angle helps ensure that the correct layer of skin is reached.

After the injection, it is important not to press on or massage the site, which could push the medication into

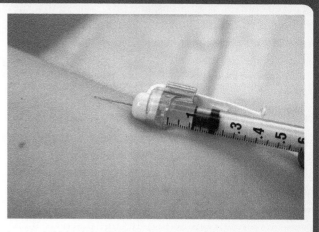

Intradermal injections are given at a 10- to 15-degree angle.

the tissues or out of the injection site. It is also undesirable to apply a bandage to the site, because a bandage might cause redness or swelling that could result in an inaccurate reading. The needle is immediately discarded into a **sharps container** (a puncture-resistant, leakproof disposable container for sharp items, such as needles and scalpels).

Depending on the type of test, the length of time required for a reaction, and the policies of the particular workplace, the medical assistant may read the test results and check the injection site or may tell the patient to return to the office at a particular time or check the results at home. Then the medical assistant documents the procedure, site, results, and any instructions to the patient in the medical record.

up to date and arranged in an orderly way. Medical assistants should be comfortable and skilled at handling several tasks at once. They need to be able to set priorities, choosing what needs to get done first and planning a logical sequence for all tasks. At the same time, they should be prepared to shift priorities when the situation demands it.

Several other personal characteristics are important. Medical assistants need good interpersonal skills, or the ability to get along well with others. They also must be comfortable working as members of a team. In addition, medical assistants should be able to pay close attention to detail and to remain calm in stressful or emergency situations.

Employment Opportunities and Trends

The Bureau of Labor Statistics (BLS) projects that the demand for medical assistants will grow 34 percent from

2008 to 2018, making it the nation's sixteenth fastest-growing occupation. Helping to drive this growth is the rising number of group practices, clinics, and other health care facilities that need support personnel. Medical assistants, who can handle both administrative and clinical duties, are ideal for such settings. In addition, demand for medical assistants is high because they work mostly in primary care, a growing sector of the health care industry.

Other trends in health care also contribute to creating more jobs for medical assistants:

- The need for health care workers of all kinds will increase due to the growth and aging of the population and technological advances in medicine. These advances provide more options for diagnosis and treatment and allow people to live longer.
- As people continue to develop medical conditions like diabetes and obesity, the need for health care services will increase.

- To care for additional patients, doctors will continue to need more medical assistants.
- The pressure of cost control will prompt health care facilities to substitute less expensive workers, such as medical assistants, for higher-wage workers, where the law allows.

In 2008, medical assistants held about 483,600 jobs. Roughly 62 percent worked in physicians' offices. Another 13 percent worked in hospitals. Eleven percent worked in the offices of other health care practitioners, such as chiropractors, optometrists, and podiatrists. Most of the rest were employed in outpatient care centers, nursing and residential care facilities, and other health care settings.

The BLS predicts excellent job prospects for medical assistants, both from newly created jobs and from the need to replace workers who leave the occupation. Applicants with formal training, experience, and certification should have the best job opportunities.

Professional Organizations

Medical assistants are not required to join a national organization in order to work. Membership in a professional organization, however, has many benefits, including:
- access to educational seminars
- access to continuing education units
- subscription to professional journals
- access to annual conventions
- group insurance plans
- networking opportunities

Information about professional organizations can be obtained by visiting their web sites, talking to instructors, or contacting a local chapter.

Two national professional organizations for medical assistants are the AAMA and AMT. The mission of the AAMA is to help medical assistants improve their knowledge, skills, and professionalism; to protect their right to practice; and to promote effective health care delivery through its professional credential. The organization has more than 325 local chapters in 43 states. Local chapters and state societies provide opportunities for networking and for continuing education through seminars and workshops. The AAMA's professional journal, *CMA Today*, includes articles that provide continuing education. Additional benefits include a national conference and discounts on self-study courses.

Founded in 1939, AMT has more than 41,000 members, including medical assistants and other allied health personnel. It places a strong emphasis on continuing education through its annual convention, state society meetings and seminars, and online learning. The organization encourages professional development through participation in state and national meetings and boards. It also offers a career center with an online job bank.

CHECK POINT

1 What are a medical assistant's work responsibilities?

SURGICAL TECHNOLOGISTS

Surgical technologists perform a variety of tasks so that operations proceed smoothly and safely. They work with surgeons, anesthesiologists, and nurses as vital members of the operating room team.

History of the Profession

Surgeons have had assistants throughout history, but the modern profession of surgical technology dates to after World War II. Many operating room technicians, as they were then called, came from the military, which had trained its own technicians during the war. Civilian technicians were trained on the job, with standards varying widely.

Various groups, including technicians and operating room nurses, worked to make the operating room technician a recognized professional with universal training standards. In 1969, the Association of Operating Room Technicians was formed; later, the group was renamed as the Association of Surgical Technologists (AST). In 1972, the AMA approved a set of recommended educational standards, and an accreditation review committee was formed. The AST established a certification program, code of ethics, and standards of practice. It participates in the accreditation review committee and helps define a core curriculum for accredited schools.

Education, Training, and Legal Requirements

To become a surgical technologist, a person must have a high school diploma or GED and must complete a training program. Training programs last from nine months to two years and lead to a certificate, diploma, or associate's degree. Programs are offered by community and junior colleges, vocational schools, universities, hospitals, and the military. Applicants may need to take the ACT exam or a health profession exam. As of 2010,

455 surgical technologist programs are accredited by CAAHEP.

Training programs combine classroom instruction, mock surgery, and supervised work in hospitals as part of a surgical team. Course work includes the following:
- anatomy and physiology
- medical terminology
- microbiology (the study of microscopic forms of life)
- pharmacology
- physical environment and safety standards
- sterile techniques
- surgical procedures
- patient care and safety
- legal, moral, and ethical issues
- communication skills
- skills for professional behavior

Students also learn how to sterilize instruments and how to transport patients and position them on the operating table. They learn how to prevent and control infection and care for wounds. Students are taught to handle surgical equipment, drugs, solutions, and supplies. They must become familiar with many different types of surgical instruments and understand how they are used. Newer medical technology, such as laser or endoscopic surgery, may also be covered.

Surgical technologists are not licensed, though state law may limit the scope of their work. Certification is also not required, but most employers prefer to hire certified technologists.
- The CST (certified surgical technologist) credential is awarded by the National Board of Surgical Technology and Surgical Assisting. To earn this credential, candidates must graduate from an accredited CAAHEP program and pass an exam.
- The National Center for Competency Testing (NCCT) awards the Tech in Surgery–Certified, or TS-C (NCCT), credential. To take the exam, candidates must meet one of the following requirements: (1) have completed a training program recognized by the U.S. Department of Education; (2) have completed any training program and gained one to two years of experience doing the job; (3) have at least seven years of experience doing the job in the previous ten years; or (4) belong to one of several other health care occupations and have extensive experience doing the work of a surgical technologist.

Both certifications must be renewed after several years through continuing education or an exam. Surgical technologists need to keep up with changes in technology, new surgical techniques, and other developments in the field through continuing education and other means.

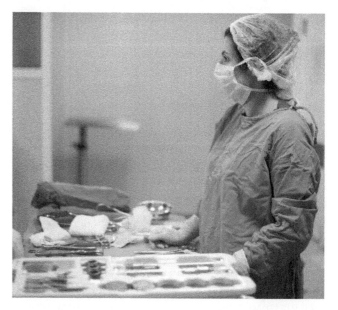

Surgical technologists keep track of surgical equipment before, during, and after surgery.

Work Responsibilities

Most of a surgical technologist's work can be divided into three phases: before, during, and after an operation.

Before an Operation

Before an operation, a surgical technologist prepares the operating room, gathering the necessary supplies and equipment. He or she checks all equipment to make sure it is working properly and places instruments, other supplies, and equipment exactly where they will be needed during the surgery. The surgical technologist helps count sponges, needles, and instruments. This important task is done again both during and after surgery to make sure nothing is left inside the patient.

When the patient arrives in the pre-operative area, a surgical technologist provides emotional support if the patient wants or needs it and may check charts and monitor vital signs. He or she transports the patient to the operating room and helps position the patient on the operating table. It is the surgical technologist's responsibility to prep the patient, by washing the site where the surgeon will make the incision (cut), shaving the area, if necessary, and wiping it with disinfectant.

Before assisting with an operation, surgical technologists *scrub* (thoroughly wash their hands and forearms) and put on sterile gowns and gloves. They may help other team members put on their gowns and gloves.

Next, a surgical technologist puts sterile drapes over the patient to create a sterile field, a germ-free area around the patient where an operation is performed. To protect the patient from infection, the surgical technologist must maintain the sterile field before, during, and after the operation until the patient is transported to the recovery area.

During an Operation

During an operation, a surgical technologist may pass instruments, equipment, and supplies to the surgeon and surgical assistant. The technologist may hold *retractors*, instruments used to pull back skin; use sponges or suction to clear fluids from the operation site; cut sutures; and set up drains and tubing. He or she may monitor vital signs and operate equipment. It is also the surgical technologist's responsibility to take care of any specimens collected during the operation. The technologist labels these specimens, records them, and sends them for analysis. A technologist also may prepare dressings and apply them to the incision site.

After an Operation

After an operation, a surgical technologist takes the patient to the recovery room. Surgical technologists also remove the used instruments, equipment, and supplies from the operating room, dispose of them appropriately, and set up the room for the next patient.

Typical Tasks of a Surgical Technologist

- Establish a sterile field
- Open sterile supplies
- Perform a surgical scrub
- Assist with draping a patient
- Receive drugs or solutions in the sterile field
- Pass instruments to the surgical team
- Help with drug, needle, and instrument counts
- Collect waste and sharps containers
- Inspect for room readiness
- Restock unused supplies

Personal Characteristics of Surgical Technologists

Surgical technologists have very responsible positions. People considering this occupation should have a strong sense of responsibility and should be conscientious about their work.

Surgical technologists must be good organizers and skilled at paying attention to detail. Tasks like arranging the operating area and setting up instruments and equipment require these skills.

SPOTLIGHT ON SKILLS Typical Task: Open a Sterile Pack

Position: Surgical Technologist

Many of the basic supplies and equipment for a surgical procedure may be packaged together in a sterile surgical pack. Opening these packs properly is essential for preparing and maintaining a sterile field. Surgical technologists are taught to open a sterile pack in a specific way.

First, the technologist verifies the procedure to be performed and retrieves the appropriate pack. The technologist checks the label for the contents, expiration date, and any tears, stains, or moisture, which could mean contamination. Then the technologist places the package, with the label facing up, on a clean, dry, flat surface, such as a Mayo or surgical stand.*

After washing his or her hands, the technologist carefully removes the package's sealing tape, taking care not to tear the wrapper. Many disposable packages are wrapped in clear plastic film that will become the sterile field. The first flap of the folded wrapper is loosened by pulling it up, out, and away, letting it fall over the far side of the table or stand. That way, there's no need to reach across the sterile field again. The side flaps are opened in a similar way, using the left hand for the left flap and the right hand for the right flap. It is important to touch only the outer surface, not the sterile inner surface.

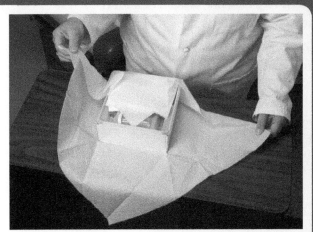

Maintaining a sterile field while opening a sterile pack.

Next, the technologist grasps the outer surface of the remaining flap and pulls it down and toward him or her. The outer surface of the wrapper is against the surgical stand, and the sterile inside of the wrapper forms the sterile field. The steps are repeated for packages with a second inside wrapper (which also will provide a sterile field). The contents of the pack are now ready for use in surgery.

*Sterile fields are set up on stands holding sterile instruments and supplies, as well as at the operation site.

Accuracy and precision are two other important qualities. Counting sponges, needles, and instruments, for example, requires these abilities. Surgical technologists must be careful, steady workers.

People in this occupation must have initiative. They should know their own jobs thoroughly and do tasks without having to be told. They also must understand the jobs of other members of the surgical team, as well as the surgical procedure being performed. That way, they can anticipate what is needed and be ready with that item.

Surgical technologists must be accurate listeners. They need to respond quickly and correctly when a surgeon asks them for an instrument or when another team member gives them instructions. During a surgical procedure, everyone must work quickly and efficiently to keep the patient as safe as possible.

Like medical assistants, surgical technologists should be good team players. They need to be able to work well with the other members of the surgical team. The ability to stay calm and think clearly during stressful or emergency situations is also important.

Surgical technologists need manual dexterity, or skill at working with their hands, to handle surgical instruments properly and quickly. Being in good physical condition is also important, because surgical technologists spend a lot of time on their feet.

Employment Opportunities and Trends

Like medical assisting, surgical technology is a rapidly growing occupation. The Bureau of Labor Statistics predicts that this career will grow 25 percent between 2008 and 2018, adding 23,200 new jobs. One factor leading to this growth is an expected increase in the number of surgeries performed due to general population growth and the rising proportion of older people in the population. Older people generally require more surgeries than younger ones.

A second reason for job growth is improvements in medical technology. Technological advances will result in new surgical procedures, thus increasing the need for surgical technologists.

In 2008, most surgical technologists—about 71 percent—worked in hospitals. Others were employed in physicians' offices and outpatient care centers. Some worked in dentists' offices where outpatient surgery is performed. A few worked directly for surgeons as part of special surgical teams, such as transplant teams.

The BLS predicts that most surgical technologists will continue to work in hospitals. However, it expects much faster job growth for technologists in physicians' offices and outpatient care centers, where pay is higher.

Surgical technologists who are certified will have the best job opportunities.

Professional Organization

The professional organization for surgical technologists is the AST. Its main purpose is to ensure that surgical technologists have the knowledge and skills required to deliver the highest quality of care. The AST works to advance the profession by helping set accreditation standards and by lobbying at the state and national levels. Membership benefits include free and discounted continuing education opportunities; a career center where members can search for jobs and post professional profiles; a subscription to *The Surgical Technologist*, the organization's professional journal; and an annual national conference.

CHECK POINT

2 What personal characteristics should a surgical technologist have?

PHYSICIAN ASSISTANTS

A physician assistant, or PA, examines patients, diagnoses illnesses, arranges treatment, and performs many other tasks that doctors typically do. However, a PA must perform these tasks under the supervision of a physician. Physician assistants provide primary care in rural settings, inner-city clinics, and other places where doctors are sometimes in short supply. In a busy medical practice, a physician assistant can free up a physician by assuming responsibility for routine tasks. In 2009, *Money* magazine ranked physician assistant second among its 50 best jobs in America, based on factors such as salary and job

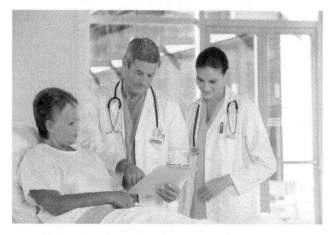

Under the supervision of physicians, PAs examine patients, diagnose illnesses, arrange treatment, and perform many other tasks that doctors typically do.

satisfaction. It was also named one of the 50 best careers of 2010 by *U.S. News and World Report*.

History of the Profession

Physician assisting is a young occupation that began in the 1960s. As with surgical technology, the first members came from the ranks of *corpsmen*, enlisted men trained by the military to provide first aid and basic medical care. The career was born when doctors urged that a new mid-level health care professional be created. A shortage of primary care physicians, particularly in some geographic locations, was the primary reason for this need.

In 1964, Surgeon General William Stewart asked Dr. Richard A. Smith to develop a training program for PAs. The resulting MEDEX (Medical Extension) model called for the use of students and graduates in communities without adequate medical services. The following year, a separate pilot program at Duke University Medical Center enrolled the first four PA students, all former Navy corpsmen.

In the next 15 years, the occupation developed rapidly. Universities established degree programs, and in 1969, the American Association of Physician Assistants (AAPA) was founded. Articles in popular magazines attracted ex-corpsmen to the new occupation and helped make it more acceptable to the public. The AMA and other professional organizations, as well as private groups and the federal government, helped to promote and develop it. Processes for accreditation and certification were established. In 1973, the first national certifying exam was administered. Insurance companies started approving payment for the services of PAs, and states began allowing certified PAs to practice.

Since then, the profession has continued to grow. The PA's role has expanded, and PAs are used in an increasing number of health care settings. By 2009, nearly 74,000 PAs were in practice, according to an estimate by the American Academy of Physician Assistants (AAPA).

Education, Training, and Legal Requirements

To become a PA, a person must complete an accredited education program and pass a national exam. These are the requirements to obtain a license, which is required for practice by every state and the District of Columbia. Applicants must have completed a minimum of two years of college and, for nearly every program, must have some work experience in health care. According to the AAPA, applicants usually have a B.A. or B.S. degree and have worked in the field for about four years.

A college student planning to apply to a PA education program should take classes in biology, chemistry, mathematics, psychology, English, and the social sciences. Applicants include registered nurses and members of other allied health occupations, such as emergency medical technicians (EMTs), paramedics, physical therapists, and respiratory therapists.

Programs are typically full time and usually last at least two years. The average length, according to the AAPA, is about 26 months. Typical classroom subjects include the following:

- biochemistry (the study of chemical processes in organisms)
- pathology (the science of the causes and effects of disease)
- anatomy
- physiology
- microbiology
- pharmacology
- physical diagnosis
- clinical medicine
- geriatric and home health care
- disease prevention
- medical ethics

Students also receive clinical training through clerkships, or rotations, in hospitals and clinics. This training covers areas such as emergency medicine, family medicine, geriatrics, internal medicine, obstetrics and gynecology, pediatrics, psychiatry, and surgery.

Education programs are accredited by the Accreditation Review Commission on Education for the Physician Assistant (ARC-PA). As of 2009, 148 entry-level programs were offered. Most programs are in schools of allied health, academic health centers, medical schools, and four-year colleges. A few are in community colleges, the military, and hospitals. The commission maintains a list of accredited programs. Of these programs, 120 offer the option of a master's degree. Most of the remaining programs award a bachelor's degree, with a few conferring an associate's degree or a certificate.

All PAs must pass the Physician Assistant National Certifying Examination, administered by the National Commission on Certification of Physician Assistants (NCCPA). Only graduates of accredited PA education programs may take the exam. A successful grade earns the credential "Physician Assistant-Certified."

To keep their certification, PAs must pass a recertification examination every six years. In addition to the exam, PAs must complete 100 hours of continuing medical education every two years through courses, journal reading, independent study, and other means. An alternative to the traditional exam is an open-book exam. PAs who select this option must also earn 100 credits through taking courses, teaching, publishing, or other approved activities.

Physician assistants may choose to specialize in emergency medicine, surgery, or another area. Specializing requires additional education. Physician assistants can complete postgraduate programs in critical care, internal medicine, neonatology (care of newborns), occupational medicine, primary care, psychiatry, surgery, and other specialties.

Work Responsibilities

Physician assistants always work under the supervision of a physician or surgeon and within their scope of practice. Their responsibilities vary according to state law, experience, training, and the decisions of their supervisor. Typically, PAs have these responsibilities:

- taking medical histories
- completing physical examinations
- advising patients on diet, exercise, and other means of staying healthy
- interviewing and examining sick people
- diagnosing diseases
- discussing their diagnoses with patients

- treating patients' diseases
- ordering and analyzing lab tests, x-rays, and EKGs
- treating minor injuries, such as applying splints and casts

All states, the District of Columbia, and Guam allow PAs to prescribe some medicines.

Physician assistants work fairly independently. Nevertheless, PAs are taught to know the limits of their practice and to refer or defer to physicians when appropriate. When faced with cases that are unusual, complicated, or difficult to manage, they consult with a physician or refer the patient to one.

Typical Tasks of a Physician Assistant

- Take a complete medical history
- Perform a comprehensive physical exam
- Order and interpret basic laboratory work
- Record progress notes
- Suture cuts and wounds
- Draw blood
- Introduce catheters
- Administer IV (intravenous) medications
- Apply and remove plaster casts
- Do a vision screening

SPOTLIGHT ON SKILLS Typical Task: Adding Medications to an Intravenous (IV) Solution

Position: Physician Assistant

Hospitalized patients often receive medications intravenously. Physician assistants working in hospitals may need to add medications to an IV solution.

After gathering equipment, the physician assistant checks the patient's chart for allergies and verifies that the medication and IV fluid are compatible. Then the PA calculates the infusion rate. PAs must know the actions, safe dose ranges, purpose of administration, and adverse effects of the medication and consider whether they are appropriate for the patient.

Once these points have been researched and cleared, the medication is prepared. The PA washes his or her hands and unlocks the medication cart or drawer. This may involve entering a pass code and scanning employee identification. The PA reads the **medication administration record (MAR)** and selects the proper medication. He or she checks the label at least three times and performs calculations, if necesary. The cart or drawer must be relocked after use.

After washing hands again, the PA greets and identifies the patient, checks the patient's allergy bracelet, or asks the patient about allergies. The PA then explains the purpose and action of the medication.

For the medication to be administered, the clamp between the solution container and roller clamp on the infusion tubing must be closed and the IV pump paused, if appropriate. The PA cleans the medication port with an antimicrobial swab. He or she steadies the container, uncaps the needle or needleless device, inserts it into the port, and injects the medication. Next, the PA removes the container from the IV pole and gently rotates it to mix the medication and solution.

The PA then hangs the container, properly labeled with the dose of medication, back on the pole. The clamp is opened and the flow rate readjusted (or the pump is restarted after checking the settings for the correct infusion rate).

IV medications can have a rapid effect. For this reason, the PA must evaluate the patient for a certain period of time after administering an IV medication.

Personal Characteristics of Physician Assistants

Becoming a PA takes time and effort. People who are considering this occupation should be hard workers. They also should be self-disciplined and capable of setting goals and working on their own to reach them.

Like other health care professionals, PAs must be levelheaded and have good judgment. They must be comfortable making decisions and able to make sound decisions in emergencies. Physician assistants work with many others, including their supervising physicians, other health care professionals, and patients and their families. Therefore, they need good interpersonal skills. With patients, PAs need a good bedside manner. They need to show respect and compassion for the patient, as well as maintain professionalism.

Physician assistants must be able to speak clearly and precisely. They should be capable of talking effectively and appropriately with patients and other health care providers. Good PAs also listen carefully. When examining a patient, they are keen and careful observers. Physician assistants also must be capable readers and good writers.

Physician assistants must have integrity. They must know the boundaries of their knowledge and be ready to consult physicians and refer cases when necessary. PAs have to respect confidentiality and follow laws and ethical standards.

Finally, physician assistants must be prepared for lifelong learning. They need to realize that their education doesn't stop once they get their PA credential.

Employment Opportunities and Trends

Physician assisting is the seventh fastest-growing occupation. The BLS predicts that it will grow by 39 percent between 2008 and 2018, adding 29,200 new jobs. The bureau cites two reasons for this predicted job growth:

- the continued growth of health care industries, due to an increasing demand for health care and technological advances that make longer lives possible
- the drive to control costs, which makes PAs an attractive option, because they can provide routine services and skilled assistance in medical and surgical procedures at lower cost

Jobs for physician assistants will be available in both office settings and institutions. Hospitals, university medical centers, public clinics, and prisons are some examples. Rural and inner-city clinics will continue to look to physician assistants to help meet their medical care needs. Job

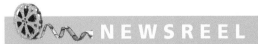

NEWSREEL

Rising Health Care Costs Mean Opportunities

One of the long-term trends that characterize the health care industry is the drive to contain costs. In clinics, hospitals, small practices, and many other health care settings, an effective strategy is to assign more responsibilities to employees who cost less, particularly routine duties or assisting work. This approach also frees up more expensive employees, like doctors, for specialized work and other duties.

Medical assistants and physician assistants benefit from this trend. State laws regulate the clinical tasks each occupation can perform to some degree. The supervising physician, however, has considerable latitude in assigning clinical tasks, and the facility plays a role, too. As a result, medical assistants and physician assistants are gaining new responsibilities and expanding their scope of duties.

opportunities for new PAs will increase as PAs retire or change occupations. In states that allow PAs to perform more services, the opportunities will be greater.

Physician assistants held about 75,000 jobs in 2008. About half worked in physicians' offices, and a quarter worked in hospitals. Most of the rest worked in outpatient care centers; the federal government; and colleges, universities, and professional schools. Some PAs were self-employed. Physician assistants also work in nursing homes, HMOs, VA medical centers, public health agencies, and almost every other health care setting.

Professional Organization

The professional organization for PAs is the AAPA. For professional development, it offers an annual conference, networking opportunities, recognition through a Distinguished Fellow program, and scholarships. The organization also provides continuing education opportunities and produces a journal and other publications.

The Physician Assistant Foundation, which is part of the AAPA, solicits member donations and sponsors fundraising events for charitable projects that provide quality health care and health care education. Two examples are free medical care for children in Namibia orphaned by HIV/AIDS and bike safety sessions and free bike helmets for children in Seattle.

The Physician Assistant Education Association represents physician assistant education programs. Its members include the faculty and staff of all accredited programs.

The association can serve as a resource for information about individual programs and the application process.

CHECK POINT

3 What education and training are needed to become a PA?

EMTs/PARAMEDICS

Emergency medical technicians (EMTs) and paramedics provide emergency medical treatment for people in their homes, at the scene of accidents, and in other locations where immediate care is required. They continue to care for these patients on their way to the hospital. The services that EMTs or paramedics provide depend on their level of training and certification. Emergency medical technicians with the highest level of training (EMT-paramedic) are called *paramedics*.

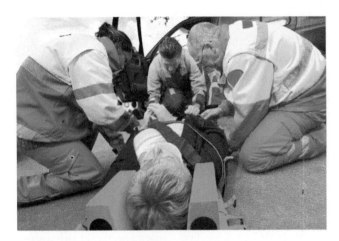

Emergency medical technicians provide care at an accident scene.

History of the Profession

Although common today, emergency medical care for victims at the scene of an accident is actually a very recent phenomenon. Before the mid-1960s, few laws regarding such care existed, and few communities had an organized system for treating and transporting sick or injured people. Often, firefighters, police officers, and volunteers took victims to the hospital. According to one account from the 1960s, fewer than half of ambulance drivers were trained to the level of Red Cross advanced first aid. Morticians provided half of all ambulance services because their hearses were big enough for stretchers.

Changes began with a report published in 1966 by the National Academy of Sciences and the National Research Council. This report was the result of a three-year investigation of the initial care that accident victims received and the emergency medical services available to them.

The report recommended the establishment of standards in three key areas:
- ambulance design and construction
- ambulance equipment and supplies
- qualifications and supervision of ambulance personnel

The report also urged states to establish policies and regulations for ambulance service and encouraged districts, counties, and cities to set up systems to deliver that service.

Congress responded with the National Highway Safety Act of 1966, which directed the Department of Transportation (DOT) to set minimum standards for ambulance and equipment design and provider training. It also directed each state to develop an emergency medical services (EMS) system.

In 1970, at the recommendation of a presidential committee, the National Registry of Emergency Medical Technicians (NREMT) was formed. Now an independent agency, NREMT develops standards and qualification levels for EMTs, offers education and training, and administers certification and recertification examinations.

The first paramedics faced obstacles in applying their skills. One was the lack of state laws permitting them to give advanced medical care. For example, in a pilot program in Los Angeles, a nurse had to ride with a paramedic on all calls. California became the first state to enact a law permitting paramedics to deliver certain types of emergency medical care. A second obstacle was opposition from some doctors and nurses who did not believe that paramedics were qualified to give adequate emergency treatment.

As states worked toward compliance with the law, the television series *Emergency!* (1972–1979) brought paramedics and emergency medical services to the public's attention. Based on the paramedic service in Los Angeles County, the show is credited with raising public support for paramedic and emergency medical services and spurring the creation of EMS systems across the country.

In 1971, DOT published a National Standard Curriculum (basic training course) for EMTs. Within six years, all states used this or a similar course for state certification.

The Emergency Medical Services Systems Act of 1973 provided additional guidelines for training and equipment. It also supplied funding for planning and starting EMS programs, as well as grants and contracts for research and studies.

In the early 1980s, the federal government turned responsibility for authorizing and funding EMS over to the states. For the next two decades, paramedic training continued to develop and improve, as did ambulance services, emergency rooms, and government systems for providing emergency medical care.

ZOOM IN

The Golden Hour

People often refer to the quiet, pleasant time after work, or after young children have been put to bed, as the "golden hour." In emergency medicine, however, the golden hour is the period immediately after a victim sustains a life-threatening injury or experiences the sudden onset of a critical illness. This is the period during which a majority of victims could be saved if they get the treatment they need. "Only 60 minutes," says the New Jersey Trauma Center at The University Hospital in Newark, from the moment of injury to notify the police; dispatch an ambulance to the scene; transport the victim to a hospital; summon the appropriate surgical and support staff; and perform the necessary life-saving surgery. Without an organized, regionalized system of emergency medical care, it is easy to imagine how that Golden Hour could tick away before each element could be completed."

The golden hour can be more than an hour, or it can be less. The victim's condition determines how quickly life-saving treatment is needed. Still, the basic principle—the need for quick, effective emergency medical care—is the same.

Education, Training, and Legal Requirements

To become an EMT or a paramedic, a person must complete a formal training program. Applicants need a high school diploma or GED and a driver's license. Training is offered at three levels, with certification required by all states at each level. All levels of EMTs must be able to perform the skills taught at the lowest level. Each level includes both classroom instruction and work in a hospital or clinic or in the field.

- **EMT-Basic.** These training programs, offered by hospitals, fire and police departments, community colleges, and other organizations, follow the DOT National Standard Curriculum. Classroom instruction generally takes about 110 hours. Students also work with experienced EMTs in the field or at emergency rooms or clinics. At the basic level, EMTs learn to assess, lift, and move patients; administer CPR; control bleeding; give oxygen; treat shock, burns, poisoning, and allergic reactions; and use an automatic defibrillator. They also learn how to deliver babies, calm people, deal with emotionally disturbed patients, and apply splints and bandages. Graduates of approved programs must pass a written and practical examination administered by the state or NREMT.

- **EMT-Intermediate.** Training requirements for this level, which is being phased out in some locations, vary by state. EMT-Intermediate has two nationally recognized sublevels, EMT-Intermediate 85 and EMT-Intermediate 99. These levels usually require 30 to 350 hours of additional training based on scope of practice. Candidates learn to perform tasks at a higher level, such as advanced patient assessment, and they learn additional skills, such as how to use a manual defibrillator, start an IV, and insert an endotracheal tube (a tube placed in the *trachea*, or windpipe).

- **EMT-Paramedic.** This is the most advanced level of training. Subjects are studied in much greater depth than at the lower levels. Paramedics can give many more medications than EMTs at the lower levels. They can use advanced life support systems and supplies and provide advanced emergency services. The National Standard Curriculum calls for hospital and field work, with students progressing in the field to serve as team leaders. Candidates then do a field internship. EMT-Paramedic programs—usually one to two years long—are offered by community colleges and technical schools. These programs may lead to an associate's degree. Upon passing the NREMT exam, graduates are certified as paramedics.

The NREMT registers (or certifies) EMTs at each level. In most states and the District of Columbia, NREMT registration is required for some or all levels of certification. Other states have their own certification exams or let EMTs or paramedics choose which exam to take.

EMTs and paramedics must be recertified, usually every two to three years. Generally, they must be working as an EMT or paramedic, have current CPR certification (and, for paramedics, current advanced cardiac life support certification), and take an exam or a refresher course and additional continuing education courses.

Work Responsibilities

EMTs and paramedics respond by ambulance to emergency calls, typically from 911 dispatchers. Knowledge of the area and road conditions that might affect their choice of route, such as construction or traffic, is important. Often, EMTs and paramedics are the first qualified personnel to arrive at the scene. They have to assess the situation swiftly. If they find multiple victims, they must determine the priority of care.

EMTs and paramedics must evaluate a patient's illness or injury quickly and try to get information about the person's medical history. They talk to the victim, if possible, or to people who know the victim. They look for medical

ID bracelets or other clues. Information about allergies, diabetes, and other conditions can help determine what has caused a critical illness and can affect how an illness or injury is treated.

EMTs and paramedics provide many different types of emergency care. For example, they may perform CPR, clear blocked airways, stabilize a fracture, or treat a collapsed lung. They give some types of treatment on their own, using established procedures. For others, they follow specific instructions from a physician given by radio. Their level of certification partly determines the care EMTs or paramedics are allowed to provide.

Typical Tasks of an Emergency Medical Technician (EMT)

- Recognize hazards and potential hazards
- Assess a patient's breathing
- Do a rapid trauma assessment
- Provide oxygen by a face mask
- Suction an airway
- Use an automated external defibrillator
- Start an IV
- Run and read an EKG
- Attach a cardiac monitor and a pulse oximeter
- Insert an artificial airway
- Stabilize impaled objects
- Administer certain medications

Once patients have been stabilized, it is safe to transport them. Not all patients are taken to a medical facility. Minor injuries may be treated on the scene, and the patient may be allowed to leave afterward. Patients treated in their homes may be well enough to stay there. Those who do need to go to a hospital are lifted onto stretchers, which are placed in ambulances and secured. When a life-threatening illness or injury can't be treated effectively on the scene and time is an essential factor, the EMT or paramedic may decide to "load and go"—transporting the victim immediately. Some paramedics are part of helicopter crews, transporting critically ill or injured patients to trauma centers.

EMTs and paramedics generally work in two-person teams. In these teams, one person drives the ambulance and the other monitors the patient and provides any care needed. A physician continues to direct this care by radio. During the drive, the EMTs or paramedics also radio the medical facility's emergency department, giving them the number of patients, their condition, and the estimated arrival time.

At the medical facility, EMTs and paramedics may help take patients to the emergency room and assist with the first steps in their care. They also provide any information about the patients that they can. Afterwards, EMTs and paramedics check in with their dispatchers and get ready for the next call. They restock supplies and make sure the ambulance is clean and ready to go.

Personal Characteristics of EMTs/Paramedics

To manage the high stress in their jobs, emergency medical technicians and paramedics must be emotionally steady. They must be able to make quick decisions and to stay calm and clear-headed in dangerous situations. The ability to calm and reassure patients, family members, and bystanders is valuable.

Workers in this occupation need excellent communication skills. The National Standard Curriculum for

SPOTLIGHT ON SKILLS Typical Task: Provide Oxygen by Continuous Positive Airway Pressure (CPAP)

Position: EMT/Paramedic

EMTs and paramedics often have to help patients who are having difficulty breathing. For severe respiratory distress, continuous positive airway pressure, or CPAP, is an alternative to inserting an endotracheal tube. A CPAP device provides sufficient air pressure to prop airways open, easing breathing and improving gas exchange in the lungs.

The patient is placed in a seated position. The EMTs or paramedics then apply a cardiac monitor and a pulse oximeter, which measures the amount of oxygen in the arterial blood. They set up the CPAP system and explain the procedure to the patient. They start airflow, verify that oxygen is flowing to the mask, and place the mask over the patient's mouth and nose. They gradually increase the pressure, following a set of standards. Every few minutes, vital signs and pulse oximetry are taken.

If the patient improves, CPAP continues until arrival at the hospital, with an EMT or paramedic notifying the hospital in advance that CPAP is being used. If the patient does not improve or worsens, CPAP is stopped and another method of supplying air to the lungs is employed.

EMT-Basic includes specific instruction on radio communications, verbal reports to hospital staff, and written care reports. Emergency medical technicians and paramedics must be able to communicate information about a patient clearly, both orally and in writing. They must be able to listen carefully and speak clearly and accurately to patients and other emergency personnel.

Emergency medical technicians and paramedics must be comfortable working independently and as part of a team. They also must have good leadership skills. These workers should be in good physical condition and able to lift and carry heavy loads. Finally, EMTs and paramedics should be willing and able to improve their knowledge and skills.

Employment Opportunities and Trends

The BLS predicts that employment for EMTs and paramedics will grow by 9 percent between 2008 and 2018. The bureau points to three factors prompting this growth:

- As with other occupations profiled in this chapter, more jobs will be available for EMTs and paramedics because the number of older adults is rising. Older adults are more likely to require emergency medical services, thus creating more EMT jobs.
- EMTs and paramedics are spending more time with each patient, due to emergency room overcrowding. With overcrowding, it can take longer to transfer a patient's care to the hospital emergency department. Overcrowding also means that the nearest hospital sometimes cannot admit a patient, so the EMTs and paramedics must continue providing care while the patient is moved to a more distant hospital.
- More and more, hospitals are specializing in treating particular illnesses or injuries. When patients are transferred to another hospital, they usually must travel in an ambulance and be monitored by paramedics and EMTs en route.

Several other factors will create job opportunities. Turnover will occur as EMTs and paramedics change occupations when they lack opportunity for advancement or seek better pay or benefits. There also will be more full-time, paid positions as unpaid volunteers are replaced. The amount of training and time that being an EMT or a paramedic requires makes recruiting and keeping unpaid volunteers increasingly difficult, although rural and smaller metropolitan areas will continue to need part-time, volunteer EMTs. Jobs in local government—in fire and police departments and independent rescue squads—will be the hardest to come by because salaries and benefits for these jobs are generally better. EMTs and paramedics with advanced education and certification are likely to have the best job opportunities.

In 2008, EMTs and paramedics held about 210,700 jobs. Most career EMTs and paramedics were employed in metropolitan areas. About 45 percent worked for ambulance services, 29 percent in local government, and 20 percent in hospitals.

Professional Organization

The professional organization for paramedics and EMTs is the National Association of Emergency Medical Technicians (NAEMT). The organization advocates for paramedics and EMTs on a national level. It provides three major courses throughout the country: PreHospital Trauma Life Support, Advanced Medical Life Support, and Emergency Pediatric Care. Membership benefits include networking opportunities, free and discounted courses, conference and journal discounts, and free publications. In addition, the NAEMT offers scholarships and an awards program. Paramedics and EMTs also can join various state, city, and county associations, some of them union associations.

CHECK POINT

4 What employment opportunities are available for EMTs and paramedics?

Chapter Wrap-Up

Don't forget to visit the Point companion website for additional study resources!

CHAPTER HIGHLIGHTS

- Medical assistants perform administrative and clinical tasks to keep physicians' offices and other health care facilities running smoothly. Many medical assistants complete a one- to two-year medical assisting program.
- Medical assisting is one of the nation's fastest-growing occupations, with excellent job prospects. Applicants with formal training, experience, and certification should have the best job opportunities.
- Surgical technologists perform a variety of tasks before, during, and after operations so that the operations proceed smoothly and safely. They are vital members of the operating room team. Training programs for surgical technologists last from nine months to two years.
- Surgical technology is a rapidly growing occupation. Most surgical technologists will continue to work in hospitals, but much faster job growth is expected for physicians' offices and outpatient care centers. Surgical technologists who are certified will have the best job opportunities.
- Physician assistants examine patients, diagnose illnesses, arrange treatment, and perform many other tasks that doctors typically do, under the supervision of a physician. Becoming a PA requires completing an accredited education program and passing a national exam.
- Physician assisting is the seventh fastest-growing occupation. The BLS projects job growth of 39 percent from 2008 to 2018.
- Emergency medical technicians and paramedics provide emergency medical treatment for critically ill and injured people at the scene of accidents and other locations and during transport to a medical facility. To become an EMT or a paramedic, a person must complete a formal training program and be certified. Training is offered at three levels.
- The BLS predicts that employment for EMTs and paramedics will grow by 9 percent between 2008 and 2018. Those with advanced education and certification should have the best job opportunities.

REVIEW QUESTIONS

Matching

1. _____ Assists with physical exams
2. _____ Performs a comprehensive physical exam
3. _____ Gets supplies for those working in the sterile field
4. _____ Usually requires 30 to 350 hours of additional training based on scope of practice
5. _____ Requires study of advanced life support tasks

   a. Physician assistant **b.** Surgical technologist **c.** EMT-Intermediate **d.** Medical assistant
   e. EMT-Paramedic

Multiple Choice

6. One of this professional's most important tasks is maintaining a sterile field.
   a. physician assistant
   b. surgical technologist
   c. EMT/paramedic
   d. medical assistant

7. These professionals combine administrative and clinical tasks.
   a. physician assistants
   b. surgical technologists
   c. EMTs/paramedics
   d. medical assistants

8. These professionals are trained and certified at one of three levels.
   a. physician assistants
   b. surgical technologists
   c. EMTs/paramedics
   d. medical assistants

9. This profession requires the most schooling.
   a. physician assisting
   b. surgical technology
   c. EMTs/paramedics
   d. medical assisting

10. Which is NOT a benefit of membership in a professional organization?
    a. access to educational seminars
    b. automatic certification
    c. subscriptions to professional journals
    d. networking opportunities

Completion

11. _____ tasks generally involve examining and helping treat patients.

12. Materials used to close wounds are known as _____.

13. Puncture-resistant, leakproof disposable containers for items like needles and scalpels are known as _____.

14. _____ is the science of the causes and effects of disease.

15. MAR stands for _____.

Short Answer

16. People often confuse medical assistants and physician assistants. Explain the basic difference between these two occupations.

    _____

    _____

17. Describe the surgical technologist's role on the operating room team.

    _____

    _____

18. How is a physician assistant different from a physician?

    _____

    _____

19. Medical assistants, surgical technologists, and physician assistants free up other medical professionals for more specialized work by performing routine tasks. Give two examples for each occupation.

    _____

    _____

20. Identify the three levels of EMTs, and describe the basic differences between them.

    _____

    _____

INVESTIGATE IT

1. Bioethics and medical ethics are often in the news. Look for an article or case study related to bioethics or medical ethics in a newspaper or magazine or on a web site. A good resource is the Bioethics page at the Markkula Center for Applied Ethics at Santa Clara University (http://www.scu.edu/ethics/practicing/focusareas/medical). Choose a specific case involving ethics and then identify the issue, the individuals or companies involved, and the different points of view.

2. Choose a technological change that likely will affect an occupation in this chapter. Two examples are electronic medical records and the handheld computers used for taking notes on patients. Describe the change. Then explain how the change will affect how people in one of the occupations do their work.

3. Emergency medical services have a fascinating history. Take some time to learn more about this history. Here are some possible topics:
   - cardiopulmonary resuscitation (CPR)
   - the 911 system
   - how the combat medical model was applied to civilian emergency treatment (initial treatment, transport, and emergency room)
   - trauma centers
   - air care

   Write a brief report on your findings.

RECOMMENDED READING

Canning P. *Paramedic: On the Front Lines of Medicine*. New York: Ballantine Books, 1997.

Canning P. *Rescue 471: A Paramedic's Stories*. New York: Ballantine Books, 2000.

Dillon T. "Healthcare Jobs You Might Not Know About." *Occupational Outlook Quarterly* 52;2 (Summer 2008):28–37. Available at: http://www.bls.gov/opub/ooq/2008/summer/art03.pdf.

Joint Commission on Allied Health Personnel in Ophthalmology. Available at: http://www.jcahpo.org.

Sacks T. J. *Opportunities in Physician Assistant Careers*. New York: VGM Career Books, 2002.

U.S. News Staff. "Best Careers 2010: Physician Assistant." *U.S. News and World Report*. December 28, 2009. Available at: http://www.usnews.com/money/careers/articles/2009/12/28/physician-assistant-2.html.

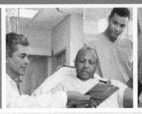
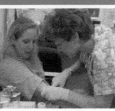

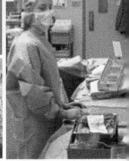

Patient Care: Nursing

CHAPTER OBJECTIVES

After careful study of this chapter, you should be able to:

✳ State the education, training, and legal requirements for becoming a registered nurse, licensed practical nurse, and certified nursing assistant.

✳ Describe the typical work responsibilities in each of these nursing professions.

✳ List personal characteristics desirable in someone who wishes to be a registered nurse, licensed practical nurse, or certified nursing assistant.

✳ Identify employment opportunities and key trends for these occupations.

KEY TERMS

advanced practice nurse
certified nursing assistant
  (CNA)

in-service education
licensed practical nurse
  (LPN)

nurse practice acts
nursing

registered nurse (RN)

Nursing can be broadly defined as caring for people who are ill, injured, or unable to care for themselves in some other way. The profession offers steady employment, opportunities that suit many different career interests, solid paths for advancement, and the ability to change employers with relative ease. This chapter profiles three different nursing professionals: registered nurses, licensed practical nurses, and certified nurse assistants.

REGISTERED NURSES

Registered nurses (RNs) have the most education and the widest scope of practice of the three nursing occupations. Registered nursing is also the largest nursing occupation—in fact, it is the nation's largest health care occupation. The Bureau of Labor Statistics (BLS) singles out this occupation, along with a few other health care careers, because of the high number of job openings it is expected to continue to generate. This vigorous demand, along with the diverse work settings and flexible working arrangements available with this career, prompted *U.S. News and World Report* to name registered nursing as one of its best careers of 2010.

History of the Profession

Nursing has a long history. In ancient civilizations, women tended their families during sickness by providing physical care and herbal remedies. During the early Christian period, women called deaconesses made the first organized visits to sick people, and members of male religious orders provided nursing care and buried the dead.

In the Middle Ages, people traveling on pilgrimages lacked access to family members for care when they become ill or injured. In hospitals built for pilgrims nursing became a respected vocation. Both male and female religious orders devoted to nursing were founded during this period.

At the beginning of the 16th century, many monasteries and convents closed, leading to a tremendous shortage of people to care for the sick. Many women who had committed crimes were recruited into nursing instead of serving jail sentences. These nurses received low pay and worked long hours in unfavorable conditions.

In the 18th and 19th centuries, social reforms changed the role of nurses. During this time modern nursing began to take shape. Many aspects of the nursing profession are based on the beliefs of Florence Nightingale. Nightingale elevated the status of nursing to a respected occupation, improved the quality of nursing care, and founded modern nursing education.

Born in England in 1820, Nightingale was well educated and traveled extensively and undertook nurse's training. During the Crimean War in 1853 Nightingale led a team of nurses she had trained to Turkey to care for wounded British soldiers. After the war, she returned to England, where she established a training school for nurses and wrote books about health care and nursing education. Nightingale and other historically important nurses are shown in Figure 19-1.

Nightingale's work and the care provided by nurses like Clara Barton during the U.S. Civil War focused attention on the need for educated nurses in the U.S.

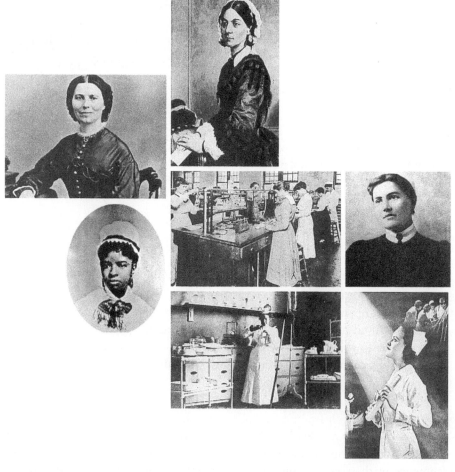

Figure 19-1 These images of nursing include Florence Nightingale, Clara Barton (founder of the American Red Cross), Isabel Hampton Robb (the first president of the American Nurses Association), and Mary Mahoney (the first black professional nurse in the U.S.). (*Courtesy of the Center for the Study of the History of Nursing, University of Pennsylvania*)

Schools of nursing were established in hospitals, based on many of Nightingale's beliefs. At first, the training was mainly through apprenticeships. As students and later as graduates, female nurses were under the control of male hospital administrators and physicians.

After World War II, nursing education improved further. Universities and colleges set up schools of nursing and based their programs on educational objectives. Both men and women earned nursing degrees. During this period, states developed and adopted a national licensing exam for nurses.

Today, nursing includes a specific body of knowledge, practice in a wide variety of health care settings, and recognition of the role of nurses in promoting health. Increased emphasis on education as the basis for nursing practice has led to the growth of nursing as a professional discipline.

Education, Training, and Legal Requirements

Three main types of approved educational programs lead to licensure as an RN: diploma programs, associate's degree programs, and bachelor's degree programs.

Diploma and Degree Programs

Diploma programs, offered by hospitals, take about three years to complete. The first schools established to educate nurses were diploma programs, and they were the main source of graduates until the 1960s. In recent years, the number of diploma programs has decreased considerably. Graduates of diploma programs have a sound foundation in the biological and social sciences, with a strong emphasis on clinical experience in direct patient care.

An associate's degree in nursing, or ADN, is earned at a community or junior college, generally in two to three years. ADN programs prepare nurses to care for patients in various settings, including hospitals, long-term care facilities, and home health care settings. Graduates are technically skilled and well prepared to carry out nursing roles and functions.

Most bachelor's degree nursing programs lead to a bachelor of science in nursing, or BSN. These programs take about four years to complete. Individuals who already hold a bachelor's degree in another field may enroll in accelerated BSN programs lasting from a year to a year and a half. In either case, the major in nursing is built on a general education base, with a concentration on nursing at the upper level. Students work with members of a health care team, use research to improve practice, and have a foundation for graduate study. BSN nurses practice in a wide variety of settings.

All three types of programs include both classroom work and supervised clinical experience in hospitals and other health care facilities. Students take courses in anatomy, physiology, microbiology, chemistry, nutrition, psychology and other behavioral sciences, and nursing practice.

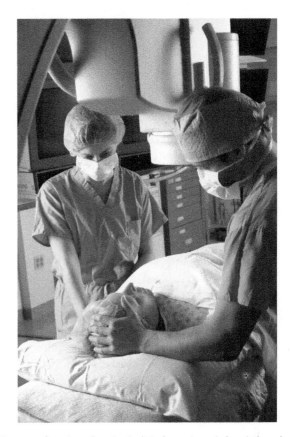

A key part of nursing education is clinical experience in hospitals and other health care facilities.

Further Education

RNs who want more education have several options. Many working RNs with a diploma or associate's degree choose to return to school for a bachelor's degree. Many participate in an RN-to-BSN bridge program, which can be completed while working as an RN. Students can also enroll in accelerated master's degree programs (awarding both the BSN and the master's of science in nursing, or MSN), which generally take three to four years to complete.

A bachelor's, master's, or doctoral degree increases opportunities to advance and opens additional career paths. A bachelor's degree is required for many administrative, managerial, and community health positions. A master's degree is the minimum for all of the advanced practice nurse specialties described in the "Newsreel" feature later in this chapter.

Many hospitals and health care agencies provide on-site education and training for nurses and others employees, a practice called in-service education. This training might teach employees a specific nursing skill, such as how to use new equipment or how to provide care for specific diseases. Many of these in-service education services offer continuing education hours for licensure renewal.

Licensure and Certification

Graduates of all three diploma or degree programs take the NCLEX-RN, the licensing examination for registered nurses. Although it is a national examination, it is administered by each state, and nurses are licensed by individual states (or the District of Columbia or U.S. territories). Other licensure requirements vary by state. The practice of nursing is regulated in each state through state laws known as nurse practice acts.

All RNs must renew their licenses periodically. In some states, renewal requires continuing education. Colleges, hospitals, voluntary agencies, and private groups offer continuing education through courses, seminars, and workshops.

Certification is available in many specialty areas. Some states require nurses to be certified in a specialty in order to practice it. Nurses in advanced practice nurse specialties typically choose to obtain national certification in their specialty or are required to do so. Among other benefits, certified nurses earn an average of $9,000 more than nurses who aren't certified.

Certification is offered by many professional associations, including two primary ones: the American Association of Critical-Care Nurses (AACN) and the American Nurses Association (ANA). To be certified, an RN must be licensed and, generally, must have completed a bachelor's degree, a graduate program, or a set number of hours working in a specialty area. In addition, the RN needs a certain number of continuing education hours, depending on the type of certification sought. Certification must be renewed every three years for the AACN and every five years for the ANA. Renewal options generally include continuing education, practice hours, passing an exam, or some combination of those options.

Work Responsibilities

The main responsibility of most registered nurses is the care and treatment of patients, often in a hospital. A shift typically begins with reviewing the day's assignments and receiving a report from nurses on the previous shift. RNs review the plan of care for each patient to whom they're assigned. They also develop these plans or contribute to them.

RNs who supervise other nurses and nursing assistants delegate some nursing duties to them. During a shift,

Typical Tasks of a Registered Nurse
• Administer medications
• Perform tests and analyze the results
• Start and discontinue IVs
• Care for wounds
• Give patients oxygen
• Take vital signs
• Administer a tube feeding
• Insert a catheter
• Suction airways
• Prepare a sterile field
• Provide preoperative and postoperative care
• Assist with range-of-motion exercises
• Administer a blood transfusion
• Give a bed bath

RNs continue to monitor their patients, recording any important observations and changes. Before leaving at the end of their shift, they make sure incoming staff are aware of their patients' conditions and needs.

RNs often describe themselves as patient advocates, representing patients' interests or guiding patients in protecting their own rights. They may work as intermediaries between patients and physicians. They talk with social workers and other health care professionals to help arrange the services patients need. They offer advice and emotional support to patients' families. They also instruct families on how to care for patients when they return home. In addition, RNs teach patients about their medical problems, how to care for themselves, and how to improve their health.

Specialties

RNs can choose several different specialties. Some specialties focus on a particular setting. Two familiar examples are emergency or trauma nurses, who work in emergency rooms, and critical care nurses, who work in intensive care units. RNs can also specialize in treating certain health conditions. Addictions nurses, for instance, care for patients seeking to overcome addictions to alcohol, tobacco, drugs, and other substances. Diabetes management nurses help patients manage their disease by teaching them how to eat a nutritious diet, check blood sugar, and give themselves insulin injections. A third area of specialization is specific organs and body systems. For example, cardiovascular nurses care for patients who have heart disease or who are recovering from heart attacks. A fourth type of specialization focuses on well-defined populations, such as newborns (neonatal nurses), children (pediatric nurses), or older patients (geriatric nurses). Some RNs combine specialties.

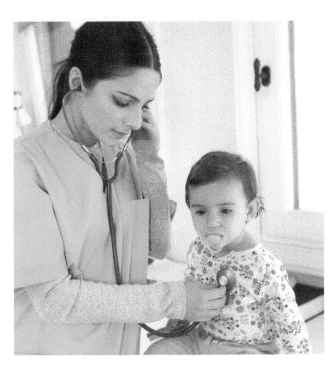

Pediatrics is one area of nursing specialization.

Most RNs work as staff nurses, as part of a health care team. Some RNs, however, choose to become advanced practice nurses. These RNs have more extensive education and training and a broader set of work responsibilities, which may include providing primary care. You can learn more about advanced practice nurses in the "Newsreel" feature later in this chapter.

Some RNs do not work directly with patients. They may be infection control nurses, forensics nurses, informatics nurses, or case managers, for example. Few occupations offer as many opportunities to specialize and as wide a range of career choices as RN.

Personal Characteristics of Registered Nurses

The desire to help others draws many people to health care careers. Having nurses with a caring, sympathetic attitude obviously benefits patients, and this attitude benefits RNs as well. It helps them put the demands of the

SPOTLIGHT ON SKILLS Typical Task: Give Oral Medication to a Patient

Position: Registered Nurse

Patients are often given medications to swallow in the form of a tablet, capsule, pill, or liquid. This method is preferred by many patients and is the easiest to administer.

Before giving an oral medication, the nurse checks the medication order against the original physician's order and clarifies any inconsistencies. He or she checks the patient's chart for allergies. The nurse must know the actions, safe dose ranges, purpose of administration, and adverse effects of the medication and consider its appropriateness for the patient.

Next, the nurse retrieves the medication. After washing his or her hands, the nurse unlocks the medication cart or drawer. With an automated medication dispensing system, the nurse may need to enter a pass code and scan his or her employee identification. The nurse reads the medication administration record (MAR) and selects the proper medication. The nurse compares the label with the MAR, checks expiration dates, and performs calculations if necessary.

Then the appropriate amount of medication is prepared. After this is done, the nurse rechecks the label against the MAR and checks to be sure that the patient will get the medication at the correct time.

Now the medicine can be administered. The nurse identifies the patient and checks the patient's chart for drug allergies. Before administering the medicine, the

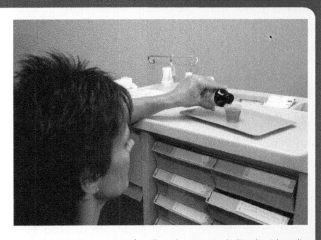

Correct dosage is important for all medications, including liquid medication for oral administration.

nurse explains its purpose and action. The nurse assists the patient into an upright or lateral position to make swallowing easier. With most medications, the nurse offers water or another permitted fluid. He or she must remain with the patient until the medication is swallowed. Unless the nurse has seen the patient swallow the drug, it cannot be recorded as administered. Medication should never be left at the patient's bedside.

The nurse checks on the patient within 30 minutes after giving the medication, or at a time appropriate for the drug, to observe the patient's response.

job into perspective and gives them a feeling of satisfaction in their work.

RNs need to be detail-oriented and good at organizing. They must be able to sift through the many different needs of patients and other responsibilities and prioritize them. Being organized is important in carrying out nursing functions as well. Even the simplest tasks consist of a series of steps that must all be followed carefully and in a certain order to get the desired results and to help ensure the patient's and caregiver's safety.

At the same time, RNs need to be flexible. The workload can be unpredictable, and priorities can change with little or no notice. This type of work environment calls for the ability to reset priorities quickly and completely.

Good judgment is another personal characteristic of effective nurses. During a workday, many situations can arise that require the ability to make careful, considered decisions. Nursing is emotionally demanding work. Therefore, emotional steadiness is also valuable.

Nurses must have a high degree of personal responsibility. Patients' health, and sometimes their lives, can depend on a nurse's ability to handle responsibility.

Most RNs work as part of a health care team. They may interact with physicians, other RNs, licensed practical nurses, nursing assistants, therapists, lab personnel, and other staff members. RNs must be able to work and communicate with the people on their team and other medical staff in an effective, professional manner.

Employment Opportunities and Trends

In 2008, registered nurses held about 2.6 million jobs. Some 60 percent of registered nurses worked in hospitals, and another eight percent worked in physicians' offices. Home health care services and nursing care facilities each employed 5 percent. Most of the rest worked in employment services, government agencies, social assistance agencies, and educational services. About one in five registered nurses worked part-time.

The BLS projects strong employment growth of 22 percent for this occupation from 2008 to 2018. Three trends will drive this growth:

* Improvements in medical technology that make more health problems treatable
* An increased emphasis on preventive care
* The growth in the number of older adults

In some settings, job growth for RNs will be even higher: 48 percent for physicians' offices, 33 percent for home health care services, 25 percent for nursing care facilities, and 24 percent for employment services. In terms of the number of new jobs, registered nursing ranks first among all occupations, with an anticipated 581,500 jobs to be added from 2008 to 2018.

Employment growth in hospitals will be slower, at 17 percent. This reflects slower growth in the number of hospital patients, shorter hospital stays, and more procedures

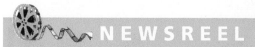

NEWSREEL

Opportunities in Advanced Practice Nursing

The ANA reports that well over 200,000 nurses in the U.S. are advanced practice nurses—registered nurses with graduate education who work independently or directly with physicians. Three of the specialties in advanced practice nursing are certified nurse practitioner, certified nurse-midwife, and certified nurse anesthetist.

* Nurse practitioners combine the caring function of nursing with the physician's functions of diagnosis and treatment. Nurse practitioners serve as primary care providers and specialists in hospitals, clinics, urgent care facilities, public health departments, nursing homes, and many other settings. According to the American Academy of Nurse Practitioners, the nation's 125,000 nurse practitioners see almost 600 million patients each year.
* Nurse-midwives have been delivering babies in the U.S. since the 1920s. They also care for women during and after pregnancy and during menopause, do gynecological exams, advise on family planning and other health-

related topics, and serve as primary care providers. There are more than 7,000 certified nurse-midwives, and they work in hospitals, HMOs and other managed care medical facilities, obstetrics/gynecology practices, birth centers, public health clinics, and private practice.

* According to the American Association of Nurse Anesthetists, 44,000 nurse anesthetists administer about 32 million anesthetics in the U.S. each year. These advanced practice nurses work in every setting where anesthesia is given. They are the primary anesthesia providers in rural hospitals and for military personnel on the front lines. Nurse anesthetists earn some of the highest salaries among nursing specialties. In 2008, annual compensation exceeded $163,000.

The BLS projects that from 2008 to 2018, advanced practice nurses will be in high demand, especially in inner cities, rural settings, and other medically underserved areas. According to the ANA, consideration is being given to requiring a doctoral degree for advanced practice nurses.

being done in outpatient clinics, where brisk job growth is expected. Still, because hospitals have a relatively high turnover among nurses, they're expected to offer attractive benefits, such as signing bonuses, family-friendly work schedules, and subsidized training.

With such high job growth rates, the BLS projects that job opportunities for nurses during 2008–2018 will be excellent. RNs with a bachelor's degree or higher will have even better prospects.

Professional Organization

Membership in a professional nursing organization has many benefits. These include opportunities to network with other nurses and to keep current with issues and trends.

The professional organization for RNs is the ANA. It is formed from the state nurses' associations to which individual nurses belong. Founded in 1896, the ANA sets standards of practice, encourages research to advance nursing practice, and advocates on behalf of nursing at the state and federal levels. ANA membership includes subscriptions to several professional journals and discounts on certification, online continuing education, conferences, and educational events.

CHECK POINT

1 What are the three main types of educational programs for RNs?

2 What are the four types of specialties that RNs can pursue?

LICENSED PRACTICAL NURSES

Licensed practical nurses (LPNs) perform many of the routine tasks of nursing under the direction of a physician or RN. These nurses are called *licensed vocational nurses* (LVNs) in Texas and California. BLS anticipates very good job opportunities for LPNs from 2008 to 2018.

History of the Profession

For centuries, women have given practical nursing care to family members, neighbors, and people in their community. The first formal training program for practical nursing in the U.S. probably began in 1892. Established through the YWCA (Young Women's Christian Association) in Brooklyn, New York, this three-month program focused on developing skills for home care of children and family members who were older, chronically ill, or disabled.

A few similar programs followed, and by 1930, there were 11 practical nursing schools. Practical nursing as a profession expanded greatly during and after World War II because of a shortage of registered nurses, efforts by RNs to advance their profession, studies that urged creation of a system of formally trained practical nurses, and increased federal funding for vocational education after the war.

In 1941, the Association of Practical Nurse Schools was founded. Later known as the National Association for Practical Nurse Education and Service (NAPNES), it developed the first planned curriculum for practical nursing. By the late 1940s, the number of schools for practical nurses had more than tripled to 36. In just six more years, an additional 260 opened.

The process of state licensure started in the late 1930s. In 1938, New York became the first state to require practical nurses to be licensed. Seven years later, 19 states and one territory had laws regarding the profession, although New York remained the only state to require licensure. By 1955, all states had licensure laws.

Accreditation of training programs by the National League for Nursing (NLN) began in 1966. In 1979, the NLN published a list of competencies for graduates of practical/vocational nursing programs. In 1996, the National Council of State Boards of Nursing, in collaboration with NAPNES, offered the first certification exam for LPNs in long-term care.

Education, Training, and Legal Requirements

Practical or vocational nursing programs teach graduates to give bedside nursing care. Most programs are offered by technical and vocational schools, as well as community and junior colleges. Some high schools, hospitals, colleges, and universities also offer programs. Acceptance generally requires a high school diploma or the equivalent.

Most practical nursing programs last about a year and include both classroom study and supervised clinical practice. Clinical work usually takes place in a hospital but sometimes in another health care setting. Classes cover a variety of subjects:
- Basic nursing concepts
- Anatomy and physiology
- Medical-surgical nursing
- Pediatric nursing
- Obstetric nursing
- Pharmacology
- Nutrition
- First aid

All states and the District of Columbia require practical nurses to be licensed. To get a license, a candidate must graduate from a state-approved program and take the NCLEX-PN. Some states have additional licensing requirements. In some states, license renewal requires a certain number of hours of continuing education.

Work Responsibilities

LPNs do many of the hands-on tasks typically associated with nursing and provide basic nursing care. In their role of providing—They—help patients with personal hygiene, dressing, and sometimes eating. LPNs record how much a patient eats and drinks and any reactions to medications. They observe patients and talk with them about how they're feeling. Any changes or important information about a patient's condition is reported.

LPNs also collect laboratory samples, perform routine tests, or assist physicians and RNs in administering tests. Other frequently performed tasks are monitoring and cleaning medical equipment.

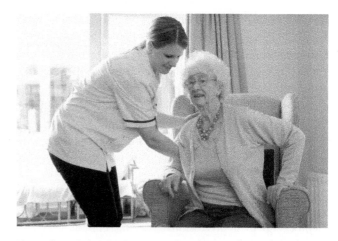

Licensed practical nurses have many duties, many of them hands-on with patients.

While the work of LPNs frequently overlaps with the work of RNs, it differs. LPN training is skills-based. RNs have more classroom education, and they learn more about nursing theory. They also have a wider scope of

SPOTLIGHT ON SKILLS Typical Task: Clean a Wound and Apply a Dry, Sterile Dressing

Position: Licensed Practical Nurse

Cleaning and dressing wounds is a common nursing task. It begins with reviewing the physician's order or nursing plan of care, gathering supplies, identifying the patient, and explaining the procedure. Wound care and dressing changes may cause pain for some patients. If an analgesic is appropriate, the nurse checks the physician's orders and administers it, allowing enough time for it to take effect before undertaking the rest of the procedure.

When the patient is ready, the nurse washes his or her hands and sets the bed at a comfortable working height. The nurse assists the patient to a comfortable position that provides easy access to the wound area, covering any other exposed area with a bath blanket.

The nurse must check the position of drains, tubes, or other devices before removing the dressings, a process which is done slowly and carefully to prevent tissue damage and minimize pain. Gloves protect the nurse from contaminated dressings and prevent the spread of microorganisms.

The nurse closely examines the dressings and wound site, noting any drainage, the size of the wound, and its appearance. The nurse assesses pain and checks sutures, Steri-strips™, staples, and drains or tubes. All of this information must be documented when the nurse completes the procedure.

Before cleaning the wound, the nurse prepares a sterile work area, using a sterile cleaning solution. The nurse cleans the wound as ordered by the physician, working from the area of least contamination to most contamination. After the wound has been cleaned, the nurse dresses it again.

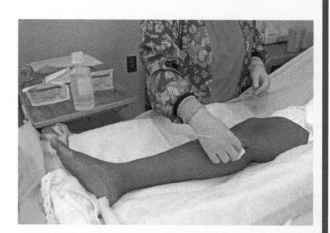

Cleaning and dressing a wound.

When the nurse has finished cleaning the wound, he or she must properly dispose of all materials and supplies. In addition, the LPN, sometimes the RN, must record any observations about the patient's condition in the patient's record.

practice. In some states, LPNs can do more advanced tasks, such as giving prescribed medicines and starting an intravenous line (IV). But generally RNs are trained and licensed to perform more advanced nursing procedures. When an LPN works under an RN, the RN is responsible for the LPN's actions.

Depending on where they work, LPNs can have a variety of other assignments. For example, at a hospital, they may do triage and initial assessments. Those who work in obstetrics help to deliver and care for babies. At a nursing care facility, they might supervise nursing assistants and develop patient care plans. In a physician's office, their work could include making appointments and other administrative duties. In home health care, LPNs might teach family members how to perform simple nursing tasks.

Typical Tasks of a Licensed Practical Nurse

- Take vital signs
- Change dressings
- Record food and fluid intake and output
- Help patients get out of bed and walk
- Give a blanket bath
- Treat bedsores
- Administer medicines (which requires a pharmacology course in some states)
- Draw blood
- Give IV therapy
- Provide preoperative and postoperative care

Personal Characteristics of Licensed Practical Nurses

LPNs typically spend many hours providing bedside care. They need empathy—having some understanding of how a patient is feeling—to adjust their approach and perform their tasks in a way that benefits a particular patient. Because nursing is sometimes stressful, LPNs should be steady emotionally.

LPNs should be observant and quick to note any changes in a patient's condition that should be recorded or communicated to an RN or physician. They should also be skilled at oral communication. This includes being able to talk easily with patients about their needs, their medical history, and how they are feeling, as well as the ability to report briefly and clearly on a patient's condition to an RN or physician.

An LPN's work often requires patience. Giving a patient a blanket bath, coaxing a nursing home resident to try something new, helping someone get out of bed, or giving a fourth injection in the course of a few hours are all common nursing tasks. Patients sometimes react with anger or frustration at these tasks, even though the tasks are necessary. The nurse must be able to handle these situations without letting negative emotions spill out.

LPNs must understand their role in a health care team. They should be capable of following orders and working under supervision. LPNs should be careful listeners, able to grasp instructions the first time they are given. They should also be comfortable asking questions when those instructions aren't clear.

Employment Opportunities and Trends

In 2008, there were more than 753,000 LPNs employed in the U.S. Twenty-five percent worked in hospitals, 28 percent worked in nursing care facilities, and 12 percent were in physicians' offices. Others were employed by home health care services, employment services, residential care facilities, elder care facilities, outpatient centers, and government agencies.

The BLS projects 21 percent employment growth for LPNs during 2008–2018, with the addition of 155,600 new jobs. The Bureau expects rapid growth for this profession in most health care settings, particularly those that serve older adults. It has identified two settings as having the best opportunities in the future:

- *Home health care services.* Strong growth will result from the rising number of older people who need health care and who wish to be cared for at home and from technological advances that allow people to live longer.
- *Nursing care facilities.* These facilities will gain more clients (and need more staff) because of the increasing number of older people requiring long-term care and the number of discharged hospital patients needing short-term care.

The number of LPNs should increase faster in physicians' offices and outpatient care centers than in hospitals, as procedures once done only in hospitals are increasingly performed in those facilities. Still, hospitals will continue to be one of the largest employers of LPNs.

Professional Organizations

Two national professional organizations for licensed practical nurses are NAPNES and the National Federation of Licensed Practical Nurses (NFLPN). NAPNES, which was founded by practical nurse educators, develops practice and education standards for LPNs and related occupations. It represents them in national meetings that review and set nursing policy and educates legislators and government agencies on LPN practice and education. Individual members have the right to vote on organizational issues, receive a professional journal, and can enjoy opportunities for networking, such as private online forums and chat rooms.

NFLPN is the only professional organization governed entirely by LPNs. It promotes high standards of education and practice; monitors legislation; represents LPNs before Congress and regulatory bodies; speaks on their behalf at national nursing meetings; and works with other national nursing, medical, and allied health organizations. Membership is based on the three-tier concept of local, state, and national enrollment. Benefits include continuing education courses, a national convention, scholarships, and a career center for LPNs and prospective employers.

Both organizations offer national certification programs in specialty areas: pharmacology and long-term care (NAPNES) and IV therapy and gerontology (NFLPN).

CHECK POINT

3 How does the training for LPNs differ from that of RNs?

4 In which two settings will employment opportunities for LPNs be best in the future?

CERTIFIED NURSING ASSISTANTS

Certified nursing assistants, or CNAs, perform simple, basic nursing functions and care for patients' personal needs under the direction of an LPN or RN. Sometimes known by other titles, such as certified nurse assistant, nursing assistant or nursing aide, CNA ranks ninth among those occupations that the BLS projects will add the most jobs between 2008 and 2018.

History of the Profession

Some of the same factors that led to the development of licensed practical nursing in the U.S. also contributed to the growing profession of nursing assistants. Studies around the time of World War II recommended delegating more basic nursing tasks to auxiliary personnel, meaning aides or assistants as well as LPNs. As nursing education after the war improved, hospitals that had previously assigned student nurses to perform this type of work began training aides to do it instead.

Over the next few decades, nursing assistants worked in long-term care facilities and hospitals. Often, they weren't trained in health care and gave care that was less than optimal. In the 1980s, in response to public concerns, Congress asked the U.S. Institute of Medicine to study how to

better regulate quality of care in nursing homes certified by Medicare and Medicaid.

Among the Institute's many recommendations was to require formal training of nursing assistants who wanted to work in nursing homes. This recommendation became part of the Omnibus Budget Reconciliation Act (OBRA) passed in 1987. The law required all states to set up training programs for nursing assistants and administer competency tests. Qualified candidates would be certified nursing assistants. The law also required annual in-service education.

The CNA occupation is continuing to develop. Various professional organizations at the state and national level are advocating for higher standards of professionalism and better benefits and working conditions.

Education, Training, and Legal Requirements

To become a certified nursing assistant, a candidate must complete a state-approved training program and pass a competency test. Training programs, which must be a minimum of 75 hours, are available at vocational schools, community colleges, the Red Cross, and health care facilities. Topics covered include the following:
- Anatomy and physiology
- Body mechanics
- Bathing, dressing, and other personal care skills
- Nutrition
- Safety and emergency procedures
- Communication and skills
- Documentation skills
- Infection control
- Patient room upkeep
- Patient/resident rights

The competency test includes both a written component and an assessment of practical skills. In some states, experienced health care workers or people trained in a related field can take the exam without training. Candidates who pass the exam are certified, and the state places their names on a registry. To remain certified, CNAs must complete a minimum of 12 hours of in-service education each year.

Some states accept the federal minimum of 75 hours of training. Others require more hours, and some states impose additional requirements. The state nurse aide registry or state licensing board can provide information about a particular state's standards. In all states, certified nursing assistants are required to work under the supervision of an RN or LPN.

Work Responsibilities

CNAs provide patients with hands-on, personal care. They assist with personal hygiene, serve meals, and help patients eat and dress. They help patients move about in bed and answer their calls for assistance. CNAs also have light housekeeping duties, such as making beds and tidying up rooms.

CNAs may care for patients in a variety of other ways. For example, they may take vital signs, help patients get in and out of bed and walk, and transport them by wheelchair or stretcher. They might give skin care or help with range-of-motion exercises.

In addition to working directly with patients, CNAs often assist other medical staff in their work. For example, they might help set up equipment and move and store supplies. They may also assist LPNs, RNs, and physicians in procedures.

In nursing care facilities, CNAs often have more contact with patients than other members of the health care team. Therefore, they're in a good position to observe changes that a supervisor may need to know about.

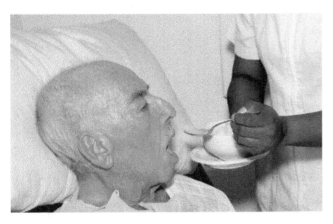

Certified nursing assistants often work directly with patients.

Typical Tasks of a Certified Nursing Assistant

- Feed patients and measure and record food intake and output
- Bath patients and help them with toilet needs
- Help patients dress
- Turn and reposition patients in bed
- Move patients to or from bed
- Apply dressings
- Collect specimens
- Supervise patients as they exercise
- Clean rooms

Personal Characteristics of Nursing Assistants

Empathy is an important personal quality for nursing assistants because they spend so much time interacting directly with the people in their care. Their patients have different backgrounds, personalities, attitudes, moods, and needs. The ability to understand people and their particular situations and feelings is valuable to both the patient and the caregiver.

Patience and emotional strength are other assets. A nursing assistant's work is repetitive and often time-consuming. A patient's progress may be slow, or a patient may be difficult to deal with. Despite disruptions to the routine, such as when a staff member is sick, the work must still get done. This occupation can be emotionally demanding, so a nursing assistant needs to be emotionally strong.

Nursing assistants usually work in a team environment, with nurses, physicians, and other medical staff. Therefore, cooperation is an important quality. Nursing assistants should be respectful, professional in appearance and attitude, and willing members of the team.

Nursing assistants must also be responsible. When they are with a patient or resident, they are responsible for that person's safety and comfort. They have many duties that must be carried out carefully and accurately, with minimal supervision. Because they work so much with patients and residents, nursing assistants may observe changes and situations related to a patient's health and safety that others aren't aware of and that need to be addressed.

Employment Opportunities and Trends

The BLS places nursing assistants in a category called *nursing aides, orderlies, and attendants.* The BLS projects that employment growth for these workers from 2008 to 2018 will be faster than average, at 19 percent. This will be due mostly to growth of the older population and its need for long-term care. In addition, earlier discharges of patients from hospitals seeking to control costs will give nursing care facilities more clients. Technology that saves lives and helps people to live longer will also contribute to the need for long-term care. As a result of these trends, more jobs will be created in nursing and residential care facilities than in hospitals. Strong growth is also expected in elder care centers, and hospitals will remain a major employer.

Nursing aides, orderlies, and attendants held 1,469,800 jobs in 2008. About 41 percent worked in nursing care

SPOTLIGHT ON SKILLS Typical Task: Assist a Patient with Turning in Bed

Position: Certified Nursing Assistant

Frequently, nursing assistants must help patients who are weak and cannot move unaided. Good lifting techniques and assistive equipment can help ensure that patient handling and movement are safe for both the assistant and patient.

First, the bed is set at an appropriate and comfortable working height, with the head adjusted to a flat position or as near to one as the patient can tolerate. This position facilitates the turning maneuver and minimizes strain when lifting the patient.

Next, the nursing assistant lowers the nearest side rail and positions a friction-reducing sheet or drawsheet (a small or standard-size folded sheet used to help move a patient) under the patient. The sheet or drawsheet is used to move the patient to the edge of the bed, opposite the side to which the patient will be turned. Then the assistant raises the rail on that side of the bed and moves to the opposite side of the bed.

Standing on the side of the bed toward which the patient will be turned, the nursing assistant first lowers the side rail. He or she then places the patient's arms across the patient's chest and crosses the patient's far leg over the nearest leg. This facilitates the turning motion and protects the patient's arms.

Next, the nursing assistant stands opposite the center of the patient's body, with feet spread to about shoulder width and one foot ahead of the other. The assistant flexes his or her knees so that the leg muscles will be used to do the pulling. This is a stable position with good body alignment that enables the use of large muscle masses to turn the patient, which avoids straining the lower back.

Now the nursing assistant positions his or her hands on the patient's far shoulder and hip and rolls the patient toward himself or herself. This maneuver supports the patient's body and makes use of the assistant's weight to aid in turning. Alternatively, the patient can be moved by using the friction-reducing sheet or drawsheet to gently pull the patient over on a side. The assistant then places a pillow or other support behind the patient's back and pulls the shoulder blade forward and out from under the patient.

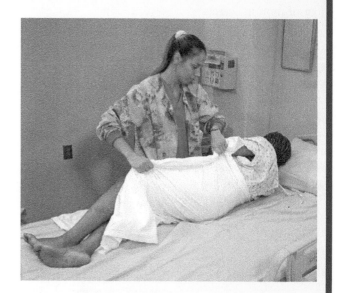

Moving a patient with a drawsheet.

After turning, the patient is made comfortable by placing pillows or other supports under the leg and arm as needed. The pillow under the patient's head is readjusted, and the head of the bed is elevated as needed for comfort. The bed is set at the lowest position, with the side rails up.

---

facilities, and 29 percent worked in hospitals. Because of the occupation's projected strong growth, coupled with high turnover, the BLS foresees excellent job opportunities for people wanting to become CNAs.

Professional Organizations

Founded in 2006, the National Association of Health Care Assistants has a membership of more than 35,000 health care assistants and caregivers from 29 states and the District of Columbia. It provides development training and mentoring programs and advocates on issues related to caregivers and long-term care. Membership benefits include educational opportunities, a news magazine, a national convention, and a national awards program.

CHECK POINT

5 What personal characteristics should certified nursing assistants have?

Don't forget to visit thePoint companion website for additional study resources!

CHAPTER HIGHLIGHTS

- Registered nursing is the largest nursing occupation and the nation's largest health care occupation. To become an RN, a person must complete an approved diploma, associate's degree, or bachelor's degree program and pass a national exam. For many administrative, managerial, and community health positions, a bachelor's degree is required.
- BLS projects that in the near future, more jobs will be added for registered nurses than for any other occupation. It anticipates robust growth, especially in physicians' offices, home health care services, nursing care facilities, and employment services.
- Licensed practical nurses perform many of the routine tasks of nursing under the direction of a physician or RN. To become an LPN, a person must graduate from a state-approved school and pass a national exam. Most practical nursing programs last about a year.
- BLS projects significant employment growth for LPNs in the future. Many jobs will be available in home health care services and nursing care facilities.
- Certified nursing assistants perform simple, basic nursing functions and care for patients' personal needs under the direction of an LPN or RN. To become a CNA, a person must complete a state-approved training program and pass a competency test.
- Nursing assistants, aides, and orderlies rank ninth among all occupations in expected job growth. Nursing and residential care facilities and hospitals will be top employers.

REVIEW QUESTIONS

Matching

1. _____ Working as a trauma or critical care nurse
2. _____ Delivering babies
3. _____ Serving as a primary care provider
4. _____ Caring for patients' personal needs
5. _____ Doing many of the hands-on tasks typically associated with nursing

   a. Certified nursing assistant   **b.** Nurse-midwife   **c.** Licensed practical nurse
   d. Nurse practitioner   **e.** Registered nurse

Multiple Choice

6. What regulates the practice of nursing?
   - **a.** international standards and codes
   - **b.** federal guidelines and regulations
   - **c.** state nurse practice acts
   - **d.** institutional policies

7. Which is the largest group of health care providers in the U.S.?
   - **a.** physicians
   - **b.** registered nurses
   - **c.** licensed practical nurses
   - **d.** certified nursing assistants

8. Which professional typically performs light housekeeping duties as well as patient care?
   - **a.** certified nursing assistant
   - **b.** licensed practical nurse
   - **c.** registered nurse
   - **d.** geriatric nurse

9. Which nursing occupation offers many opportunities to specialize?
   - **a.** certified nurse anesthetist
   - **b.** certified nursing assistant
   - **c.** licensed practical nurse
   - **d.** registered nurse

10. The need to better regulate the quality of care in nursing homes led to formal training programs for
    - **a.** nurse practitioners
    - **b.** registered nurses
    - **c.** licensed practical nurses
    - **d.** certified nursing assistants

Completion

11. _____ is caring for people who are ill, injured, or unable to care for themselves in some other way.

12. On-site education and training provided by employers is known as _____.

13. Modern nursing is based on many beliefs of this historical figure: _____.

14. A nurse anesthetist is a type of RN known as a/an _____.

15. A/an _____ works under the supervision of an LPN or RN.

Short Answer

16. Compare the educational requirements for the three nursing occupations.

    _____

    _____

17. What are some key differences in the work of a registered nurse and a licensed practical nurse?

    _____

    _____

18. Why must LPNs be observant and good at oral communication?

    _____

    _____

19. Give three examples of tasks that certified nursing assistants typically perform.

    _____

    _____

20. Briefly explain the requirements for licensure or certification for the three nursing occupations in this chapter.

    _____

    _____

INVESTIGATE IT

1. Visit the web site DiscoverNursing.com at http://www.discovernursing.com. Read several of the profiles of nurses, and write a paragraph about the different types of work they do, why they like their jobs, or what they like about them. Also browse the Nursing Careers section of the site (under the "What" tab). Find a career that interests you and write a paragraph about that career.

2. Watch a movie or episode of a television show, new or old, with one or more nurses as characters. Some examples are *Atonement*, *M*A*S*H*, *One Flew Over the Cuckoo's Nest*, *Grey's Anatomy*, *ER*, and *China Beach*. How accurately do you think the movie or television show portrays nurses and their work? What, if anything, does it tell you about society's perceptions of nurses?

3. Suppose that you were to create a timeline of American nursing. Choose an event or person that should be included in that timeline. Write a paragraph explaining your choice.

RECOMMENDED READING

Culkin J. *A Final Arc of Sky: A Memoir of Critical Care*. Boston: Beacon Press, 2009.

D'Antonio P et al. *Nurses' Work: Issues Across Time and Place*. New York: Springer, 2006.

Gordon S. *Life Support: Three Nurses on the Front Lines*. Ithaca, NY: ILR Press, 2007.

Heron E. *Tending Lives: Nurses on the Medical Front*. New York: Ivy Books (Ballantine/Random House), 1998.

Johnson & Johnson Services, Inc. DiscoverNursing.com. Available at: http://www.discovernursing.com.

LPN Café. Available at: http://www.lpncafe.ca. Accessed October 19, 2010.

Nursing Assistant Resources on the Web. Available at: http://nursingassistants.net.

U.S. News Staff. Registered Nurse. In: The 50 Best Careers of 2010. *U.S. News and World Report* [serial online]. Posted December 28, 2009. Available at: http://www.usnews.com/money/careers/articles/2009/12/28/registered-nurse.html.

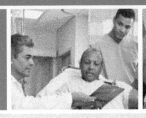
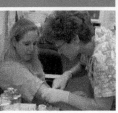
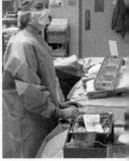
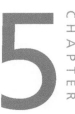

Patient Care: Dental

CHAPTER OBJECTIVES

After careful study of this chapter, you should be able to:

✴ State the education, training, and legal requirements for becoming a dentist, dental hygienist, and dental assistant.

✴ Describe the typical work responsibilities of each profession.

✴ List desirable personal characteristics of dentists, dental hygienists, and dental assistants.

✴ Identify employment opportunities and key trends for these occupations.

KEY TERMS

bridge

crown

dental assistant

dental hygienist (DEN
 tăl hī JĔ nist)

dentures

oral

oral hygiene (ŌR ăl
 HĬ jēn)

periodontal (PER ē ō
 DON tăl)

root canal

More than many other parts of the body, teeth and gums require frequent care to maintain good health. Daily brushing and flossing help prevent painful tooth decay and gum disease. In addition, scientists are finding that dental and periodontal (gum and bone) health impacts people's overall health. For instance, research suggests that bacteria that enter the bloodstream through unhealthy gums are associated with a wide range of medical problems from diabetes to cardiovascular disease.

In addition to daily personal care, regular checkups and cleanings can greatly reduce a person's risk of developing oral (mouth) diseases. The dental health care team that provides these services includes dentists, dental hygienists, and dental assistants.

DENTISTS

Dentists are doctors who care for people's teeth and gums. They educate patients to prevent dental problems, detect and treat diseases, repair and replace teeth that have been damaged or lost, and improve the appearance of teeth with straightening or whitening procedures.

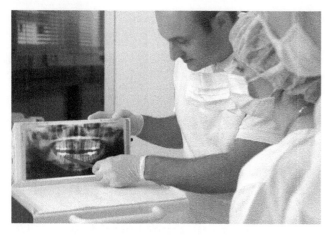

Dentists care for patient's teeth and gums.

History of the Profession

People have always suffered from dental problems. Toothbrushes, made from twigs, show that even thousands of years ago, people understood the need to keep their teeth clean. More than 2,000 years ago, the Etruscans (people of ancient Italy and Corsica) fashioned crowns (caps for broken or weak teeth) and bridges (artificial teeth or crowns attached to adjoining teeth). Over time, the practice of dentistry evolved into the form familiar to us today.

Early History

Some of the earliest dentists practiced in ancient Egypt, where teeth were one of several specialties that a doctor could choose to pursue. The first dentist known to historians was the Egyptian Hesi-Re, who died about 2600 BC. The ancient Romans were great believers in oral hygiene, or keeping one's mouth clean. They used a variety of tooth-cleaning powders and provided dinner guests with fancy toothpicks to clean their teeth between courses. In Rome, India, and Islamic cultures, physicians or surgeons performed dentistry as part of their medical duties.

The Middle Ages, the Renaissance, and the 17th Century

In medieval Europe, monks provided most medical treatment, including dental care. Barbers who visited monks gradually became their surgical assistants. When the Roman

Catholic Church eventually forbade monks from providing medical and dental care, barbers were ready to take over. Barber-surgeons extracted teeth and performed other procedures as part of medical care.

A renewed interest in scientific studies during the Renaissance advanced the understanding of human anatomy, including dental anatomy, and the practice of surgery. Along with other developments, this eventually led to the recognition of dentistry as a separate area of science.

Dentistry in the U.S.

In colonial America, physicians provided dental services. The most effective of these services was extraction with an instrument that looked like a key. Traveling toothdrawers, surgeon-dentists, barbers, and even blacksmiths performed extractions. Some advertised their services in newspapers, including the patriot Paul Revere. Revere performed the first identification of a corpse based on dental evidence when he identified the body of Dr. Joseph Warren from a bridge he had made for him.

In 1840, the first dental college was established in Baltimore, and the first national organization of dentists was formed. There was also a substantial increase in the publication of dental literature, including the professional journal the *American Journal of Dental Science*. Progress continued in the last half of the century. In 1859, 26 dentists meeting in Niagara Falls, N.Y., formed the American Dental Association (ADA). This group remains the leading national professional organization for dentists today. By 1880, there were 28 dental schools; 20 years later, there were 57.

In the 20th century, more gains followed. One important change was a movement that ensured professional standards. Private schools with widely varying educational standards flourished at the time. The lack of standards was resolved through efforts of the ADA, tightening state laws, and a 1926 landmark report on dental education that highlighted the problems in some of these schools. These factors led to the establishment of a system of accredited dental schools affiliated with universities and with curriculum standards.

In 1928, the ADA formed the National Board of Dental Examiners to create a national exam. Five years later, the first National Board dental examinations were given. Dental specialties were established, and dental technology continued to advance.

Education, Training, and Legal Requirements

To become a dentist, a person must graduate from an accredited dental school, which is usually a four-year program. As of 2010, 58 schools were accredited by the Commission on Dental Accreditation. Admission to dental school is quite competitive. Applicants must meet these requirements:

- Complete at least two years of college-level, pre-dental education. Each dental school has a list of required classes. According to the ADA, these generally include eight hours each of biology with a lab, physics, English, general chemistry with a lab, and organic chemistry with a lab.
- Take the Dental Admission Test (DAT).

While only two or three years of college may be required, most dental school applicants have at least a bachelor's degree.

Dental school generally begins with two years of classroom and laboratory instruction in basic health sciences, with a focus on dental topics. These are examples of typical courses:

- Anatomy and physiology
- Biochemistry
- Microbiology
- Laboratory techniques
- Pharmacology
- Histology (the study of tissues)

During the first two years of dental school, students also learn basic principles of diagnosing and treating tooth and gum diseases. They may practice on models or manikins initially and begin treating patients later in the second year.

In the last two years of dental school, students treat patients under the supervision of licensed dentists. They work in hospitals, outpatient clinics, community clinics, or other settings. Students also take classes that will be useful in managing a practice, such as communication skills and business management.

Most dental schools award the D.D.S. degree (doctor of dental surgery). Some award the equivalent D.M.D. (doctor of dental medicine).

Dentists are licensed by the states. All states and the District of Columbia require dentists to be licensed in order to practice. In most states, candidates must have graduated from an accredited dental school and must pass both a written and a practical exam. In many states, students may take the National Board Dental Examination to fulfill or partly fulfill the written requirement. Dentists must renew their licenses every one to three years, depending on state rules. In nearly every state, renewal requires continuing education.

Most dentists are general practitioners. However, some choose to specialize in one of the areas described in the "Work Responsibilities" section below. All 50 states

and the District of Columbia license dentists to practice in nine specialties. To specialize, dentists must complete two to four years of additional education in the specialty. They may also need to do a postgraduate residency, typically lasting up to two years, and pass an exam.

Work Responsibilities

Dentists examine people's teeth and gums to determine whether they are healthy. Sometimes using x-rays, they identify and treat cavities, gum disease, and other dental problems. Dentists fill cavities, repair fractures, and extract teeth. When people have broken teeth or teeth that must be replaced, dentists fit them with crowns, dentures (appliances to replace missing teeth), and other appliances. Dentists also straighten teeth with braces and retainers. They put protective sealants on children's teeth, and they perform surgery to correct gum disease. Besides diagnosing and correcting problems, dentists advise people on how to keep their teeth healthy with brushing, flossing, and other care.

Like physicians, dentists record notes of their examinations in their patients' records. They can use these notes to determine the adequacy of home care and to monitor conditions that require attention.

Typical Tasks of a Dentist

- Examine a patient's teeth, gums, and mouth
- Interpret an x-ray
- Formulate a plan of treatment
- Administer an anesthetic
- Fill a cavity
- Apply a crown
- Perform a root canal
- Extract a tooth
- Apply braces
- Insert a dental implant

Dentists may work with patients with special needs, such as pregnant women, patients with illnesses or injuries, and very young children. Dentists must be aware of the particular needs of these patients and be prepared to address them. With children, for example, they may need to explain carefully and slowly what they're going to do in order to set the patient at ease.

Dentists can specialize in the nine areas of care detailed in Table 5-1 (following page).

Personal Characteristics of Dentists

After college, dentists may join a practice. More often, however, they start their own office and begin seeking patients. Either way, establishing oneself in the profession

Table 5-1 Nine Dental Specialties

Specialty	Work Involved
Orthodontics	Straightening teeth with braces and retainers (the largest specialty)
Oral and maxillofacial surgery	Surgery on the mouth and jaws
Pediatric dentistry	Dental treatment of children
Periodontics	Care of the gums and bones supporting the teeth
Prosthodontics	Replacement of broken parts of teeth or missing teeth with crowns, bridges, dentures, or other fixtures
Endodontics	Treatment of the interior of the tooth, such as the root canal (the pulp-filled cavity in the root of a tooth), including replacement of infected or inflamed pulp in a root canal with artificial material
Dental public health	Promotion of oral health and disease prevention
Oral and maxillofacial pathology	Diagnosis and treatment of oral diseases
Oral and maxillofacial radiology	Use of imaging to diagnose head and neck diseases

takes hard work and time. A person considering this occupation should be self-disciplined and should have a strong work ethic.

Like many other medical professionals, dentists need to be good problem solvers, able to consider the different information about a patient's condition and determine the cause of a problem. Their work requires attention to detail, patience, thoroughness, and the ability to focus on a task, as well as good manual dexterity.

A dentist's success relies strongly on the loyalty of patients and staff. Several qualities help to develop that loyalty. One is strong communication skills. Dentists must be good listeners. They should also be able to explain dental problems to patients in a way that is easily understood and give clear instructions and recommendations. Another important quality is the ability to get along well with others. Dentists interact with many different people, including patients, dental hygienists, dental assistants,

SPOTLIGHT ON SKILLS Typical Task: Probe and Measure a Pocket

Position: Dentist

A *pocket* is a space between an inflamed gum and the surface of a tooth. The use of a probe is the only accurate, dependable method to assess and measure pockets.

To probe a pocket, a dentist holds the side of the probe tip flat against the tooth surface and slides the probe along the tooth surface down to the base of the pocket. The dentist may feel roughness as the probe is passed down the side of the tooth and must evaluate the topography and nature of the tooth surface. With slight pressure, the tension of the attached periodontal tissue at the base of the pocket can be felt. The dentist uses the minimum amount of pressure needed to gauge the health of the attached tissue.

To read the depth of a pocket, the dentist brings the probe to a position as nearly parallel with the long axis of the tooth as possible. A pocket is measured from the *gingival margin* (the border of the gum that surrounds but is not attached to the tooth) to the attached periodontal tissue.

The dentist counts the millimeters that show on the probe above the gingival margin and subtracts that number from the total number of millimeters shown on the probe.

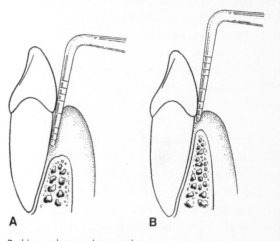

Probing and measuring a pocket.

office staff, and other dentists. Successful dentists display a proactive, caring attitude toward their staff and patients.

A positive attitude also helps. Dentists set the tone for their office staff. A positive attitude can earn the goodwill of patients and establish good working relationships with colleagues.

Employment Opportunities and Trends

The Bureau of Labor Statistics (BLS) reports that in 2008, dentists held about 141,900 jobs. Some 85 percent were in general practice. Orthodontists made up five percent; oral and maxillofacial surgeons, five percent; and the other specialties, the rest. Nearly all dentists were in private practice. According to the ADA, about 75 percent of these dentists were sole proprietors, with nearly 15 percent in a partnership. A few worked in hospitals and physicians' offices.

Most beginning dentists take over an existing practice (for example, when a dentist retires) or start their own. Some spend one or two years working for dentists who are already practicing, gaining experience and saving money to open their own practice.

From 2008 to 2018, the BLS projects that the number of dentists will grow by 16 percent. There will be 22,100 new jobs, 18,400 of which will be in general dentistry. This growth will result from an increased demand for services due to several factors:

- Population growth, especially the population that is older. Older Americans will need more complicated dental work, such as dentures, and will tend to retain more teeth than in the past and, therefore, need more care.

- Preventive care for younger people
- Increasing dental coverage among private insurance companies
- The rising popularity of cosmetic dental services, such as braces and whitening

The projected growth, which is faster than the average, won't match the demand for dental services, according to the BLS. If that is the case, skilled dentists should be quite busy.

Improvements in technology will allow dentists to do more work, and they will hire more dental hygienists and dental assistants to provide some dental care. The BLS predicts good job prospects, many from vacancies created when older dentists retire or shift to part-time work.

Professional Organization

The national professional organization for dentists is the ADA. It is the largest dental association in the U.S., representing more than 157,000 members as of 2010. The ADA advocates for the dental profession and oral health. It monitors policy issues in Congress, state legislatures, regulatory agencies, and foreign governments. Medicaid, issues affecting small businesses, student financial aid, tobacco control, advertising by professionals, licensure, and scope of practice are some of the issues addressed by the ADA. The organization's goals include advancing standards for oral health care and educating the public about better oral health.

Other activities of the ADA include the following:

- Through its Commission on Dental Accreditation, establishing standards for and accrediting dental education

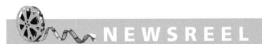 **NEWSREEL**

Oral Pathology

Every dental checkup includes a thorough examination of the mouth for evidence of disease. Dentists and dental hygienists are trained to detect not just common problems like tooth decay or gum disease, but a wide range of diseases that affect the mouth and other parts of the body. The first signs of some medical problems—osteoporosis or AIDS, for example—can appear in the mouth.

In oral pathology classes, dental professionals learn to identify diseases, or narrow the possibilities, from signs such as the appearance of a lesion or ulcer or a characteristic swelling or inflammation. General dentists treat some diseases themselves; for others, they refer the patient to a specialist. Diseases that affect the teeth,

tongue, gums, jaw, and lining of the mouth may be referred to an oral and maxillofacial pathologist for final diagnosis and treatment.

Examples of oral diseases include stomatitis, a viral illness; burning mouth or burning tongue syndrome; a yeast infection known as oral candidiasis; recurrent canker sores; and various bone diseases.

The ADA recently concluded a three-year public awareness program on oral cancer. Although the number of new cases and deaths among the general public has been falling slowly for many years, the number of new cases among adults under age 40 has been rising significantly. The goals of the campaign were to boost public awareness of oral cancer and to highlight the dentist's role in identifying the disease.

programs, including general and specialist dentistry, dental assisting, and dental hygiene programs

- Issuing the Dental Admission Test and National Board Dental Examinations
- Developing standards for dental products and testing them for safety and effectiveness
- Conducting scientific research

Dentists who join the ADA are enrolled in the national association, as well as 53 state or territorial associations and 545 local dental societies. Member services include continuing education opportunities; publications, including *The Journal of the American Dental Association*; advice on business management; and opportunities to network at local, state, and national meetings and online.

CHECK POINT

1 Name and briefly describe the nine dental specialties.

DENTAL HYGIENISTS

When people have a dental checkup, the first professional they see, and the one who spends the most time with them, is usually a dental hygienist. Dental hygienists provide a wide range of services focused on preventing and treating tooth and gum disease and promoting good oral hygiene and health. They usually work under the supervision of a dentist.

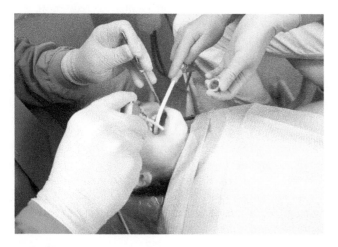

Dental hygienists promote good oral hygiene and health.

History of the Profession

The history of dentistry shows that even many centuries ago, people understood that there was a connection between caring for their teeth and preventing dental disease. However, the scientific explanation wasn't known until the 1890 publication of *Microorganisms of the Human Mouth* by Willoughby D. Miller. In his book, Miller, a dentist with a degree in chemistry, physics, and applied mathematics, developed the basic theoretical understanding of dental decay.

Interest in oral hygiene among dentists had been growing for some time. Civic-minded dentists spoke or wrote about the importance of brushing, flossing, and *prophylaxis* (professional cleaning and polishing). However, Miller's book opened a new field to dentists: *preventive dentistry*. Preventive dentistry focuses on preventing dental disease through professional cleaning and polishing of teeth and teaching patients to care for their teeth and mouths. The book also prompted a worldwide movement to promote regular brushing and flossing.

Alfred C. Fones, a dentist in Bridgeport, Connecticut, coined the term *dental hygienist* and became known as the father of dental hygiene. After hearing a lecture on prophylaxis in 1896, he became keenly interested in oral hygiene and implemented it in his practice. In comparing his patients with those of his father, with whom he shared an office, Fones found that his patients had healthier mouths. However, it proved difficult for Fones to find time for thorough cleaning and polishing when he had cavities to fill, teeth to pull, and other demanding tasks. As a result, Fones taught his assistant and cousin, Irene Newman, to clean teeth, using teeth he had extracted for practice.

In 1913, Fones opened the first oral hygiene school. The first class consisted of 34 women, many of whom were nurses, physicians' wives, and teachers. Courses included tooth anatomy, histology, and clinical practice. Lectures were delivered by dentists and dental instructors from Yale and Columbia universities and from around the world. The Bridgeport Board of Education hired most of the first graduating class to clean schoolchildren's teeth.

The new occupation grew rapidly. In 1916, Columbia University started the first university-based hygienist program. The next year, Connecticut became the first state to license dental hygienists, with the first license granted to Irene Newman. Several other states quickly followed. Dental hygienists began forming state professional associations. In 1923, dental hygienists in California formed the national association for dental hygienists, the American Dental Hygienists' Association (ADHA), winning the approval of the ADA and inviting into its membership dental hygiene organizations and alumni "with well known merits and high standards."

Licensing and education standards soon followed. By 1951, all states required dental hygienists to be licensed. In 1947, the ADHA and the ADA established accreditation standards for dental hygiene programs. Accreditation began in 1952. In 1962, the first National Board Examination for Dental Hygienists was administered.

Education, Training, and Legal Requirements

In nearly every state, a person must graduate from an accredited dental hygiene program to become a dental hygienist. Most programs grant an associate's degree. Some offer a certificate, a bachelor's degree, or a master's degree. Dental offices usually require a minimum of an associate's degree or certificate.

According to the ADHA, entrance requirements for accredited programs generally include a high school diploma or equivalent; high school courses in math, chemistry, biology, and English; and a college entrance test such as the SAT or ACT. Programs include both academic classes and supervised clinical instruction. Students take general education courses, such as speech and psychology, as well as science and dentistry-related courses in three areas:

- *Basic science*: General chemistry, anatomy, physiology, biochemistry, microbiology, pathology, nutrition, and pharmacology
- *Dental science*: Dental anatomy, head and neck anatomy, oral pathology, radiography, pain control, and dental materials
- *Dental hygiene science*: Oral health education and preventive counseling, patient management, clinical dental hygiene, community dental health, and medical and dental emergencies

In addition to coursework, students spend an average of more than 650 hours in supervised clinical work.

The practice of dental hygiene is regulated by the states through state dental practice laws. All states require dental hygienists to be licensed. In almost every state, obtaining a license requires graduating from an accredited dental hygiene program and passing both a written exam and a clinical board exam. The written exam is a national exam administered by the ADA's Joint Commission on National Dental Examinations (JCNDE). The clinical exam is administered by state or regional testing agencies. Most states require students to pass an additional exam on legal issues relating to dental hygiene practice.

Alabama is the only state that does not require the ADA written examination for licensure. Instead, candidates must take courses, be trained on the job in dentists' offices, and pass a written exam administered by the state. Indiana differs from the other states in the title given to licensed dental hygienists, calling them RDHs (registered dental hygienists) or LDHs (licensed dental hygienists).

Dental hygienists must renew their license periodically, every one to five years depending on the state. Almost all states require continuing education as a condition of renewal.

Work Responsibilities

Dental hygienists clean people's teeth. They remove plaque and other materials from the teeth and from below the gum line, and they polish teeth, removing stains. Dental hygienists examine a patient's mouth, looking for evidence of tooth decay, gum disease, and other problems. They take x-rays and sometimes develop them. Dental hygienists also apply fluoride treatments, sealants, and other materials to prevent cavities. In addition, they make casts or impressions of patients' teeth that dentists can then use for creating dentures, crowns, or bridges. Dental hygienists document their work in paper records or on a computer, and they may schedule return appointments for their patients.

Dental hygienists can perform a variety of additional tasks, depending on the state in which they practice. They may be allowed to inject local anesthetics, such as novocaine and lidocaine, and to give other anesthetics, such as nitrous oxide. Dental hygienists may also prepare and place fillings, remove sutures, apply *periodontal dressings* (bandages placed on the gums following dental surgery), and smooth and polish crowns and other metal restorations.

An important part of dental hygienists' work is teaching patients about good home care. For example, they may demonstrate how to brush and floss teeth, check young patients' brushing skills at each visit, and advise patients about dietary habits that will improve their dental health. Because smoking is related to oral health, they sometimes run smoking cessation programs. Like dentists, they may need to take special care with patients with particular needs, such as children.

Typical Tasks of a Dental Hygienist

- Remove plaque, calculus, and stains
- Take and process x-rays
- Apply cavity-preventive agents
- Use a periodontal probe
- Apply topical fluoride
- Apply a light-cured sealant
- Make a *maxillary* (upper jaw) preliminary impression
- Apply a *rubber dam* (a piece of latex that isolates a tooth for work while protecting the surrounding teeth)
- Finish and polish an *amalgam restoration* (a mercury and silver alloy filling)
- Place a stainless steel crown

SPOTLIGHT ON SKILLS Typical Task: Polish Teeth with a Rubber Cup Attachment

Position: Dental Hygienist

During a dental checkup, the hygienist usually polishes a patient's teeth to remove stains. A common method of polishing is to use a low-power handpiece with a soft rubber cup at the end.

Before polishing, the dental hygienist looks closely at a patient's teeth to determine where stain removal is needed. He or she then fills the rubber cup with a polishing agent and distributes it over the surfaces to be polished. To stabilize and control the teeth during polishing, a *finger rest* is established by placing the third finger of the hand holding the instrument on a tooth or teeth. The hygienist brings the rubber cup almost in contact with the tooth surface and then activates the power source.

Using the slowest rpm, the dental hygienist applies the revolving cup at a 90-degree angle to the tooth surface for one or two seconds, using light pressure so that the edges of the rubber cup flare slightly. The cup is then moved to an adjacent area on the tooth surface. The hygienist uses a patting or brushing motion, turning the handpiece to adapt the rubber cup to fit each surface of the tooth. He or she replenishes the supply of polishing agent on the cup as needed.

Teeth are polished in *quadrants*. (The upper teeth form one arch, and the lower teeth, a second arch; each arch is divided into two quadrants.) Polishing starts with the far surface of the tooth farthest back in a quadrant and moves forward. For each tooth, the dental hygienist works from the gingival third (the gum line) of the tooth toward the incisal third (the top).

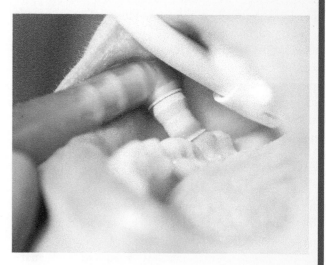

Cleaning with a rubber cap attachment.

Personal Characteristics of Dental Hygienists

Dental hygienists need to be good at detail work. Giving a thorough, careful examination and cleaning requires this quality. So do many other tasks that hygienists perform, from making impressions or ensuring that a filling fits right to properly updating the patient's record after the exam. Manual dexterity is also required for this type of work.

At the same time, dental hygienists need to be efficient and well-organized. They often see many patients in the course of a day. Doing their work well, while keeping to a schedule, requires these characteristics.

Dental hygienists need good people skills. Some patients like to sit quietly while they're having dental work done. Others enjoy conversation. Hygienists should be able to tell what a patient prefers and accommodate that preference. Being able to remember details about patients, such as their jobs, interests, and children's names, makes interactions more pleasant.

A few other qualities are desirable for this work. One is patience, especially when working with nervous patients and young children. Dental hygienists should be flexible and able to adjust easily when a patient is late or needs unanticipated care or when the office is short-staffed. It is also essential for them to be able to work well with the rest of the dental office—the dentists, other hygienists, dental assistants, and administrative staff.

Employment Opportunities and Trends

In 2008, dental hygienists held 174,100 jobs. Because some held more than one job, the number of jobs actually exceeds the number of hygienists. (Opportunities for a flexible work schedule are a feature of this occupation.) Nearly all hygienists worked in dentists' offices.

The BLS anticipates growth of 36 percent for this occupation from 2008 to 2018, with nearly 63,000 new jobs being created. As a result, dental hygiene ranks first among all occupations requiring an associate's degree in terms of employment growth. It is among those health occupations with the fastest growth.

This high rate of job growth will result from an increased demand for dental services created by an expanding population; the fact that older people increasingly keep more of their teeth; and a growing focus on preventive care. To meet this demand, dentists will need to hire additional hygienists.

The BLS thinks that job prospects for dental hygienists from 2008 to 2018 will be favorable but will vary by location. In areas with several dental hygiene programs, competition for jobs may be keen.

Professional Organization

The professional organization for dental hygienists is the ADHA. It has a three-tier structure of local and state groups and the national association. At the national level, the ADHA monitors legislation and federal activities; represents the profession before Congress; and works with state associations to advocate on issues such as scope of practice, education, and licensing. The ADHA promotes dental hygiene education and research, offering fellowships, grants, and other types of funding through its Institute for Oral Health.

Membership in the national association automatically enrolls a hygienist in local and state associations. These associations offer continuing education programs and opportunities for networking. Other membership benefits include a nationwide employment assistance program.

CHECK POINT

2 What personal characteristics should dental hygienists have?

DENTAL ASSISTANTS

Dental assistants perform a wide variety of tasks to keep a dental practice running smoothly. Like medical assistants, some dental assistants do both clinical and administrative work, and some employers ask them to work in a dental laboratory as well. Dental assistants always work under a dentist's supervision.

History of the Profession

The person generally credited with founding the profession of dental assisting was Dr. C. Edmund Kells, a New Orleans dentist. Dr. Kells was an inventor and innovator. He was the first person in the U.S. to take dental x-rays, and he invented an *aspirator* (a device for removing fluid and other materials by suction) for dental and medical surgery that is still used today.

Throughout the 1800s, dentists occasionally employed men as apprentices or general assistants. In 1885, Dr. Kells hired a female assistant to replace his male assistant who had

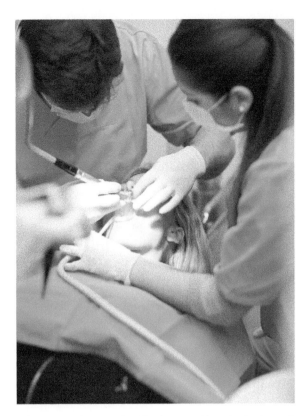

Dental assistants always work under the supervision of a dentist, and may assist in procedures.

left the office. One advantage of having female assistants was that it made it more socially acceptable for female patients to come to the dental office alone, without being escorted by a male relative. As the practice of hiring female assistants spread, it became common to see a sign in the front window of a dental office that declared "Lady in Attendance."

These early dental assistants provided some of the same services as dental assistants today. An important function was that of *chairside assistant*—working closely with the dentist as he or she performs a procedure, as a surgical technologist does with a surgeon. Other duties included cleaning instruments, preparing materials, and managing the office.

One of these early dental assistants was Juliette Southard, hired by Dr. Henry Fowler in 1921 to assist in his dental practice in New York City. That year, Southard and some of her associates founded one of the first dental assisting societies, the Education and Efficiency Society. It eventually became the American Dental Assistants Association (ADAA), the national professional association for dental assistants today.

The ADAA has been active in the development of both educational programs and certification standards. In 1930, the organization formed a committee to develop educational guidelines and training courses. In 1944, it created another committee to develop standards and a competency exam. The first 140-hour training course was adopted in 1946. In 1948, the ADAA established a Certifying Board, now known as the Dental Assisting National Board (DANB), and developed an accreditation process for training programs. Today, programs are accredited by the ADA's Commission on Dental Accreditation.

Education, Training, and Legal Requirements

Some dental assistants are trained on the job, but most attend dental assisting programs offered by community and junior colleges, trade schools, technical institutes, and the military. Most programs last about a year and award a certificate or diploma. Community and junior colleges offer two-year programs that lead to an associate's degree. As of 2009, the Commission on Dental Accreditation had approved 281 programs.

To be admitted to a program, a candidate must have a high school diploma or equivalent. Some programs require applicants to have taken computer and science courses. Helpful high school courses include biology, chemistry, health, and office practices.

Accredited dental assistant programs must include coursework in general education, biomedical science, dental science, clinical sciences, and clinical practice. The following are examples of required classroom subjects:
- Oral and written communication
- Oral health education
- Anatomy and physiology
- Microbiology
- Oral pathology
- Nutrition
- Pharmacology
- Dental materials
- Chairside assisting
- Dental radiology
- Psychology
- Practice management

Programs also include clinical practice with a dentist.

Most states regulate the duties that dental assistants may perform. In some states, dental assistants must have a license or be registered to take x-rays or to perform certain advanced tasks, such as polishing teeth, which are often known as "expanded functions." Obtaining such a license may require attending an accredited dental assisting program or passing a written or practical exam. Continuing education is usually a condition for renewal of that license. Some states let dental assistants perform any duty a dentist assigns them. Individual state requirements may be checked at the DANB web site.

DANB offers two broad credentials for dental assistants: Certified Dental Assistant (CDA) and Certified Orthodontic Assistant (COA). It also provides competency certifications in two specialty areas: radiation health and safety and infection control. Candidates must pass an exam to qualify. As of 2009, 37 states and the District of Columbia recognized or required passing a DANB exam to meet state regulations or to perform advanced tasks. These credentials can also help in getting jobs.

Work Responsibilities

Dental assistants may help care for patients, do office tasks, or work in a dental laboratory. In their role of caring for patients, dental assistants prepare the examination room before patients arrive. They use sterile techniques to make sure surfaces and instruments are germ-free and may use sterilizing procedures for the entire office. Dental assistants prepare materials that will be used during the exam or procedure. They retrieve the patient's records and arrange the materials and instruments properly.

Dental assistants question patients about their dental history, escort them to the examination room, and prepare them. Their responsibilities may include helping the patient feel comfortable before, during, and after treatment. They may also take, develop, and mount x-rays.

During an exam or procedure, assistants perform chairside duties such as handing instruments and materials to the dentist. They also use compressed air and suction to keep the patient's mouth clean and dry.

Dental assistants may perform a number of other clinical tasks. For example, they may prepare materials used in taking impressions of teeth, and they may even take the impressions. Dental assistants may also prepare materials used for crowns and other restorations. Dental assistants may remove sutures, apply anesthetics that are painted on or rubbed into gums, apply cavity-preventing treatments to teeth, and remove extra cement after a filling.

In some offices, dental assistants advise patients on how to keep their teeth and gums healthy. They also instruct patients who have had dental surgery on home care.

Dental assistants who have office duties may make and confirm appointments, answer phones, greet patients, keep treatment records, manage billing, oversee inventory, and order supplies. In laboratories, dental assistants may make casts of teeth and mouths from impressions; clean and polish removable appliances; and make temporary crowns.

In some states, dental assistants with the proper training and experience can do additional "expanded functions" tasks, such as polishing teeth, placing rubber dams, and making sports mouth guards. They may also act as surgical technologists for minor dental surgery, setting up a sterile field and handing the dentist instruments.

Typical Tasks of a Dental Assistant

- Open the office according to a daily routine
- Prepare the dental treatment room
- Set up instrument trays
- Seat the patient
- Take and develop x-rays
- Hand instruments to the dentist
- Instruct patients in oral hygiene
- Clean and polish removable appliances
- Complete health history records
- Prepare bank deposits

Personal Characteristics of Dental Assistants

Dental assistants must be reliable. The dentist and other employees in a practice depend heavily on dental assistants. Dental assistants should be comfortable working under supervision, and they should work well with others.

Good communication skills are also important. Dental assistants work closely with dentists, patients, and other members of the staff. Being a good listener and being able to talk easily with patients and to communicate clearly with fellow employees are assets. Like dental hygienists, dental assistants also need manual dexterity.

Employment Opportunities and Trends

In 2008, dental assistants held more than 295,000 jobs, nearly all them in dentists' offices. More than a third of dental assistants worked part-time. Some held more than one job, and many had variable work schedules.

The BLS projects that employment of dental assistants will grow by 36 percent from 2008 to 2018. This places it among those health occupations with high employment growth. An estimated 105,000 new jobs will be added.

The same factors that will spur employment growth for dentists and dental hygienists will increase dental assistant employment as well. Job prospects will be excellent, according to the BLS. Some dentists will favor assistants who are qualified to perform advanced tasks.

Professional Organization

The ADAA is the oldest, largest professional organization representing dental assistants. It places a strong emphasis on education. As noted earlier, DANB, the organization's certifying board, offers credentials, and these credentials are recognized or required in 37 states. The ADAA provides home-study continuing education courses on basic dental care, treatment of diseases and conditions, radiology, practice management, pharmacology, infection control and occupational safety, and hazardous materials. Membership enrolls a person in the national association and also in state and local associations, where available.

SPOTLIGHT ON SKILLS Typical Task: Apply Compressed Air

Position: Dental Assistant

A common task of dental assistants is applying compressed air to clear saliva and debris from a tooth surface or to dry the surface. Appropriate, timely application of air facilitates examination procedures, makes the treatment area easier to see, and prepares the teeth or gums for certain procedures, such as applying cavity-preventive agents.

Applying air properly requires holding the compressed air syringe in a particular way. The dental assistant uses a *palm grasp* around the handle, holding it in the palm by cupped index, middle, ring, and little fingers and placing the thumb on the release lever or button on the handle.

Technique is equally important. The dental assistant tests the air flow so that the strength of flow can be controlled

and makes relatively short, gentle applications of air. Several actions and situations must be avoided, including:

- Sharp blasts of air on sensitive areas of teeth or unfilled cavities
- Application of air directly into a pocket. This could force *biofilm* (a surface film containing microorganisms and other biological substances) from under the gum line into the tissues, sending bacteria into the blood.
- Forceful application of air, which can direct saliva and debris out of the mouth and contaminate the working area and clinician
- Directing air toward the back of the patient's mouth, which may cause coughing
- Startling the patient. The dental assistant should warn patients when air is to be applied.

ZOOM IN

Expanding Horizons

The demand for dental assistants is strong, but what about professional satisfaction and growth? Opportunities are there, if a dental assistant looks for them. Here are three keys to expanding a dental assistant's professional horizons:

- **Continuing education.** The role of dental assistants is expanding rapidly as the profession advocates for increased responsibilities and states add to the duties dental assistants can perform. New technologies and the needs of dental offices also prompt the delegation of higher-level tasks to dental assistants. Through workshops, online or home education courses, conferences, and webinars, dental assistants can position themselves to take advantage of these opportunities.

- **Becoming active in professional associations.** Through state or local professional associations, dental assistants can lobby their state government for changes in regulations; apply for scholarships; and network and find mentors to help guide their professional development. They can also actively seek other opportunities for professional growth. For example, Dental Assistants Recognition Week is an annual event that focuses on both recognition and educational charitable work by dental assistants through associations, schools, or dental practices.
- **Certification.** Even when a state doesn't require it, certification confers professional advantages. It is nationally recognized, and it can lead to better jobs and higher pay.

Members enjoy a number of benefits, including opportunities for free or discounted continuing education and a subscription to *Dental Assistant*, a professional journal.

CHECK POINT

3 What are "expanded functions" in dental assisting, and what must dental assistants do in order to perform these functions in some states?

Don't forget to visit thePoint companion website for additional study resources!

CHAPTER HIGHLIGHTS

- Dentists are doctors who care for people's teeth and gums. Dentists must be licensed to practice. In most states, getting a license requires graduating from an accredited dental school (usually a four-year program) and passing a written and a practical exam. Admission to dental school requires the DAT and at least two years of college-level pre-dental education.
- Dental hygienists clean and polish teeth, teach patients about oral hygiene, and perform a variety of other tasks. All states require dental hygienists to be licensed, which nearly always requires graduating from an accredited dental hygiene program and passing both a written and a clinical board exam.
- With a projected growth rate of 36 percent, dental hygiene ranks first among occupations requiring an associate's degree in terms of employment growth. Job prospects will be favorable from 2008 to 2018 but will vary by location.
- Dental assistants perform a wide variety of tasks to keep a dental practice running smoothly. They may do clinical, administrative, and/or dental laboratory work, depending on their employers' needs. Most dental assistants attend dental assisting programs, which typically last a year.
- Job prospects for dental assistants are excellent. The BLS projects that employment will grow by 36 percent from 2008 to 2018, and an estimated 105,000 new jobs will be added.

REVIEW QUESTIONS

Matching

1. _____ Prepare and install braces and retainers
2. _____ Clean and polish patients' teeth
3. _____ Hand instruments and materials to the dentist
4. _____ Identify and treat cavities, gum disease, and other dental problems
5. _____ Specialize in the care of the gums and bones supporting the teeth

   a. Dentist   **b.** Dental assistant   **c.** Dental hygienist   **d.** Orthodontist   **e.** Periodontist

Multiple Choice

6. When people have a dental checkup, the first professional they see, and the one who spends the most time with them, is usually
   a. a dentist
   b. a dental assistant
   c. a dental hygienist
   d. an orthodontist

7. Endodontists specialize in
   a. promotion of oral health and disease prevention
   b. replacement of missing teeth
   c. treatment of the interior of teeth, including root canals
   d. use of imaging to diagnose head and neck diseases

8. Which statement about dentists is NOT true?
   a. Most dentists specialize in a certain area of care.
   b. Dentists need to be good business managers.
   c. A typical dentist has six to eight years of college or professional education.
   d. The professional organization for dentists is the ADA.

9. Which of the following is a typical work responsibility of dental hygienists?
   a. repairing cracks in teeth
   b. applying fluoride treatments and sealants
   c. making crowns
   d. opening the dental office

10. Which statement about dental assistants is NOT true?
    a. Dental assistants always work under a dentist's supervision.
    b. Most dental assisting programs are one-year programs.
    c. All states require dental assistants to be licensed.
    d. Nutrition, microbiology, and oral pathology are typical classroom subjects in dental assistant programs.

Completion

11. Keeping one's mouth clean is known as _____.

12. A dental assistant who works closely with a dentist during a procedure is performing the function of _____.

13. The largest specialty for dentists is _____.

14. Professional cleaning and polishing of the teeth is known as _____.

15. A cap that is placed on a broken tooth is known as a/an _____.

Short Answer

16. Compare and contrast the education and training of dental hygienists and dental assistants.

    _____

    _____

17. How are dental assistants like medical assistants? How are they like surgical technologists?

    _____

    _____

18. What are the two main job responsibilities of dental hygienists?

    _____

    _____

19. Give three examples of administrative tasks that dental assistants typically perform.

    _____

    _____

20. Briefly summarize the personal characteristics that dental hygienists need to have.

    _____

    _____

INVESTIGATE IT

1. What does current scientific evidence say about the link between gum disease and other medical problems, such as obesity or diabetes? Read an article about a recent research study. The following web site might be helpful: http://www.sciencedaily.com.

2. Both the ADA web site (http://www.ada.org) and the ADHA web site (http://www.adha.org) have sections devoted to public or oral health, and the ADA site has a section, "ADA News," with videos called "Dental Minutes" on dental technology and research. Visit one of these sites and read, watch a video, or listen to a podcast about a topic that interests you. These are some suggested topics:
   - The effect of diet, smokeless tobacco, or cigarettes on oral health
   - Whitening treatments
   - Intra-oral cameras
   - Perio screening and computers
   - Tooth farms

3. Perform Internet research to answer one or more of the following questions. Determine the important words or phrases in the questions below and use those as your search criteria.
   - What was the tooth worm theory, and when was it finally debunked?
   - When did the U.S. start adding fluoride to drinking water, and what prompted it to do so?
   - What is four-handed dentistry?
   - When did people start using toothpaste in a tube? What are some examples of other substances people have used to brush their teeth?

RECOMMENDED READING

Aetna, Inc. Simple Steps to Better Dental Health. Available at: http://www.simplestepsdental.com/SS/ihtSS/r.WSIHW000/st.31819/t.31819/pr.3.html.

Aulie N. *Career Diary of a Dental Hygienist.* Washington: Garth Gardner; 2007.

Goforth S. Test-Tube Teeth. [The Why Files website]. February 19, 2004. Available at: http://whyfiles.org/shorties/147tooth.

Kendall B. *Opportunities in Dental Care Careers.* Chicago: VGM Career Books; 2001.

Reece T. A Reason to Smile. *Career World.* February/March 2009;37(5):20–22.

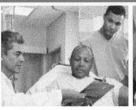
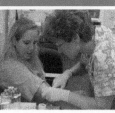
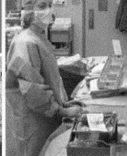

Laboratory and Pharmacy Services

6 CHAPTER

CHAPTER OBJECTIVES

After careful study of this chapter, you should be able to:

* State the education, training, and legal requirements for becoming a clinical laboratory technologist, clinical laboratory technician, laboratory assistant, pharmacist, and pharmacy technician.

* Describe the typical work responsibilities of each profession.

* List desirable personal characteristics of clinical laboratory technologists, clinical laboratory technicians, laboratory assistants, pharmacists, and pharmacy technicians.

* Identify employment opportunities and key trends for these occupations.

KEY TERMS

bacteriology (bak TĔR ē OL ŏ jē)

cytology (sī TOL ŏ jē)

histology (his TOL ŏ jē)

mycology (mī KOL ŏ jē)

parasitology (PAR ă sī TOL ŏ jē)

pharmaceutical (fahr mă SŪ ti kăl)

pharmacology (fahr mă KOL ŏ jē)

quality assurance (QA)

quality control (QC)

virology (vī ROL ŏ jē)

The occupations profiled in the previous three chapters involve direct patient care. People in the occupations described in this chapter, however, do not always work directly with patients. Yet the services they provide serve to analyze and detect, which are vital in protecting and restoring patients' health. The tests performed by laboratory personnel help physicians prevent and diagnose diseases, gauge the progress of diseases, and assess a patient's response to treatment. Pharmacists and pharmacy technicians provide the medications needed to prevent, treat, and manage diseases. Physicians, nurses, and other health care practitioners rely on the timely and accurate services of laboratory and pharmacy personnel.

CLINICAL LABORATORY TECHNOLOGISTS

Taking samples for tests—blood, urine, throat swabs, and so on—is part of many visits to physicians or hospitals. The health care professionals who perform the tests and analyze the results are often clinical laboratory technologists. Sometimes called *medical technologists* or *clinical laboratory scientists*, these health care workers perform a wide array of tests on tissues, body fluids, and cells. These tests can show whether a person has a particular disease or condition, how well a treatment is working, and whether blood is safe to be used for transfusion.

History of the Profession

The first clinical laboratories were established in the late 1800s and early 1900s. The discovery of the bacteria that caused tuberculosis and other epidemic diseases, and the development of tests for detecting these bacteria, demonstrated the importance of laboratory work. The pathologists who ran these laboratories started training assistants, often women, to perform many of the simpler tasks and procedures, which gave the pathologists time for more complex work.

During World War I, qualified laboratory personnel were in short supply, as the number of laboratories increased and as pathologists and bacteriologists left private industry jobs for the armed services. Technicians took on some of the pathologists' and bacteriologists' responsibilities in the lab, performing simple tests and reporting the results.

After the war, many programs to train laboratory technologists arose. To help standardize their education, the American Society for Clinical Pathology (ASCP) created a Board of Registry (BOR) in 1928 to certify laboratory technicians and later a Board of Schools (BOS) to accredit educational programs. Graduates who passed the BOR's accrediting exam came to be referred to as *medical technologists* and had the designation MT (ASCP). In 1933, medical technologists formed their own professional organization, now known as the American Society for Clinical Laboratory Science (ASCLS).

As clinical laboratory science continued to develop, educational requirements for medical technologists increased. In 1973, the function of accreditation passed to the National Accrediting Agency for Clinical Laboratory Sciences (NAACLS). Master's and doctoral programs were introduced to train medical technology faculty, and states began to license medical technologists. Over the past ten years, the name for professionals in this occupation has been gradually changing from *medical technologists* to *clinical laboratory technologists* or *clinical laboratory scientists*, terms that are thought to more accurately describe their work.

Education, Training, and Legal Requirements

Most clinical laboratory technologists have a bachelor's degree in medical technology or a life science. Entry-level positions typically require a bachelor's degree. For some jobs, however, a combination of education and on-the-job and specialized training is acceptable.

The Clinical Laboratory Improvement Amendments (CLIA) are a set of federal quality standards for all laboratory testing to ensure the accuracy, reliability, and timeliness of patient test results, regardless of where the test is performed. CLIA divides laboratory tests into three levels based on the complexity of the testing method:

- Waived, or low-complexity, tests, such as simple blood glucose or pregnancy tests
- Moderate-complexity tests, such as microscopic urinalysis and throat cultures
- High-complexity tests, such as manual cell counts

CLIA requires all laboratory personnel who perform highly complex tests to have at least an associate's degree. ASCLS recommends that students interested in becoming clinical laboratory technologists take classes that will give them a solid foundation in biology, chemistry, and math.

Both universities and hospitals offer medical technology programs that combine academic classes with clinical experience. Options include a 3+1 program (three years of academic classes followed by a one-year clinical internship, usually at a hospital), a 4+1 program (a bachelor's degree plus a one-year clinical internship), and coursework with shorter clinical experiences (five to six months, for example). State requirements influence the options schools can offer. Master's and doctoral programs in clinical laboratory science are also available. As of 2010, NAACLS accredited 215 clinical laboratory scientist and medical technologist programs.

Curriculum requirements of NAACLS-accredited programs include:

- Scientific content (as a prerequisite or as part of the curriculum) in areas such as anatomy and physiology, immunology, microbiology, and statistics
- Instruction on preparing for laboratory tests, performing them, and analyzing the results in areas such as hematology, chemistry, urinalysis, and immunology
- Quality assurance (QA)—a plan for ensuring high quality performance in all areas of a laboratory's technical support functions—and quality improvement

- Safety and government regulations and standards
- Communication and teamwork skills
- Ethics and professionalism
- Educational techniques and vocabulary sufficient for training or educating other personnel
- An understanding of research design and practice, to evaluate published studies in an informed way
- An overview of laboratory operations, including human resources and financial management

Many programs also offer or require courses in management, business, education, and computer applications. In their clinical work, students perform laboratory tests, often rotating through the different departments of a hospital to gain exposure to different types of tests.

Some states require clinical laboratory technologists to be licensed or registered. Requirements vary but generally include a bachelor's degree and an exam. A state's department of health or board of occupational licensing can provide information about requirements.

Professional certification is optional, but it gives a technologist a strong advantage in the job market. Clinical laboratory technologists can seek both general and specialized certifications. The following organizations offer professional credentials:

- American Medical Technologists (AMT)
- ASCP
- Board of Registry of the American Association of Bioanalysts
- National Credentialing Agency for Laboratory Personnel

Work Responsibilities

Clinical laboratory technologists prepare specimens, perform tests on them, and interpret the results. They test body fluids and tissues, looking for bacteria, viruses, and other microorganisms. They scrutinize cells under a microscope, checking for changes and abnormal cells that can indicate diseases such as cancer. They test the chemical content of samples, checking such things as the glucose or cholesterol levels in the blood or how a patient is responding to a new drug treatment. In addition, clinical laboratory technologists type and cross-match blood for transfusions.

Increasingly, clinical laboratory technologists use complex instruments and equipment in their work. Two examples are automated cell counters, which count and size blood cells, and chemistry analyzers, which can perform up to 30 or more tests on proteins, electrolytes, and other substances in body fluids. Some tests are still performed manually, however.

In larger labs, such as those in hospitals, clinical laboratory technologists often specialize in particular types of tests:

- Clinical chemistry technologists prepare specimens and analyze DNA, cells, and chemicals and hormones in blood.
- Microbiology technologists examine and identify bacteria, viruses, fungi, parasites, and other microorganisms.
- Blood bank, or immunohematology, technologists collect blood, type it, test it for diseases and other medical problems, and prepare it for transfusions.
- Immunology technologists test for diseases that involve the body's immune system to help determine if the system is functioning properly.
- Cytotechnologists study cells, looking for cancer and changes that signal pre-cancerous conditions, infections, and other diseases.
- Molecular biology technologists do complex testing on cell samples.

After testing and examining a specimen, clinical laboratory technologists analyze the results, interpret them, and communicate them to the pathologist or researcher running the lab or to the physician who ordered the test. They may also enter test results into a computer.

A very important part of the clinical laboratory technologist's work is checking for accuracy. Test results must be checked carefully to ensure that the conclusions or diagnoses on which they are based are sound. Clinical laboratory technologists also routinely check that instruments are working properly and that data are being recorded correctly.

Clinical laboratory technologists do a lot of detective work as they perform tests and analyze the results. When results are unusual and unexpected, they have to find out why. Was it the way the sample was obtained? Was there a problem with the lab equipment or with the test materials? Was the data analyzed incorrectly?

Another common responsibility of clinical laboratory technologists is quality control. A laboratory's quality control (QC) program monitors each phase of the laboratory process. Technologists need to make sure that chemicals and other materials used for tests are of acceptable quality and that instruments are working accurately. They may also establish and monitor quality assurance and quality improvement programs.

Clinical laboratory technologists with a strong educational background and work experience may perform more complex tests, and they may have other responsibilities as well. For instance, a technologist may be in charge of all lab work ordered during his or her work shift or in a particular section of a lab. Clinical laboratory technologists may train

SPOTLIGHT ON SKILLS Typical Task: Care for a Microscope

Position: Clinical Laboratory Technologist

Microscopes are delicate, expensive instruments. To ensure that they are kept in good working order, they must be maintained according to the manufacturer's standards.

Before doing maintenance on a microscope, the clinical laboratory technologist washes his or her hands, gathers supplies, and puts on gloves to avoid transferring skin oils to the microscope's optical surfaces. The optical surfaces are cleaned with lens cleaner and lens paper. Tissue and gauze cannot be used because they might scratch the lenses.

Beginning with the eyepieces, the technologist places a drop or two of lens cleaner on a sheet of lens paper and wipes each piece thoroughly. Then he or she moves to the three or four *objective lenses* (the different-power lenses through which specimens are examined), using new sheets of lens paper moistened with lens cleaner. The technologist starts with the lowest-power lens and continues to the highest-power lens, to ensure that the cleanest areas are cleaned first. The *oil objective*, a lens with oil on it, is cleaned last so that oil from that lens isn't carried to the other lenses. Using new, dry lens paper, the technologist wipes each eyepiece and objective lens again to prevent distortion from any cleaner that might remain.

Next, the technologist cleans the light source and the *condenser*—the part that concentrates the light rays to focus on the slide—using a new sheet of lens paper moistened with lens cleaner for each of these pieces.

After that, the technologist washes the non-optical surfaces of the microscope, using gauze with a mild soap solution or an alcohol wipe. He or she then rinses the washed areas, using another piece of gauze moistened with water.

After storing the cleaned microscope, the technologist documents the cleaning on the maintenance log sheet for that microscope and sanitizes the work area.

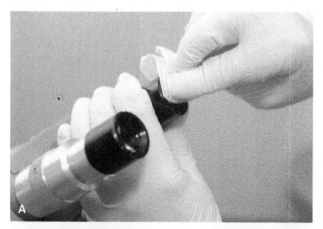

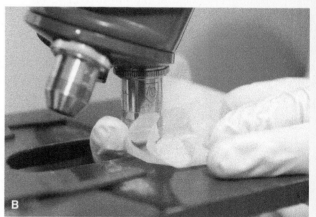

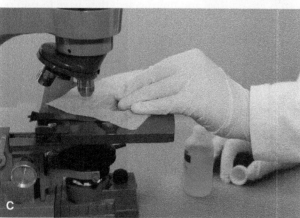

Three steps of microscope care: cleaning the eyepiece, the lenses, and the condenser.

and supervise other laboratory workers. They may also develop new tests under supervision and evaluate them.

Typical Tasks of a Clinical Laboratory Technologist

- Perform venous and skin punctures for blood collection
- Prepare reagents (chemicals used to produce a reaction) and other supplies and equipment for tests
- Perform complete blood counts
- Examine cells using a microscope
- Analyze test results
- Enter test results into a computer and report abnormal results immediately
- Calibrate laboratory equipment
- Run daily quality control checks on testing equipment
- Train subordinates in new techniques
- Design and develop research experiments

Personal Characteristics of Clinical Laboratory Technologists

Clinical laboratory technologists have many important responsibilities. How well they do their jobs can literally mean the difference between life and death for a patient. People who choose this occupation must be responsible and reliable. A commitment to thorough, high-quality, accurate work is essential.

People who are good at problem-solving make good clinical laboratory technologists. Workers in this field often characterize their jobs as detective work—analyzing samples, for example, and tracking down the source of a problem. Their work requires them to bring together and apply their knowledge of physiology, diseases, and testing. Clinical laboratory technologists are typically people who like challenges and who set high standards for themselves.

Tests sometimes have to be done under time pressure. Clinical laboratory technologists should be capable of working well under pressure, able to focus on a complex test and perform it swiftly but carefully.

Clinical laboratory technologists communicate constantly, in person, on the phone, and in writing, with laboratory personnel, physicians, nurses, researchers, and others. Therefore, they should have good communication skills, in both speaking and writing.

These workers often have a lot of independence in their work. Clinical laboratory technologists should be self-starters and capable of working on their own.

Employment Opportunities and Trends

In 2008, clinical laboratory technologists held 172,400 jobs. Sixty-one percent of these jobs were in hospitals.

Another 15 percent were in medical and diagnostic laboratories, and seven percent were in physicians' offices. Most of the remaining jobs were in colleges, universities, and other educational institutions; ambulatory care services, such as outpatient care centers; and state and local government.

The BLS projects that employment growth for this occupation during 2008–2018 will be 14 percent. The Bureau identifies several reasons for this level of growth. More tests will be required to meet the needs of the growing population. The volume of tests will also increase as new tests continue to be developed.

From 2008 to 2018, the BLS predicts that about 20,500 new jobs will be added. Hospitals will continue to be the main employer. Employment will also grow rapidly in medical and diagnostic laboratories, physicians' offices, and other ambulatory care services. The BLS anticipates that job opportunities will be excellent.

Professional Organization

The ASCLS represents laboratory personnel, including clinical laboratory technologists. It advocates for laboratory occupations, monitors legislation, and acts as a liaison to Congress and federal and state agencies, weighing in on issues such as licensure and scope of practice. The organization encourages grassroots involvement by members at regional, state, and local levels. The ASCLS also emphasizes standards setting, professional and continuing education, and personal and professional development. Its goals include cost-effective, high-quality, accessible laboratory services for health care clients.

Membership benefits include online courses, audioconferences, and workshops that fulfill recertification or license renewal requirements; scientific assemblies (groups that provide opportunities for a variety of professional activities, from writing articles to helping to develop laboratory standards); an annual meeting and exposition; and scholarships and research grants. National, regional, state, and local associations offer opportunities for networking and social events.

CHECK POINT

1 What education and training are needed to become a clinical laboratory technologist?

CLINICAL LABORATORY TECHNICIANS

Clinical laboratory technicians, also known as *medical laboratory technicians*, perform tests on tissues, cells, and body fluids, typically working under the supervision of

ZOOM IN

What's What in the Lab

Blood, tissue, and cell samples are sent for testing to different laboratories or to different departments in a large laboratory. Each laboratory or department specializes in certain areas. Some of these specialties are described below.

- **Blood bank technology.** At blood banks, a variety of tests are performed on donated blood to determine its characteristics and ensure its safety. Laboratory personnel check the ABO blood type and Rh status. They also look for red blood cell antibodies that could cause a reaction in the recipient. Technologists also check platelets for bacteria, and they test for a variety of communicable diseases, including hepatitis B and C, HIV types 1 and 2, human T lymphotropic virus, syphilis, West Nile virus, and increasingly, Chagas' disease, a parasitic infection that can damage the heart and be fatal.

- **Cytotechnology.** Cytology is the study of the structure of cells. Cytotechnologists examine cells microscopically, looking for changes or abnormal cells that indicate viral or bacterial infections, cancer, or precancerous conditions. For example, a Pap smear taken during a gynecological exam is tested in this way. Cellular examination is a key method of detecting cancer early, when it is often easier to treat. Cytotechnologists work in many laboratory settings, including hospital, private, and university laboratories.

- **Hematology.** Hematology labs or departments perform blood tests. A common example is a complete blood count, a screening test used to diagnose and manage many different diseases. This test includes counts of red and white blood cells, *hematocrit* (the percentage of red blood cells), and several other procedures. Another common example is the prothrombin time (PT) test, which shows the time it takes for a sample of

blood to clot. This test is used to diagnose bleeding problems and to check whether blood thinning medication is working.

- **Histology.** The study of the microscopic structure of tissue is called histology. Histology labs or departments deal with tissue samples taken from living patients and during autopsies. The tissues are sized, dried, and then embedded in wax so they can be easily cut into sections and stained for study. A sample taken during surgery may need to be analyzed while the patient is still on the operating table. This situation might arise when an unexpected disease is found during surgery or if the surgeon wants to make sure that the correct tissue for study has been removed. In these cases, the tissue is flash-frozen and quickly sliced, stained, and analyzed. Histological study is used in the diagnosis of cancer and other diseases.

- **Microbiology.** Microbiology labs or departments identify the various microorganisms that cause disease. Technologists and technicians use samples of blood, urine, stool, sputum, and other specimens to grow and test microorganisms. These laboratories or departments sometimes run tests to determine which drug treatment would be most effective against a particular microorganism. Microbiology may include bacteriology (the study of bacteria), virology (the study of viruses), mycology (the study of fungi and yeasts), and parasitology (the study of parasitic protozoa and worms).

- **Immunology.** Immunologists perform a variety of simple and highly specialized tests to determine whether the immune system is functioning as it should and to screen for a variety of disease processes and conditions that involve the immune system. Examples are tests for AIDS, measles, allergies, and pregnancy.

---

a clinical laboratory technologist, laboratory manager, or other professional. Their work is essential in helping physicians to diagnose, treat, and prevent disease. Clinical laboratory technician was named one of the 50 best careers of 2010 by *U.S. News and World Report*, due in part to the relatively low cost of education, opportunities for advancement, low stress, and good wages.

History of the Profession

The occupation of clinical laboratory technician emerged in the 1960s. Advances in scientific knowledge and new technologies were bringing new tests, new procedures,

and automated equipment into the laboratory. Educators in medical technologist training programs saw the need for a new category of laboratory personnel that would perform some of the medical technologist's more technical functions, allowing medical technologists to take on new and expanded responsibilities.

Other factors aided the development of this new occupation. One of them was the increasing popularity of two-year community and junior colleges, which had begun to offer programs preparing students for health occupations. Another was the federal Allied Health Personnel Training Act, passed in 1966, which provided federal funding for allied health programs.

In 1969, the American Association of Junior Colleges and the National Council on Medical Technology Education published guidelines for educational programs for medical laboratory technicians, and the BOR offered the first certification exam. Both the guidelines and the exam needed refinement, however. In 1971, the ASCP established a committee to recommend standards for two-year schools, accredit medical laboratory technician programs, and prepare certification exams. The committee submitted "Essentials for an Approved Program for Associate Degree Medical Laboratory Technicians" to the AMA, which approved them and published them in 1972. In 1973, the American Society for Medical Technology (ASMT, now the ASCLS) approved entry-level competencies for medical laboratory technicians.

Today, the NAACLS accredits clinical laboratory technician programs, and several organizations offer optional certification.

Education, Training, and Legal Requirements

Most clinical laboratory technicians have an associate's degree from a community or junior college or a certificate from a hospital, a vocational or technical school, or the armed forces. A few of these workers learn their skills on the job. CLIA requires clinical laboratory technicians who will perform highly complex tests to have at least an associate's degree.

As of 2010, there were 196 accredited clinical laboratory technician programs. The curriculum for an accredited program must include general education courses, basic sciences, math, and professional courses, including practical clinical experience. It must also cover these items:

- Laboratory methodologies, including problem-solving and troubleshooting techniques
- Specimen collection, processing, and analysis
- Use of laboratory results in diagnosis and treatment
- Communications
- Quality assessment
- Laboratory safety and regulations
- Information processing
- Ethical and professional conduct
- Professional development

In some states, clinical laboratory technicians must be licensed or registered. People interested in this occupation should check with their state department of health or board of occupational licensing to learn the requirements.

Like clinical laboratory technologists, clinical laboratory technicians don't have to be certified. Certification does offer advantages in getting jobs, however. Four organizations offer certification:

- AMT
- ASCP
- Board of Registry of the American Association of Bioanalysts
- National Credentialing Agency for Laboratory Personnel

Work Responsibilities

Clinical laboratory technicians collect specimens for testing, prepare them for study (culturing and staining bacteria, for example), conduct the tests, and do some analysis of the results. Their exact responsibilities vary, depending on the rules of their employer.

Entry-level clinical laboratory technicians are qualified to perform routine tests in all areas of the laboratory. Some tests are done manually, and some use complex instruments and equipment, such as chemistry and coagulation analyzers. Typically, clinical laboratory technicians perform less complex tests than clinical laboratory technologists, often working from a set of established procedures. But they may perform more complex tests, depending on their experience, state regulations, and the laboratory setup.

Technicians monitor tests carefully. They're expected to recognize basic problems and to use established procedures to correct them without being told. When tests are complete, they analyze the results. The amount of analysis they do varies. Generally, they make sure the results conform to specifications and relate them to common diseases and conditions. The next step is to record the findings by entering them in a computer or writing them on paper. When the results indicate a possible medical problem, technicians may report it directly to a supervisor.

Clinical laboratory technicians may work in different areas of the laboratory or specialize. For example, phlebotomists draw blood from patients for testing (see Chapter 7, "Diagnostic and Imaging Services"). Histotechnicians cut and stain tissue specimens for analysis.

A common responsibility of clinical laboratory technicians is care of laboratory instruments and equipment. They may set up and adjust instruments and equipment, clean them, maintain them, and troubleshoot malfunctions and other problems. Other responsibilities may include cross-matching blood; care of specimens, including labeling, recording, sorting, prioritizing, and storing; and training new employees.

SPOTLIGHT ON SKILLS Typical Task: Inoculate a Culture

Position: Clinical Laboratory Technician

A common means of diagnosing diseases is to take a sample of a body substance, such as sputum, and place it in a *culture*—a medium that will support the growth of microorganisms, including those likely to cause disease. As these microorganisms grow, they can be readily identified. The procedure of introducing a specimen into a culture is called *inoculating* a culture.

To prepare for the procedure, the clinical laboratory technician washes his or her hands, puts on protective equipment, such as gloves, and gathers supplies, including the specimen on a swab, a disposable *loop* (a tool with a small loop at the end), and a Petri dish containing culture medium. The technician labels the Petri dish with the patient's name, the date, and other information. The information needs to be on the "medium" side of the dish, because that side is always placed upward to keep condensation from dripping onto the culture.

Taking the cover off the Petri dish, the technician places it on the work surface with the opening facing up to prevent contaminating the interior with any substance from the work surface. He or she streaks the specimen swab across half of the dish containing the culture. Disposing of the swab, the technician takes up the loop, passes it a few times through the streaked specimen, and then draws a bit of the specimen onto the clean surface of the medium. He or she pulls the loop out gradually, thinning bits of the specimen to isolate colonies. This is done because large groups of colonies close together are more difficult to identify than isolated colonies.

When finished, the technician disposes of the equipment and supplies, washes his or her hands, documents the procedure, and sanitizes the work area.

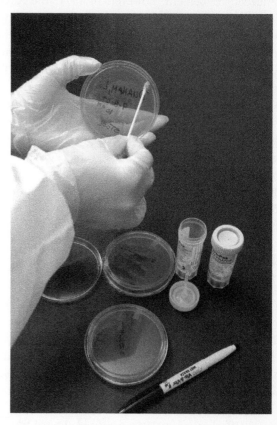

Preparing a culture.

Typical Tasks of a Clinical Laboratory Technician

- Collect a throat specimen
- Draw blood by finger stick
- Make a peripheral blood smear
- Perform ABO and Rh blood typing
- Perform a blood cholesterol test
- Embed tissue in melted paraffin
- Weigh out chemicals and prepare reagents
- Perform basic chemical analysis of urine
- Clean and lubricate equipment
- Organize reagents and other supplies

Personal Characteristics of Clinical Laboratory Technicians

A clinical laboratory technician's job requires accuracy, good judgment, and analytical skills. Tests must be performed carefully and analyzed painstakingly. If a problem arises, it needs to be recognized and addressed. Clinical laboratory technicians must be responsible and committed to doing precise, accurate work. People who can give close attention to detail do well in this occupation.

Several other personal characteristics are also important. Tests sometimes have to be completed quickly, making the ability to work well under a tight deadline important. Many laboratories use work teams, so good teamwork and communication skills are assets.

Technicians often do much of their work independently under general supervision. People interested in this occupation should be comfortable working on their own. They should also be prepared to ask questions or check with a supervisor when they need guidance.

Employment Opportunities and Trends

In 2008, clinical laboratory technicians held about 155,600 jobs. Hospitals were the largest employers, providing

45 percent of jobs. The next three largest employers were medical and diagnostic laboratories (15 percent), physicians' offices (14 percent), and educational services (8 percent).

From 2008 to 2018, BLS projects that job growth for clinical laboratory technicians will be 14 percent. The same factors that will drive job growth for clinical laboratory technologists apply to this career.

This occupation will add 25,000 jobs from 2008 to 2018. Hospitals will continue to be the biggest employer. Employment will also grow quickly in medical and diagnostic laboratories, physicians' offices, and other ambulatory care services. Clinical laboratory technicians should enjoy excellent job opportunities.

Professional Organization

One of the organizations representing clinical laboratory technicians is the AMT. Its membership includes clinical laboratory technicians, clinical laboratory technologists, and other allied health personnel. The AMT's certification program is both nationally and internationally recognized. The organization promotes personal and professional growth and leadership skills. Continuing education opportunities are available through its annual convention, state society meetings and seminars, professional journal, and online programs. State and national committees and boards offer opportunities for networking and developing leadership skills. In addition, the AMT provides a career center with an online job bank.

> **CHECK POINT**
>
> **2** What are the typical work responsibilities of clinical laboratory technicians?

LABORATORY ASSISTANTS

Laboratory assistants, also known as *clinical assistants* or *medical laboratory assistants*, provide a variety of clinical and administrative support services. They work under the supervision of clinical laboratory technologists, pathologists, or other lab personnel.

History of the Profession

Although people have worked as laboratory assistants for centuries, the profession of clinical laboratory assistant in the U.S. emerged in the mid-1950s in response to a shortage of medical technologists, particularly in physicians' offices and laboratories in rural areas. Many technologists preferred to work in urban settings where they were able to perform a greater variety of tests and use more of their skills.

Medical technologist educators began to discuss the possibility of establishing occupational levels for laboratory personnel based on education. Soon, state medical associations started to promote the creation of formal training programs for laboratory assistants so that they could help in rural areas. These assistants would perform simple tests under the supervision of a medical technologist, and they would also handle nontechnical tasks.

In the 1960s and 1970s, steps were taken toward developing educational and certification standards for laboratory assistants. In 1962, a joint committee of the ASCP and the ASMT developed a model training program. The following year, the BOR named the first training program graduates as certified laboratory assistants. In 1967, a certifying exam administered by the BOR was made a requirement for certification. In 1973, the ASMT approved entry-level competencies for certified laboratory assistants.

Education, Training, and Legal Requirements

Laboratory assistants must have a high school diploma or the equivalent. Many are trained on the job, but some complete a formal training program. A few programs are accredited by the NAACLS, but most programs are not accredited. Programs typically last nine to 18 months and lead to a certificate. Some programs combine laboratory assistant training with phlebotomist and EKG technician training.

Laboratory assistant programs include both coursework and practical experience. Classes prepare students to work in all areas of the laboratory, taking and processing specimens, performing some tests, and doing administrative tasks. Examples of courses include:

- Laboratory assistant skills
- Introduction to health care
- Medical terminology
- Laboratory administrative skills
- Anatomy and physiology
- Medical laboratory safety
- Phlebotomy
- Computer applications
- Interpersonal communications
- Written and oral communications

Students who are considering becoming laboratory assistants should take classes in health sciences, biology, and chemistry, as well as algebra, English, and computer applications.

In some states, laboratory personnel must be licensed or registered. People interested in this occupation should check with their state department of health or board of occupational licensing. Laboratory assistants can obtain the Certified Medical Laboratory Assistant (CMLA) credential from the AMT or the National Healthcareer Association

(NHA). Some programs prepare students for phlebotomist certification as well. Certification isn't required to be a laboratory assistant, but it can help in getting jobs.

Work Responsibilities

Laboratory assistants collect samples, label them, and set up routine tests, preparing materials for analysis according to established procedures. They may also perform low-complexity tests and certain moderate-complexity tests as defined by CLIA. For moderate-complexity tests, CLIA requires that laboratory assistants have a high school diploma or the equivalent and that the laboratory provide documentation showing that the assistants have been trained to perform the test.

An important part of a laboratory assistant's work is maintaining a laboratory's storage system for specimens. Some samples require special storage procedures. Blood, for example, may need to be *centrifuged*—separated into its

component parts—and must be stored at a certain temperature. Laboratory assistants receive, sort, store, and retrieve samples. They serve as resources for laboratory personnel and health care professionals who order tests, answering questions about specimen handling and processing. Laboratory assistants may also be responsible for delivering specimens for testing in a timely manner. In addition, they're expected to recognize and report errors in specimen collection, labeling, transport, and processing.

Laboratory assistants maintain equipment and supplies. They may also be responsible for cleaning and sanitizing equipment and work areas.

Administrative responsibilities include entering patient data into a computer system, answering phones, assisting callers with inquiries, and referring calls to other personnel when necessary. Laboratory assistants are often the first level of contact for people requiring services from the laboratory. They may process orders for tests, report results, and do billing.

 SPOTLIGHT ON SKILLS Typical Task: Perform a Gram Stain

Position: Laboratory Assistant

Specimens grown on a culture may be spread on a slide for examination under a microscope. Staining the specimen can help physicians narrow the field of potential disease-causing organisms that the specimen may contain. The staining method most used in the microbiology lab is the *Gram stain*.

In a Gram stain, certain bacteria, when stained with a dye called *crystal violet*, retain the purple color and are said to be *Gram-positive*. Other bacteria stain pink or red when another type of stain, a counterstain, is applied. These bacteria are called *Gram-negative*. Often, simply knowing whether a specimen is Gram-positive or Gram-negative will enable a physician to prescribe an appropriate antibiotic while waiting for more specific tests.

Before doing a Gram stain, the laboratory assistant washes his or her hands, gathers supplies, and makes sure that the specimen has been properly fixed to the slide and that the slide is at room temperature. Then the assistant puts on gloves and places the slide on a rack for staining, with the sample side facing up.

The first step in the actual staining is to flood the slide with crystal violet. Then, holding the slide with forceps, the assistant drains off the excess dye and rinses the slide with distilled water to stop the staining process.

Next, the assistant returns the slide to the rack and floods it with Gram iodine solution. Using forceps again, he or she rinses the slide with distilled water and then rinses it slowly and gently with alcohol-acetone solution

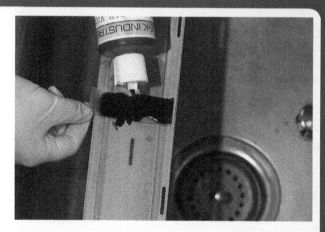
Flooding the slide with crystal violet.

until no more stain runs off. This process removes the stain from the Gram-negative bacteria and fixes it permanently to the Gram-positive bacteria. The fixing process is stopped by rinsing the slide again with distilled water.

Next, the slide is returned to the rack and flooded with counterstain, staining the Gram-negative bacteria pink or red. The assistant drains the excess counterstain, rinses with distilled water, gently blots the smear dry with absorbent paper (taking care not to disturb the specimen), and wipes the back of the slide.

After properly disposing of the equipment and supplies, the assistant washes his or her hands, documents the procedure, and sanitizes the work area.

Typical Tasks of a Laboratory Assistant

- Collect blood specimens (if trained in phlebotomy)
- Prepare, store, and dispose of specimens
- Perform blood glucose testing
- Recognize technical errors for each test performed
- Instruct patients in the proper collection and preservation of samples
- Maintain inventory control and supplies
- Prepare and stain slides for analysis
- Assemble/prepare reagents
- Take vital signs
- Follow established quality control procedures

Personal Characteristics of Laboratory Assistants

Many of a laboratory assistant's tasks require strong organizational skills and an eye for detail. Tasks that require these skills include managing the laboratory's storage system, performing tests according to procedures, and handling administrative functions, such as billing.

Laboratory assistants should be good at working both independently and as part of a team. They should be able to follow instructions and have good interpersonal and communication skills.

Work in a laboratory sometimes proceeds at a fast pace. Like other laboratory personnel, laboratory assistants should be capable of working well under time pressure. At all times, laboratory assistants must be able to work quickly and accurately.

Employment Opportunities and Trends

The ASCP conducts a survey every two years that provides information about the distribution of personnel in the laboratory workforce. Its 2009 survey found a serious shortage of personnel, which it said was caused by competition for qualified staff and lower compensation for laboratory work compared to other fields.

The survey cited other reasons for increased employment opportunities for laboratory personnel. Aging baby boomers will require more health care services in the coming years, increasing the demand for lab tests. The survey also noted low awareness of laboratory occupations.

Professional Organization

This occupation does not have its own professional organization. Some laboratory assistants belong to the ASCLS, which was described earlier.

CHECK POINT

3 What personal characteristics should a laboratory assistant have?

PHARMACISTS

Pharmacists are health care professionals authorized by law to dispense prescription medicines. People typically picture pharmacists behind the counter at a drugstore, but they're often in front of the counter too, giving flu shots, checking customers' blood pressure, and advising them on how to manage their health. In addition to working in retail pharmacies, pharmacists work in hospitals; in veterinary practices; at poison control centers; at the U.S. Food and Drug Administration, where they keep consumers informed and respond to reports of adverse drug reactions; and in nuclear pharmacies, where they prepare precise, targeted dosages of radioactive materials for cancer treatment. *U.S. News and World Report* listed pharmacy as one of its Best Careers of 2009.

History of the Profession

From ancient times, people have made medicines to treat their medical problems. Through the years, physicians, priests, monks, apothecaries, and others, as well as pharmacists, have performed that function.

During the colonial period in the U.S., people had several choices when they needed medicine. They could go to apothecaries' shops, run by doctors who *compounded*, or mixed ingredients, to make medications or by apothecaries who specialized in compounding. There were also wholesale druggists who made their own chemicals and medicines. These druggists became skilled at making true pharmaceuticals, or medicinal drugs.

Before the Civil War, most apothecaries in the U.S. were trained through apprenticeship. Apprentices worked for a practicing apothecary for an agreed-on number of years to learn their trade. In 1821, a group of apothecaries and druggists gathered in Philadelphia, intent on advancing their profession. They formed the country's first professional association of pharmacists, the Philadelphia College of Pharmacy, and opened its first college of pharmacy, which had the same name. Over the next 44 years, four additional schools of pharmacy were established, all run by pharmacists through pharmacists' associations.

After the Civil War, pharmacy education began to shift to state universities. At the University of Michigan, Dr. Albert B. Prescott changed pharmacy education from a focus on apprenticeship to a focus on academic study. He established a curriculum founded on basic science, with a full course of instruction and extensive laboratory work. Dr. Prescott's ideas were controversial, but they set the standard for future pharmacy education.

Many changes took place during the next half-century. State boards began licensing pharmacists, many more schools of pharmacy opened, and the rise of the pharmaceuticals industry signaled the beginning of the end of the pharmacist's primary role as a compounder.

In 1900, 21 pharmacy schools joined to form the American Conference of Pharmaceutical Faculties, later the American Association of Colleges of Pharmacy (AACP). In the 1920s, the AACP adopted a basic curriculum and began to require a four-year college program. In 1932, the American Council on Pharmaceutical Education, now the Accreditation Council for Pharmacy Education (ACPE), was founded. This organization began to accredit pharmacy schools, a function it continues to fulfill.

The number of years of study for a pharmacy degree, and the degrees to be awarded, continued to change. As schools worked to standardize pharmacy education, states moved to require pharmacists to have a college degree in pharmacy to be licensed. New York State was the first, in 1905.

Education, Training, and Legal Requirements

All states, the District of Columbia, and U.S. territories now require pharmacists to be licensed. To obtain a license, candidates generally must earn a doctor of pharmacy (Pharm.D.) degree from an accredited school or college of pharmacy and pass several exams. As of 2010, the ACPE had accredited 116 professional programs at colleges and schools of pharmacy in the U.S. To be admitted to a pharmacy program, applicants must have completed at least two years of undergraduate work. Most applicants have completed three or more. More than 75 percent of programs require the Pharmacy College Admission Test, or PCAT. College classes needed for admission to pharmacy programs vary widely. Undergraduates should check the requirements for the programs to which they plan to apply.

High school students may apply directly for admission to a pharmacy program by applying to the colleges and schools of pharmacy that offer either "0–6" programs or early assurance programs. In these programs, students who complete two years of undergraduate study and meet any prerequisites a school requires are guaranteed admission to the pharmacy program. Students interested in becoming pharmacists should take courses in math and science, including chemistry, biology, and physics, as well as other areas.

Pharmacy programs typically last four academic years, although some schools have accelerated programs lasting three calendar years. Program goals are to produce pharmacists who can give pharmaceutical care, develop and manage medication distribution and control systems, manage a pharmacy, promote public health, and provide drug information and education. Coursework varies, but the curriculum emphasizes these areas of instruction:

- *Pharmaceutical chemistry*, the application of chemical sciences to pharmacy
- *Pharmacognosy*, the study of natural drugs from plants and animals
- Pharmacology, understanding how drugs act in the body
- Business management
- Pharmacy practice
- A clinical component (time spent in different pharmacy practice settings, under the supervision of licensed pharmacists)

Students also take classes in mathematics, chemistry, physics, biology, English, psychology, and sociology.

Increasingly, graduates of pharmacy programs complete a residency program. Some hospitals require the pharmacists they hire to have completed residencies. Residencies last one or two years and may be taken in general pharmacy practice, clinical pharmacy practice, hospital pharmacy practice, or another area. More than 400 residency programs are offered by hospitals, community pharmacies, and other facilities.

Students who want additional clinical, laboratory, and research experience after completing a pharmacy program can pursue an M.S. or Ph.D. degree. Areas of graduate study include pharmaceutics and pharmaceutical chemistry, pharmacology, and pharmacy administration.

In all states, the District of Columbia, and U.S. territories, pharmacy school graduates must pass several tests to be licensed. Everyone must take the North American Pharmacist Licensure Exam (NAPLEX), which covers pharmacy skills and knowledge. Most states and the District of Columbia also require the Multistate Pharmacy Jurisprudence Exam (MPJE) on pharmacy law. Both exams are administered by the National Association of Boards of Pharmacy (NABP). States and territories that do not require the MPJE have their own pharmacy law exams. Some states and territories require their own exams in addition to the NAPLEX and a pharmacy law exam.

To be licensed, candidates must also complete a specified number of hours in a practice setting. That requirement is typically met while in pharmacy school.

Work Responsibilities

Today, pharmacists do little compounding. Most medications arrive from the manufacturer in prepared form.

Pharmacists receive prescriptions and fill them, and they monitor the work of the technicians who assist them. Filling prescriptions involves carefully checking drug dosages, allergies, drug interactions, and other potential problems. Pharmacists also counsel patients—in fact, in many states, they are required to counsel patients—about the drugs they have been prescribed. Counseling covers such areas as the proper use and storage of the medicine, its side effects, and possible interactions with other drugs.

Still another important part of a pharmacist's work is conferring with physicians and other health care professionals about medications, dosages, drug interactions, and side effects. Nearly all pharmacists maintain confidential computerized records of the medications that people take, to help prevent drug interactions. In health care facilities, they may plan, monitor, and evaluate drug treatment plans.

Pharmacists in community pharmacies have other responsibilities as well. They advise customers about over-the-counter medications, medical equipment, home health care supplies, and general health topics. Pharmacists may complete third-party insurance forms and other paperwork. Those who own or manage a pharmacy have additional duties related to running a business. In most states, pharmacists can give immunizations. Some pharmacies serve as centers for community health education services.

Pharmacists have a variety of career options. For instance, they can specialize in a particular type of drug therapy, such as oncology (cancer), nuclear pharmacy, geriatric pharmacy, or psychiatric pharmacy. Some do research for pharmaceutical manufacturers, helping develop and test new drugs. Some work in marketing or sales. Others are employed by health insurance companies, government agencies, managed care organizations, public health care services, or the armed forces.

SPOTLIGHT ON SKILLS Typical Task: Fill Prescriptions in a Hospital Pharmacy

Position: Pharmacist

Hospital pharmacies have standard sets of procedures to minimize the possibility of error in dispensing drugs to patients. Such procedures include multiple checks of prescription information.

In a typical sequence of steps, a pharmacist reviews the prescription order, verifying the dosage and checking the patient's record for duplicate orders, allergies, and other problems. The order is then input into the pharmacy computer system.

If a pharmacy technician completed these initial steps, a pharmacist reviews the order against the original prescription. The pharmacist also checks for the appropriateness of the drug, the dosage, any possible drug interactions, and other issues that might make the prescription a problem for the patient.

A pharmacy technician prints the label and fills the prescription, first checking the label against the medication order. The pharmacist reviews the technician's work, checking the prescription label against the medication order and the prepared prescription.

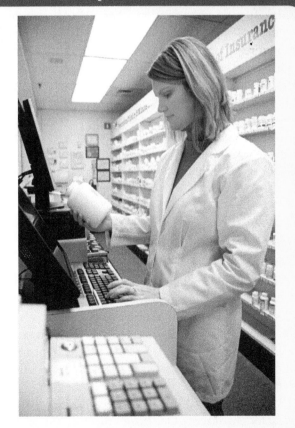

The pharmacist checks the prepared prescription against the medication order.

Typical Tasks of a Pharmacist

- Respond to a verbal prescription order
- Accurately read a prescription
- Receive a transfer prescription
- Fill a prescription for a topical compound
- Fill a prescription for an oral antibiotic suspension
- Check and sign off on a prescription prepared by a pharmacy technician
- Counsel a patient on a prescription product
- Interview and assess a patient
- Counsel a patient on a nonprescription product
- Research and respond to a medical professional about the characteristics of a medicine

Personal Characteristics of Pharmacists

A pharmacist's work involves many complex tasks. To be successful, pharmacists must be well-organized and detail-oriented. They also need to be conscientious and reliable in performing their work. Carelessly filling a prescription, or failing to detect an error in a technician's work, could cause prolonged illness or even death.

Pharmacists must make many decisions in the course of a day. To make good decisions, they should have strong analytical and problem-solving skills. Good judgment and common sense are valuable qualities.

Pharmacists interact with many different people in their work, including customers, patients, employees, physicians, nurses, and other health care professionals. Pharmacists need good communication and interpersonal skills. In community pharmacies, hospitals, and other work settings, the pharmacist is a member of a team, so good teamwork skills are also important.

Employment Opportunities and Trends

In 2008, pharmacists held nearly 270,000 jobs. About 65 percent were in community pharmacies that were either independently owned or part of a drugstore chain, grocery store, or other type of business. About 22 percent were in hospitals. A small percentage of pharmacists worked in mail-order and Internet pharmacies, pharmaceutical wholesalers, physicians' offices, and the federal government.

From 2008 to 2018, the BLS projects job growth of 17 percent for pharmacists. One factor prompting this growth will be an increased demand for prescription drugs. The middle-aged and older populations are growing, and both groups tend to use more prescription drugs than younger

people. Prescription drug use will also increase as new drugs become available and as more health insurance plans cover them. As the number of medicines grows and as drugs become more complex, pharmacists will increasingly advise patients on taking medications safely, help in drug selection and dosage, and monitor complex drug regimens.

The BLS predicts excellent job opportunities for pharmacists, mainly because of the limited capacity of Pharm.D. programs.

Professional Organization

The National Pharmaceutical Association (NPhA) is one of several professional associations for pharmacists. The NPhA represents the interests of minority pharmacists on health care and pharmacy issues. It works to advance standards of pharmaceutical care and to stimulate interest in pharmacy as a career, particularly among minority students. The organization's annual convention and regional meetings provide opportunities for continuing education and networking. A student affiliate organization was founded in 1974. The nonprofit National Pharmaceutical Association Foundation funds scholarships for members of the student organization and supports the NPhA's activities.

CHECK POINT

4 What education and training are needed to become a pharmacist?

PHARMACY TECHNICIANS

Pharmacy technicians are health care professionals who work in a pharmacy under the supervision of a licensed pharmacist. They are a valuable resource, performing many different duties. While the exact definition of their role varies depending on state law, a trained pharmacy technician generally assists in pharmacy activities that do not require a pharmacist's professional judgment.

History of the Profession

The pharmacy technician profession began with the establishment by the U.S. Army of a training program for "pharmacy specialists" in the mid-1940s. From the late 1960s to the early 1980s, several organizations worked to establish a formal system of training for pharmacy technicians. The U.S. Department of Health, Education, and Welfare worked with several professional pharmacy associations to define tasks and roles that pharmacy technicians could assume. In 1975, it used this information to establish the

American Society of Health-System Pharmacists (ASHP) education guidelines for hospital pharmacy technicians. In 1982, these guidelines were made into accreditation standards for pharmacy technician training programs, and the following year, the ASHP began accrediting programs. Both a national certification program and a model curriculum were developed in the 1990s.

Education, Training, and Legal Requirements

While some pharmacy technicians are trained on the job, most employers prefer to hire pharmacy technicians with formal training and certification. Besides having more job opportunities available to them, pharmacy technicians with certification may earn better pay and have more opportunities for promotion.

Accredited programs must provide at least 600 hours of training over a period of 15 or more weeks. Accreditation standards include a model curriculum linked to a set of goals that reflect current and anticipated pharmacy technician functions and responsibilities; development of an individualized training plan for each student; extensive laboratory experience; and an internship or externship in at least two different settings. Not all training programs are accredited.

Community colleges, vocational schools, hospitals, and the military offer pharmacy technician education programs. Programs range in length from six months to two years and lead to a diploma, certificate, or associate's degree. Coursework includes study in the following subjects:

- Introduction to pharmacy
- Medical terminology
- Pharmacology
- Pharmacy math
- Commercial pharmacy practice
- Hospital pharmacy practice
- Pharmacy law and ethics
- Computer applications
- Psychology
- Speech or interpersonal communications

Technicians must also learn medication names, actions, uses, and doses. Many programs include internships in pharmacies.

Some states require pharmacy technicians to have a high school diploma or the equivalent. Students interested in this occupation should contact their state board of pharmacy for information on the requirements in their state.

Certification is optional in most states, but some states and employers require it. Pharmacy technicians can seek certification from several organizations, including the Pharmacy Technician Certification Board and the Institute for the Certification of Pharmacy Technicians. To be certified by these organizations, candidates must pass a national exam.

Both organizations require recertification every two years. To be recertified, pharmacy technicians must meet continuing education requirements. Colleges, professional

---

SPOTLIGHT ON SKILLS Typical Task: Count Tablets or Capsules

Position: Pharmacy Technician

A common responsibility of pharmacy technicians is to fill prescriptions from bulk containers of tablets or capsules, which requires counting them. Many pharmacies use a counting tray for this purpose, because it makes counting tablets or capsules more efficient and more sanitary.

Before filling a prescription, the pharmacy technician reads the prescription carefully and calculates the correct dose, if necessary. He or she retrieves the correct stock package of medication and then double-checks the prescription for the name of the medication and the number of tablets or capsules needed.

Next, the pharmacy technician pours a small supply of the tablets or capsules into the counting tray. Using a plastic knife or spatula, the technician pushes the correct number of tablets or capsules into the tray's dispenser or well and closes the cover.

The unused tablets or capsules are poured back into the stock package (the tray has a lip at the back for this

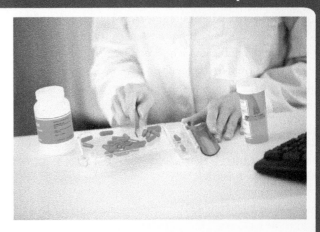

Pharmacy technicians use equipment for counting pills and tablets.

purpose), which is recapped. Then the technician pours the tablets or capsules from the dispenser or well into the prescription container and caps it. The final step is to clean the counting tray with an ethyl alcohol preparation.

organizations, pharmacy technician training programs, and other sources offer continuing education courses.

Work Responsibilities

Pharmacy technicians perform many routine tasks to help pharmacists fill prescriptions. They also do administrative work that helps keep a pharmacy running smoothly. The functions that pharmacy technicians perform vary depending on state law, the type of pharmacy, and the needs and preferences of employers. Their work with prescriptions is checked by a pharmacist for accuracy. Pharmacy technicians must refer questions about prescriptions, drug information, or health matters to pharmacists.

In mail-order and retail pharmacies, state rules and regulations govern the tasks that pharmacy technicians may perform. They can accept written prescriptions from patients, and they may accept prescriptions sent electronically from a physician's office. In some states, they can also process requests by phone. Pharmacy technicians review the information on prescriptions to ensure that it is complete and accurate. They prepare the prescriptions, counting pills, weighing and measuring materials, and sometimes compounding. They also prepare prescription labels, choose the proper containers, and label them. Once prescriptions have been filled, they price and file them. A pharmacist must check the prescriptions before they are given to patients.

Examples of administrative tasks are answering phones, operating cash registers, stocking shelves, doing inventories, preparing insurance forms, purchasing and receiving supplies, and storing medicines properly and securely. Pharmacy technicians may set up and maintain patient profiles and prepare insurance forms. They may also clean and maintain equipment in the pharmacy and work area.

Pharmacy technicians who work in hospitals, nursing homes, or assisted living facilities have additional responsibilities. For example, they prepare sterile solutions and deliver medications to nurses and physicians.

Typical Tasks of a Pharmacy Technician

- Accept a written prescription
- Count pills, tablets, or capsules and put them in a container
- Compound an ointment
- Educate a patient
- Prepare unit doses
- Prepare a prescription label
- Maintain inventory
- Complete a purchase order
- Maintain pharmacy records
- Enter an order into the computer

Personal Characteristics of Pharmacy Technicians

The pharmacy technician's job is one with a lot of responsibilities attached to it. Checking the information on a prescription carefully and filling it correctly are critical tasks. Pharmacists, who are responsible for a prescription's accuracy, must be able to rely on technicians to perform their duties conscientiously and well.

Filling prescriptions and other tasks of pharmacy technicians require an eye for detail. Pharmacy technicians need to be observant, precise, and detail-oriented. Many tasks—such as maintaining patient records, storing medicines, and taking inventories—also require good organizational skills.

Pharmacy technicians need good customer service skills because they interact with many customers and patients. A friendly, professional attitude is a plus. Particularly in hospital settings, but also in retail pharmacies, technicians will work closely with pharmacists, aides, and other technicians. Therefore, good teamwork skills are essential.

Pharmacy technicians should be good at following directions. At the same time, they need to be comfortable working independently.

Employment Opportunities and Trends

In 2008, pharmacy technicians held about 326,300 jobs. About 73 percent of these jobs were in retail pharmacies. Hospitals provided another 18 percent. A small number were with mail-order and Internet pharmacies, physicians' offices, pharmacy wholesalers, and the federal government.

The BLS projects that employment of pharmacy technicians will increase by 31 percent from 2008 to 2018 and that the occupation will add nearly 100,000 jobs. The Bureau cites two reasons for this strong growth:

- As with pharmacists, the increasing demand for prescription drugs will produce more jobs for technicians.
- Pharmacy technicians will take on additional roles. As insurers come to see pharmacies as cost-effective alternatives for some patient care, pharmacists will devote an increasing share of their time to providing that care. As a result, pharmacy technicians will have to assume new responsibilities.

With strong employment growth, pharmacy technicians will enjoy good job opportunities, especially if they have formal training and certification.

Professional Organizations

The American Association of Pharmacy Technicians (AAPT) is one of two national professional organizations for pharmacy technicians. Its mission includes representing the interests of its members to the public and health care organizations and helping technicians update their skills. The AAPT provides continuing education programs, both on a national level and through its chapters; a national convention; and a career center on its web site.

The second and largest national professional organization for pharmacy technicians is the National Pharmacy Technician Association (NPTA). Its goal is to promote professional development. NPTA advocates for the profession and conducts industry-related research. Membership benefits include a national convention; several publications;

networking opportunities through regional programs and other assemblies; a resource and support network on local, state, national, and international levels; and continuing education opportunities through seminars, workshops, conferences, video-based programs, and other means. The organization encourages member involvement through a volunteer program and various councils and committees.

CHECK POINT

5 What are the typical work responsibilities of pharmacy technicians?

Chapter Wrap-Up

Don't forget to visit the Point₊ companion website for additional study resources!

CHAPTER HIGHLIGHTS

- Clinical laboratory technologists prepare specimens, perform tests on them, check the results for accuracy, and interpret the results. They check for microorganisms in body fluids and tissues, scrutinize cells for changes and abnormalities, test the chemical content of samples, and type and cross-match blood for transfusions. They may train and supervise other laboratory workers. They may also monitor a lab's quality control program.
- Clinical laboratory technicians collect specimens for testing, prepare them for study, conduct tests, and do some analysis of the results. They typically perform less complex tests than clinical laboratory technologists, although they may perform more complex tests, depending on their experience, state regulations, and the laboratory setup. They also care for laboratory instruments and equipment.
- Laboratory assistants provide a variety of clinical and administrative support services and are often trained on the job. They collect samples, label them, and set up routine tests. They maintain a laboratory's storage system for specimens and receive, sort, store, and retrieve samples. They serve as resources for laboratory personnel and health care professionals who order tests. They also maintain equipment and supplies.
- Pharmacists are health care professionals authorized by law to dispense prescription medicines. They receive prescriptions and fill them, and they monitor the work of the technicians who assist them. They also counsel patients and confer with physicians and other health care professionals about prescribed medications. In community pharmacies, they may also give immunizations.
- Pharmacy technicians perform many routine tasks to help pharmacists fill prescriptions, and they do administrative work that helps keep a pharmacy running smoothly. While their exact role varies depending on state law, a trained pharmacy technician generally assists in pharmacy activities that do not require a pharmacist's professional judgment.

REVIEW QUESTIONS

Matching

1. _____ Counts tablets and prepares prescription labels
2. _____ Counsels patients about prescribed drugs
3. _____ May supervise other lab personnel in addition to performing tests
4. _____ Maintains a laboratory's storage system for specimens
5. _____ Performs routine tests in all areas of the laboratory

   a. Clinical laboratory technologist   **b.** Clinical laboratory technician   **c.** Laboratory assistant   **d.** Pharmacist   **e.** Pharmacy technician

Multiple Choice

6. Checking lab tests for accuracy and communicating the results to the physician who ordered them are typical responsibilities of _____.
   - **a.** clinical laboratory technologists
   - **b.** clinical laboratory technicians
   - **c.** laboratory assistants
   - **d.** pharmacy technicians

7. A clinical laboratory technician may specialize as a/an _____, who cuts and stains tissue specimens for analysis.
   a. phlebotomist
   c. immunohematologist
   b. histotechnician
   d. microbiology technologist

8. Which is NOT a task that laboratory assistants might perform?
   a. Receiving, storing, and retrieving samples
   b. Processing orders for tests
   c. Doing high-complexity tests
   d. Maintaining equipment and supplies

9. Which statement about pharmacy technicians is NOT true?
   a. They work under the supervision of a licensed pharmacist.
   b. The prescriptions they fill do not need to be checked.
   c. They can accept written prescriptions and those sent electronically.
   d. Certification is optional.

10. Which is NOT a task that pharmacists may perform?
   a. Write prescriptions
   c. Plan, monitor, and evaluate drug treatment plans
   b. Fill prescriptions
   d. Develop and test new drugs

Completion

11. _____ is the study of the structure of cells.

12. _____ is a plan for ensuring high quality performance in all areas of a laboratory's technical support functions.

13. _____ is the study of the microscopic structure of tissue.

14. _____ means mixing ingredients to make medications.

15. A laboratory's _____ program monitors each phase of the laboratory process to make sure that materials used for tests are of acceptable quality and that instruments are working accurately.

Short Answer

16. What is CLIA, and how does it affect the types of tests that clinical laboratory technologists, clinical laboratory technicians, and laboratory assistants may perform?

   _____

   _____

17. Briefly compare the work of a clinical laboratory technologist and a clinical laboratory technician.

   _____

   _____

18. What is the historical relationship among the three laboratory occupations profiled in this chapter?

   _____

   _____

19. Which steps in filling a prescription can a pharmacy technician perform?

   _____

   _____

20. What is the expected job growth rate for pharmacy technicians, and what accounts for this strong job growth?

_____

_____

INVESTIGATE IT

1. Genetic testing is in the news. Learn about one of the following types of genetic testing. Why is it done? What's the science behind it? What types of tests are performed?

   - Clinical genetic testing (for sickle cell anemia, Down syndrome, or cystic fibrosis, for example)
   - Pharmacogenomics
   - Identity testing
   - Parentage testing
   - Tissue typing
   - Cytogenetics
   - Infectious disease testing

   A good resource is "Lab Tests Online" (http://www.labtestsonline.org). If you use this web site, use at least one other resource.

2. Read about Emily's Law (at http://www.emilyslaw.org), an Ohio state law passed in 2009 that applies to pharmacy technicians. What were the circumstances surrounding the proposal and passage of this law? What does the law require? Do you think that pharmacy technicians should be regulated in this way? Why or why not?

RECOMMENDED READING

American Association of Colleges of Pharmacy. Is Pharmacy for You? Available at: http://www. aacp.org/resources/student/pharmacyforyou/Pages/default.aspx.

American Medical Association. Careers in Health Care. Available at: http://www.ama-assn.org/ ama/pub/education-careers/careers-health-care.shtml. (Profiles four of the five occupations in this chapter.)

American Society for Microbiology. What Microbiologists Do. Available at: http://www.microbe-world.org/index.php?option=com_content&view=article&id=77&Itemid=126.

Diagnostic Detectives: The Medical Laboratory Professions. Available at: http://www.medlabca-reers.msu.edu/diagnostic_content.html.

Dillon T. Healthcare jobs you might not know about. *Occupational Outlook Quarterly* [serial online]. Summer 2008;52(2):28–37. Available at: http://www.bls.gov/opub/ooq/2008/summer/art03. pdf.

Mayo Clinic. Career Exploration. Available at: http://www.mayoclinic.org/careerawareness/ careerexploration.html. (Profiles all the occupations in this chapter and includes interviews.)

Nemko M. Best Careers 2009: Pharmacist. *U.S. News and World Report* [serial online]. Posted December 11, 2008. Available at: http://www.usnews.com/articles/business/best-careers/2008/12/11/best-careers-2009-pharmacist.html.

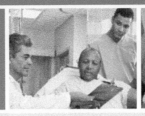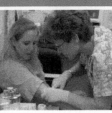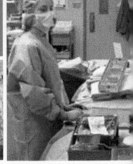

Diagnostic and Imaging Services

CHAPTER OBJECTIVES

After careful study of this chapter, you should be able to:

* State the education, training, and legal requirements for becoming a cardiographic technician, cardiovascular technologist, phlebotomist, diagnostic medical sonographer, radiologic technologist (radiographer), and nuclear medicine technologist.

* Describe the typical work responsibilities in each profession.

* List desirable personal characteristics of cardiographic technicians, cardiovascular technologists, phlebotomists, diagnostic medical sonographers, radiologic technologists (radiographers), and nuclear medicine technologists.

* Identify employment opportunities and key trends for these occupations.

KEY TERMS

balloon angioplasty (bǎ LŬN AN jē ō PLAS tē)
cardiac catheterization (KAHR dē ak KATH ě těr ī ZĂ shŭn)
echocardiography

electrocardiogram (ECG or EKG)
electrophysiology
fluoroscopy (flōr OS kŏ pē)
Holter monitor
invasive
noninvasive

nuclear medicine
pathophysiology
radionuclide (RĂ dē ō NŪ klīd)
radiopharmaceutical (RĂ dē ō FAHR mǎ sū ti kǎl)
sonography

stress test
vascular
venipuncture (VEN i PŬNGK shŭr)

The health care professionals described in this chapter work with patients and other health professionals to perform diagnostic tests and provide imaging services. Cardiovascular technologists and cardiographic technicians perform an array of procedures to help diagnose heart and blood vessel disease. Phlebotomists draw blood for laboratory testing. Diagnostic medical sonographers, radiographers, nuclear medicine technologists, and cardiovascular technologists perform imaging tests. Nearly every part of the body can be imaged, revealing such conditions as a broken bone, a defect in a developing fetus, leaking valves in the heart, and the existence and spread of cancer. The information provided by such procedures helps physicians diagnose, treat, and manage medical problems; assess the effectiveness of treatment; and monitor health.

CARDIOGRAPHIC TECHNICIANS

Cardiographic technicians perform diagnostic tests to help determine the cause and extent of cardiovascular illnesses. These technicians perform basic electrocardiograms (ECGs or EKGs), tests that record the electrical activity of the heart. With additional training, they may perform other types of tests.

History of the Profession

Electrocardiograms are invaluable tools in diagnosing and evaluating heart attacks; *arrhythmias*, or irregularities of heart rhythm; and other cardiac problems. The first EKG device, the string galvanometer, was developed by a Dutch physiologist named Willem Einthoven in 1903. His use of the device to explore the electrical properties of the heart won him the Nobel Prize.

Over the years, many improvements have been made to EKG technology. The Holter monitor, a portable EKG device that the patient carries or wears, was invented by a Montana physician named Norman Jeff Holter in 1949. Stress testing, the creation of cardiologist Robert Bruce and his colleagues, began in 1963.

As each new EKG technology moved from the laboratory to clinical settings, many more technicians skilled in operating it were needed. Cardiographic technicians and cardiovascular technologists have filled that need.

Cardiographic technicians are not regulated by the states. Their skills are usually learned on the job, and job-holders do not have their own professional organization. The recent creation of EKG training programs and the availability of two professional credentials are indicators of increasing professionalization, however. As cardiovascular technology evolves and new procedures are developed, cardiographic technicians will continue to take on added responsibilities and grow as a profession.

Education, Training, and Legal Requirements

As noted earlier, cardiographic technicians are usually trained on the job, by an EKG supervisor or cardiologist. Teaching someone to perform a basic resting EKG takes four to six weeks. Most employers prefer to train workers with experience in health care, such as nursing aides. Some students enrolled in two-year cardiovascular technology programs work part-time as EKG technicians to gain experience and meet potential employers.

There are one-year certification programs for technicians to learn how to perform basic EKGs, stress tests, and Holter monitor tests. Other training programs, including training for specialized EKG testing, can take from 18 months to two years. Students receive instruction in topics such as the anatomy and physiology of the heart, disease processes, medical terminology, legal aspects of patient contact, and medical ethics. They also get hands-on training with EKG and echocardiography equipment.

Students who are interested in becoming cardiographic technicians should take classes in algebra and the sciences. College coursework in anatomy and physiology, English, and health sciences is also helpful, as is experience working in a health care setting.

Cardiographic technicians are not licensed. However, they can choose to be certified. Two organizations award certification:

- The American Society of Phlebotomy Technicians (ASPT) awards the EKG Technician credential upon passing an exam. To sit for the exam, candidates must be ASPT members with six months of practical experience performing EKGs or graduates of an approved EKG program. To be recertified, candidates must complete six hours of continuing education units each year and renew their membership.
- Cardiovascular Credentialing International (CCI) awards the Certified Cardiographic Technician (CCT) credential to candidates who pass an exam. To renew their certification, candidates must complete 16 continuing education units every three years.

Work Responsibilities

Cardiographic technicians—also known as *electrocardiograph*, *EKG*, or *noninvasive technicians*—perform basic electrocardiograms. Noninvasive means that a procedure doesn't involve entering the body or breaking the skin. The EKG unit picks up electrical signals made by heart muscle and records them on a graph. The technician attaches electrodes to the patient's chest, arms, and legs and then operates the EKG machine. The resulting graph is printed for a physician to study and interpret. This test is performed on patients who are experiencing chest discomfort or show other

---

Typical Tasks of a Cardiovascular Technician

- Clean and maintain an EKG machine
- Place the EKG electrodes on the body
- Document the patient's medical history
- Monitor a patient's heart rhythms
- Perform a 12-lead electrocardiogram
- Document any variation from a normal tracing
- Take vital signs

signs and symptoms of possible cardiac problems. It is also done before most kinds of surgery or as part of a routine physical examination, especially on persons who have reached middle age or who have a history of cardiovascular problems.

Tests Performed by Specialized Cardiographic Technicians

With additional training, cardiographic technicians can perform three other tests: specialized EKGs, stress tests, and Holter monitor tests.

Specialized EKG Tests

Technicians who conduct specialized EKG tests must have an understanding of complex cardiac rhythms and arrhythmias. These are four examples of specialized tests:

- **Rhythm strips**—long strips recording the heart activity for a certain electrical lead or combination of leads
- **Signal-average EKGs**—more detailed EKGs that take multiple tracings over 20 minutes or so, which are then averaged by a computer
- **Event recorders**—portable EKG devices about the size of a pager that are worn from two weeks up to 60 days
- **Device interrogation**—EKGs conducted to check the function of pacemakers or other devices

Stress Tests

Physicians order a cardiac stress test to measure the response of the heart muscle to increased demands for oxygen. In this test, the patient is attached to an EKG monitor for constant tracing while performing some physical activity. Usually, the patient walks on a treadmill, but the activity may also be pedaling a stationary bicycle. If a treadmill is used, the speed or angle of the treadmill may be increased periodically.

Holter Monitor Tests

As noted earlier, a Holter monitor is a portable EKG device worn by a patient. It is especially useful in diagnosing intermittent cardiac arrhythmias or problems with pacemakers, because it records the electrical activity of the heart over a period of 24 hours or more. The patient keeps a diary of daily activities, which are coordinated with the test results.

Tasks Common to All Tests

For all tests, cardiographic technicians set up the equipment, explain the procedure to the patient, provide a gown or drape if desired, prepare the patient (for example, shave a male patient's chest before attaching electrodes), position the patient, conduct the test, document the procedure, and communicate the results to

---

 SPOTLIGHT ON SKILLS Typical Task: Apply a Holter Monitor

Position: Cardiographic Technician

The first step in Holter monitor testing is to apply the Holter monitor.

First, the cardiographic technician washes his or her hands, gathers supplies and equipment, and greets and identifies the patient. He or she explains the procedure, including how to use and care for the monitor, and reminds the patient to pursue normal activities for the duration of the test. The technician also explains the purpose of the incident diary, what information to record in it, and the need to carry it at all times.

Before applying the monitor, the cardiographic technician asks the patient to remove all clothing from the waist up and drapes the patient as needed for privacy. Next, the technician prepares the patient's skin for electrode attachment by shaving the patient, if necessary, and cleansing the area with antiseptic wipes.

To apply the electrodes, the technician exposes the adhesive backing and follows the manufacturer's directions to attach each one firmly. He or she checks the security of the attachments, positions the electrode connectors down toward the patient's feet, attaches the lead wires,

and secures them with adhesive tape. Then the technician connects the cable to the EKG machine and runs a baseline EKG.

After the baseline EKG, the technician helps the patient dress, plugs the cable into the recorder, marks the diary, and records the procedure in the patient's medical record.

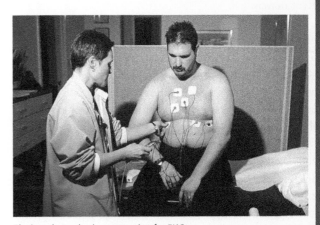

Placing electrodes in preparation for EKG.

the physician. They may also schedule appointments; review patients' files; train new employees, medical students, and other staff members; and perform various other tasks as required by employers.

Personal Characteristics of Cardiographic Technicians

Cardiographic technicians spend most of their time with patients. For that reason, they need good interpersonal skills. Technicians should have a pleasant, professional manner, and they should be able to relate to many different people.

Good communication skills are also important. Technicians must be able to give patients clear instructions, and they need to communicate with physicians and other health care personnel, in person and in writing, about test results and other important matters.

Several other personal characteristics are desirable for people in this occupation. One of them is the ability to work independently. At the same time, cardiographic technicians need to be able to follow instructions. Technicians should have good organizational skills, and they should be skilled at multitasking.

Employment Opportunities and Trends

The BLS projects rapid job growth for cardiographic technicians. For technicians and cardiovascular technologists together, employment will grow by 24 percent from 2008 to 2018. More technicians will be needed in the future due to the increase in heart disease and the needs of a larger older population, which is more prone to cardiovascular disease. Rules about Medicare and Medicaid reimbursement for medical procedures will affect demand.

Despite this strong overall growth, the BLS predicts that there will be less demand for technicians qualified to perform only basic EKGs because hospitals will train other personnel, such as nursing aides, to perform these tests. Job prospects will be better for technicians who can also perform stress tests and Holter monitor tests and who are willing to work irregular hours or relocate.

In 2008, cardiographic technicians and cardiovascular technologists held about 49,500 jobs. Roughly three-quarters of these jobs were in hospitals. The rest were in physicians' offices and medical or diagnostic labs, including diagnostic imaging centers. The BLS projects nearly 12,000 new jobs for workers in these occupations from 2008 to 2018.

Professional Organization

The Alliance of Cardiovascular Professionals (ACVP) represents more than 3,000 cardiovascular personnel from all levels and specialties, including cardiographic technicians. Its mission includes meeting the needs of cardiovascular and pulmonary providers; promoting awareness of standards; and encouraging recognition of the different cardiovascular occupations. The ACVP advocates for its members at the national and state levels and works with other organizations on health care issues.

The organization uses a variety of methods to meet the needs of the different occupations it represents. It operates specialty councils for the different occupations, and it produces more than 26 publications each year, including a newsletter sent to all members and technical publications in council areas.

The ACVP places a strong emphasis on continuing education. It offers more than 200 hours of programming each year through an annual conference, webinars, and meetings. Chapter meetings provide additional opportunities for continuing education and networking. Members can also attend certification exam review sessions and the Management Institute, which offers classes on managerial skills for members moving into managerial positions. Online resources include a job opportunities board and a message board for posting professional queries to fellow members.

CHECK POINT

1 What education and training are needed to become a cardiographic technician?

CARDIOVASCULAR TECHNOLOGISTS

Cardiovascular technologists perform diagnostic tests involving the heart and blood vessels and help treat patients with cardiac and vascular, or blood vessel, disease. Their work is done at a physician's request or under a physician's supervision.

History of the Profession

Cardiovascular technology was a 20th-century development. As noted in the previous profile, the EKG was invented by Willem Einthoven in 1903. In 1953, cardiologist Inge Edler and physicist Hellmuth Hurst were the first to use ultrasound to diagnose cardiac disease, pioneering the technique of echocardiography. In 1955, Shigeo Satomura, a professor at Osaka University, worked with several colleagues and two cardiologists to develop the first

Doppler instrument that could be used to analyze blood flow. Doppler instruments make use of the *Doppler effect*, which is the tendency of sound frequencies to increase as one object moves toward another and to decrease when the object moves away.

The technology continued to evolve and began to move into clinical settings in the early 1970s. Cardiovascular technology was officially recognized as an allied health profession by the AMA Council on Medical Education in December 1981. Four months later, a committee representing various educational institutions and professional organizations met to draft educational guidelines for accredited cardiovascular technology programs. The committee concluded its work in 1983, and two years later, the Joint Review Committee on Education in Cardiovascular Technology (JRC-CVT) was formed.

Education, Training, and Legal Requirements

A few cardiovascular technologists are trained on the job. However, most complete a two-year training program and earn an associate's degree. Some students opt for four-year programs as more of these programs become available. Qualified allied health professionals can take just one year of specialized instruction.

The JRC-CVT reviews cardiovascular technology programs for accreditation, and the programs are accredited (or not) by the Commission on Accreditation of Allied Health Education Programs (CAAHEP). As of 2010, there were 37 accredited cardiovascular technology programs in the U.S. Accreditation standards and guidelines call for a three-part curriculum consisting of core courses, specialized instruction, and clinical instruction. The core curriculum consists of the following coursework:

- An introduction to the field, including patient care techniques and the hospital environment
- General and allied sciences, including basic statistics and general math at a level approaching intermediate algebra
- Anatomy and physiology, with emphasis on the cardiac and vascular systems
- Basic pharmacology relating to cardiovascular drugs
- Basic medical electronics and medical instrumentation

Specialized instruction is provided in invasive cardiology, noninvasive cardiology, or cardiac electrophysiology. An invasive procedure is one that requires entering the body by using a tube, needle, or other device. Electrophysiology is the study of electrical activity in the body.

Clinical instruction covers the following topics:
- Cardiac and vascular pathophysiology, or changes in the body due to disease
- Patient history and physical examination
- Patient psychology, care, and communications
- CPR
- Diagnostic and therapeutic measures
- Clinical cardiac and vascular medicine and surgery
- Statistics and data management
- Physics
- Medical and legal ethics

To be admitted to a cardiovascular technology program, a student must have a high school diploma or the equivalent or belong to a related allied health profession.

Certification is voluntary. However, it is the professional standard, and most employers require it. Two organizations offer certification: the CCI and the American Registry of Diagnostic Medical Sonographers (ARDMS).

The CCI offers these certifications:
- Registered cardiac sonographer (RCS)
- Registered vascular specialist (RVS)
- Registered congenital cardiac sonographer (RCCS)
- Registered cardiovascular invasive specialist (RCIS)
- Registered cardiac electrophysiology specialist (RCES)
- Registered phlebology sonography (RPhS) (*Phlebology* is the branch of medicine that deals with veins and vein diseases.)

Two certifications are available from the ARDMS:
- Registered diagnostic cardiac sonographer (RDCS), with specialties in adult, fetal, and pediatric echocardiography
- Registered vascular technologist (RVT)

Candidates must pass one or two exams to be certified. Certification must be renewed every three years, which requires continuing education.

Work Responsibilities

Cardiovascular technologists help diagnose patients with cardiac and vascular disease. They perform ultrasound procedures, monitor patients' heart rates, review physicians' interpretations and patient files, and compare findings for an individual patient against normal findings to identify problems. They also schedule appointments, explain test procedures, and care for testing equipment. Other tasks vary widely depending on the specialty the technologist chooses. Cardiovascular technologists usually specialize in one or more of three areas: invasive procedures, noninvasive cardiology, and noninvasive peripheral vascular studies.

Invasive Procedures

Cardiovascular technologists specializing in invasive procedures are called *cardiology technologists*. Cardiology technologists assist the physician (usually a cardiologist) in performing invasive procedures, such as:

- **Cardiac catheterization.** In this procedure, a tube, or *catheter*, is inserted into a vein and guided toward the heart to reveal blood vessel blockages.
- **Balloon angioplasty.** In this procedure, a balloon attached to the end of the catheter is used to clear blockages in blood vessels.
- **Electrophysiology testing.** In this procedure, used when a patient has an arrhythmia, instruments on a catheter detect patterns in the heart's electrical activity and deliver small shocks to determine which part of the heart is causing the arrhythmia.
- **Open-heart surgery.** This term refers to any surgery to treat heart disease that involves opening the chest in order to work directly on the heart or parts of the heart.
- **Pacemaker or stent insertion.** *Pacemakers* are small devices used to regulate the heartbeat. *Stents* are tubes inserted into a blood vessel to prevent fatty deposits from closing it, which can lead to a heart attack.

Before any of these procedures, the cardiology technologist may get the room ready and prepare and position the patient. During the procedure, he or she monitors blood pressure, heart rate, and the patient's general condition and alerts the physician if something is wrong. Cardiology technologists may also collect and transcribe data.

Noninvasive Cardiology

Echocardiography is the use of ultrasound to examine the heart and blood vessels. Technologists who perform ultrasound scans of the heart are referred to as *cardiac sonographers* or *echocardiographers*. During the scan, the sonographer views the ultrasound images on a screen. He or she checks the images for subtle differences between healthy and diseased areas, judges whether the images will be useful in making a diagnosis, and chooses images to include in a report to the physician. The sonographer may photograph selected images or videotape the entire procedure.

Noninvasive Peripheral Vascular Study

A noninvasive peripheral vascular study is an ultrasound scan of the blood vessels. Cardiovascular technologists who perform these types of scans are known as *vascular technologists* or *vascular sonographers*. During the procedure, the technologist records information about blood flow through the vessels, blood pressure, oxygen saturation, and cerebral, peripheral, and abdominal circulation. The technologist provides a summary of findings to the physician who ordered the procedure.

Some cardiovascular technologists also supervise and train other technologists and students.

Typical Tasks of a Cardiovascular Technologist

- Review a patient's history
- Explain testing procedures to the patient
- Shave, clean, and numb the top of the leg
- Inject contrast medium into a blood vessel
- Choose a scanner probe
- Perform an echocardiogram
- Scan the *upper extremity* (arm, forearm, wrist, and hand)
- Take still images during a scan
- Choose images for the physician
- Review test results with the physician

Personal Characteristics of Cardiovascular Technologists

Cardiovascular technologists have a range of responsibilities that require good judgment and that must be carried out conscientiously. Physicians rely on technologists for the integrity of the diagnostic information they provide and rely on their assistance during procedures.

People in this occupation need good communication skills. They must be able to explain procedures and issue directions to patients. They also need to communicate information clearly to physicians and other health care professionals, both verbally and in writing.

Other desirable personal characteristics include the ability to follow detailed instructions and to work effectively with patients. Cardiovascular technologists may need to tailor a scan to a physician's specifications or quickly and accurately follow detailed instructions issued during an invasive procedure. A pleasant, professional manner can help to keep patients at ease before and during tests.

Employment Opportunities and Trends

Cardiovascular technologists can expect job growth of 24 percent from 2008 to 2018. As with cardiographic technicians, job growth will result from an expected increase in heart disease and an aging population, as older

SPOTLIGHT ON SKILLS Typical Task: Assist in Transesophageal Echocardiography

Position: Cardiovascular Technologist

Transesophageal echocardiography is a procedure in which a flexible tube called a TEE scope is threaded into the lower part of a patient's *esophagus* (the tube leading from the mouth to the stomach) to look at the heart, which is close by. It is used to examine the heart's structure and function, to detect heart disease, and to evaluate the effectiveness of treatment. Cardiovascular technologists may assist in this procedure.

Before the procedure, the technologist prepares the equipment; assembles supplies; and checks suction, oxygen, and basic life-support equipment. He or she confirms that the patient has not had anything to eat or drink for four to six hours prior to the procedure and obtains a brief history of drug allergies and current medications. The technologist explains the procedure, takes baseline vital signs, applies a cardiac monitor, and determines the rhythm.

Next, the technologist establishes an intravenous catheter for medications and places the patient on the left side. As the tube is inserted, the technologist helps the patient find a comfortable head position, reminds him or her to breathe regularly, and offers reassurance.

During the procedure, the technologist positions and maintains the *bite block*, a device used to protect the mouth and keep it open. He or she monitors vital signs and uses suction, if needed.

After the procedure, the technologist assists the patient during recovery, removes the catheter, and records vital signs and the patient's condition. If the patient isn't completely recovered at the time of discharge, the technologist arranges an escort.

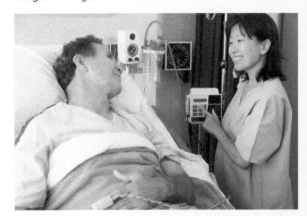

The cardiovascular technologist prepares the patient for the procedure.

people tend to have more cardiovascular problems. These factors will also affect growth:

- Noninvasive procedures, such as ultrasounds, are being performed more often than more invasive and expensive procedures.
- Vascular disease is being detected earlier due to medical advances and greater public awareness, creating a demand for more procedures.
- More jobs will be available for vascular technologists and echocardiographers as technological advances reduce the need for more costly and invasive procedures.
- Rules regarding reimbursement by Medicare and Medicaid for medical procedures will affect demand.

In 2008, cardiovascular technologists and cardiographic technicians held nearly 50,000 jobs. Hospitals were the main employer, accounting for about 77 percent of jobs. Physicians' offices and medical or diagnostic labs, including diagnostic imaging centers, provided the rest.

Technologists who are qualified to perform a range of procedures, are willing to work irregular hours, or are prepared to relocate will have the best job prospects.

Professional Organizations

Formed in 1977, the Society for Vascular Ultrasound (SVU) represents vascular technologists, echocardiographers, vascular surgeons, and other health care professionals in the vascular ultrasound field. Its mission includes representing the interests of its members and promoting quality vascular ultrasound services. The SVU monitors state and federal legislative activity and advocates for its membership before legislatures and agencies. It offers continuing education through online tests and regional programs, which also provide networking opportunities. The SVU holds an annual conference, publishes a journal, gives a scholarship and awards for member contributions to the field, and operates an online job center.

The American Society of Echocardiography (ASE), also formed in 1977, promotes excellence in echocardiography and its application to patient care. It advocates for echocardiographers before Congress and federal agencies and with private payers. The organization sponsors annual scientific sessions that feature workshops, symposiums, and classes on a wide range of topics, including cutting-edge technology. ASE University, at the organization's web site, offers additional educational opportunities and webcasts. Members can network through professional specialty councils and online discussion boards. Local societies provide networking and continuing education opportunities. Members also have access to an online career center, research and travel grants, and a professional journal. The ASE Foundation funds awards and scholarships, professional education activities, research, training, public awareness efforts, and other endeavors.

The Alliance of Cardiovascular Professionals (ACVP) represents cardiovascular technologists. For more on this organization, see the profile of "Cardiographic Technicians" earlier in this chapter.

✔ **CHECK POINT**

2 What are the typical work responsibilities of cardiovascular technologists?

PHLEBOTOMISTS

Phlebotomists are clinical laboratory technicians who collect blood samples for testing and draw blood for transfusions. The samples are used to prevent, detect, and monitor medical problems and to determine how well a prescribed drug treatment is working.

History of the Profession

From ancient times until well into the 19th century, bloodletting was a popular method of treating many different medical problems. The practice had its origins in the work of the ancient Greek Hippocrates, who believed that the body contained four humours, including blood, that had to be balanced to prevent disease and maintain health. An imbalance could cause a wide variety of diseases. If a person was judged as having too much blood, the logical solution was to take out some of the blood to restore the proper balance. This practice was known as *bloodletting*.

As the work of Louis Pasteur and other scientists showed that bacteria and viruses, rather than humours, were responsible for many diseases, the practice of bloodletting for therapeutic purposes declined. However, blood began to be drawn for the purpose of diagnosis.

The modern occupation of phlebotomy originated in the 1970s as a cost-cutting measure. Laboratory managers created lower-wage phlebotomist positions so that higher-paid clinical laboratory technologists and technicians could focus on specimen testing and analysis. The practice quickly became popular. The National Phlebotomy Association (NPA) was formed in 1978 to set a professional standard and code of ethics for phlebotomists.

The NPA administered the first national phlebotomist certification exam in 1981.

Education, Training, and Legal Requirements

To become a phlebotomist, a person needs a high school diploma or the equivalent and training in phlebotomy. Some phlebotomists learn their skills on the job, through in-house training programs at medical facilities, while others complete formal education programs. The program may be a standalone program in phlebotomy, or it may be part of another educational program. For example, some programs combine phlebotomist training with training for laboratory assistants and EKG technicians.

The National Accrediting Agency for Clinical Laboratory Science (NAACLS) approves phlebotomy programs. As of 2010, the NAACLS had approved 59 phlebotomy programs. These programs, which lead to a certificate, combine classroom instruction with a minimum of 100 hours of clinical experience, at least 100 successful unassisted blood collections, instruction in a variety of collection techniques, and contact with various types of patients. Hospitals, colleges, vocational schools, and medical laboratories offer structured programs that prepare students for national certification.

Many licensed health care professionals are trained to perform phlebotomy along with their other functions. Cross-training in phlebotomy is becoming increasingly common as health care organizations strive to control costs and improve quality.

As of 2010, only a handful of states regulated phlebotomists. Students interested in this occupation should check with their state's department of health or board of occupational licensing for details.

Certification gives an advantage in securing jobs. Organizations that certify phlebotomists include the following:

- American Certification Agency
- American Medical Technologists
- American Phlebotomy Association
- American Society for Clinical Pathology
- National Center for Competency Testing
- National Credentialing Agency
- National Healthcareer Association

Phlebotomists need continuing education to keep their knowledge and skills up to date. Many organizations sponsor workshops, seminars, and self-study programs that award continuing education units (CEUs). Most certifying and licensing agencies require CEUs or other proof of continuing education for renewal of credentials.

Employers may offer in-service education or pay for employees to attend offsite programs.

Work Responsibilities

Successfully collecting blood takes knowledge, skill, and practice. Phlebotomists expertly collect blood by a variety of methods. They must be able to collect blood from patients of all ages, from infants to older adults.

Venipuncture—drawing blood from a vein—is one of a phlebotomist's main duties. Phlebotomists must apply a tourniquet in the proper place on the patient's arm or wrist, locate a suitable vein, and insert the needle in such a way that the vein doesn't roll and blood can flow smoothly.

Another common procedure is a *capillary puncture*, or finger stick, in which a small amount of blood is obtained by pricking a finger or an infant's heel. Phlebotomists must know which fingers and which places on the fingers or heels are best to prick.

After drawing blood, phlebotomists are responsible for labeling blood samples accurately, documenting the procedures, storing blood properly, and sometimes transporting it. Phlebotomists must apply safety precautions to guard themselves and patients from blood-borne diseases.

Depending on where they work, phlebotomists may have additional duties. For example, they may perform other types of tests, such as throat cultures, urine tests, and EKGs.

Typical Tasks of a Phlebotomist

- Apply a tourniquet
- Draw blood by venipuncture
- Perform a skin test
- Obtain blood by capillary puncture
- Select additives for blood tests
- Evaluate a specimen for quality
- Enter data into a computer
- Take vital signs
- Collect a urine specimen
- Label samples accurately

SPOTLIGHT ON SKILLS Typical Task: Obtain a Blood Specimen by Capillary Puncture

Position: Phlebotomist

Capillary puncture is performed on adults when no veins are accessible, when it is desirable to save veins for procedures like chemotherapy, and for point-of-care testing. It is also the preferred method to obtain blood from infants and children, because venipuncture can damage veins and surrounding tissues.

Before taking blood, the phlebotomist checks the requisition slip to determine the tests ordered and specimen requirements, washes his or her hands, gathers supplies, and puts on gloves. He or she greets and identifies the patient, explains the procedure, and answers any questions.

Next, the phlebotomist selects the puncture site. (For adults, phlebotomists use the middle or ring finger of the nondominant hand. For children and infants, phlebotomists use one side or the other of the curved surface of the heel.) Then the phlebotomist chooses the appropriate puncture device for the site selected.

Before making the puncture, the phlebotomist makes sure that the site chosen is warm and not *cyanotic* (bluish due to lack of oxygen) or *edematous* (having accumulated watery fluid in the tissues). The phlebotomist cleanses the selected area with alcohol and allows it to air-dry.

Holding the finger or heel firmly, the phlebotomist makes a swift, firm puncture. The first drop of blood is wiped away because it may be contaminated with tissue fluid or alcohol residue. The phlebotomist collects the specimen, touching only the tip of the collection device to the drop of blood.

After the specimen is collected, the phlebotomist uses clean gauze to apply pressure on the puncture site until the bleeding stops, labels the containers, cleans up, and documents the procedure.

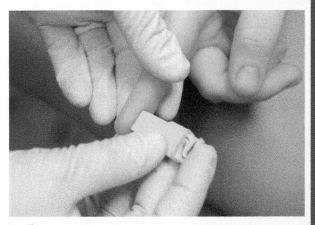

Capillary puncture.

Personal Characteristics of Phlebotomists

Phlebotomists need good interpersonal skills. They work with a wide variety of patients, so they need to be able to relate to different people, explaining how they will be collecting blood and instructing patients on what they should do to cooperate with the procedure. Phlebotomists must secure the cooperation of even very young or agitated patients. As a result, empathy and skill at calming others are useful qualities.

Another important personal characteristic for this occupation is attention to detail. Phlebotomists have many details to remember to prepare for and perform collections. If they don't do their jobs exactly right, the result could be a useless specimen or the transmission of a blood-borne disease.

Sometimes phlebotomists need to collect samples very quickly. The ability to be calm and work satisfactorily under pressure is desirable.

Employment Opportunities and Trends

The BLS classes phlebotomists with other clinical laboratory technicians. It projects 16 percent job growth for this group from 2008 to 2018, with 25,000 jobs expected to be added. The number of laboratory tests performed will increase as the population increases and as new tests are developed, but efforts to simplify some tests will enable other health care personnel and even patients to perform them. Clinical laboratory technicians should enjoy excellent job opportunities, because there will not be enough workers for the jobs available.

In 2008, clinical laboratory technicians held about 155,600 jobs. More than half were in hospitals. Physicians' offices and medical and diagnostic laboratories provided most of the rest. Hospitals will continue to be the biggest employer, but employment is expected to grow quickly in all other settings as well.

Professional Organizations

Two professional organizations that include phlebotomists in their membership are the American Medical Technologists (AMT) and the American Society for Clinical Pathology (ASCP). The AMT was described in Chapter 6, "Laboratory and Pharmacy Services." The ASCP, founded in 1922, consists of 130,000 members from various laboratory occupations. The organization strives to advance these professions through education, certification, and advocacy. It provides many continuing

education opportunities through workshops, symposia, teleconferences, e-courses, and self-study programs. It also certifies laboratory workers, including phlebotomists. The ASCP represents its members' interests before Congress, federal agencies, and state governments. It is also a respected medical publisher. Membership benefits include a variety of publications, discounts on educational programs, and an online career center.

> **CHECK POINT**
>
> **3** What personal characteristics should a phlebotomist have?

DIAGNOSTIC MEDICAL SONOGRAPHERS

Sonography is the use of high-frequency sound waves to produce images of organs and other structures in the body. Health care professionals who perform ultrasound scans are called *diagnostic medical sonographers.*

History of the Profession

The beginnings of sonography can be traced to an 1826 experiment by a Swiss physicist named Jean-Daniel Colladon. His assistant sat in a boat on one side of Lake Geneva, holding a church bell a few feet underwater. Colladon sat in a boat on the other side of the lake, holding an ear trumpet with one end submerged. The assistant struck the bell with a hammer and lit a flare. Colladon measured the time it took for the sound to reach him, becoming the first person to measure the speed of sound underwater.

This discovery stimulated efforts to explore the physics of sound waves, including the ability to determine the location and shape of a submerged object from the echoes produced when sound waves were reflected from it. After the *Titanic* sank in 1912, Reginald Fessenden, an inventor and assistant to Thomas Edison, developed a method of using echoes to detect icebergs. In response to devastating torpedo attacks on ships during World War I, physicists Robert Boyle, Paul Langevin, and others developed the hydrophone. This microphone, which could be attached to the bottom of a ship and used to detect enemy submarines, was the beginning of sonar (*s*ound *n*avigation *a*nd *r*anging).

In 1937, an Austrian neurologist named Karl Dussik and his brother Friedrich, a physicist, made the first attempt at using sound for medical imaging. After World War II, some former experts in submarine warfare turned their efforts to adapting the principles of sonar for medical purposes. Physicians, engineers, and physicists developed and applied scanning devices and procedures to image different areas of the body, revealing such conditions as breast, bowel, and brain tumors, ophthalmological problems, and neurological disease. Sonography was also used for therapeutic procedures.

The first commercial scanners became available in 1963. Over the next seven years, physicians found an increasing number and range of applications for scanners as diagnostic tools. Facing a shortage of trained personnel, commercial sonography companies hired technical specialists, as sonographers were then known, to train personnel in hospitals.

Radiologic technology was well established by that time, and some radiologic technologists began to specialize in sonography. The American Society of Ultrasound Technical Specialists (ASUTS), formed in 1969, quickly established an Education Committee to set training standards and accredit sonography schools and an Examination Committee to devise a method of credentialing sonographers. In 1975, the Examination Committee became the ARDMS and administered the first credentialing exam. The ASUTS also worked with the AMA's Manpower Division to gain recognition of ultrasound technical specialist as a distinct allied health occupation, a goal that was achieved in 1973 with the creation of the occupation of diagnostic ultrasound technologist.

From 1974 to 1979, the ASUTS worked with many medical and allied health organizations and the Department of Allied Medical Professions and Services to develop a set of standards for formal education programs. It was during this time that the term *sonographer* was coined.

Education, Training, and Legal Requirements

There are several educational routes to becoming a diagnostic medical sonographer:

- Hospitals, vocational-technical schools, colleges and universities, and the armed forces offer training programs. Some of these programs prefer candidates from other health care occupations or high school graduates with classes in math, science, and health.
- Some colleges and universities have formal two- and four-year training programs that lead to an associate's or bachelor's degree. Most people opt for a two-year program.
- Some institutions have one-year programs that typically lead to a certificate. This option is usually pursued by health care workers who want to improve their employability by learning sonography.

Employers prefer to hire sonographers who have completed an accredited program and have professional certification. The Commission on Accreditation of Allied Health Education Programs (CAAHEP) accredits diagnostic medical sonography programs. As of 2010, the CAAHEP had accredited 174 programs. Accredited programs combine classroom instruction with laboratory and clinical activities. Before beginning the core program, students take college-level classes in mathematics (algebra, statistics, or higher), physics, communication, and anatomy and physiology. Either before or during the core program, they also take classes in patient care, medical ethics and the law, medical terminology, and pathophysiology. Students may concentrate in general, cardiac, or vascular sonography. In general sonography, students are trained to use scanning instruments, recognize the normal appearance of the body parts they will scan, and recognize and identify abnormalities and disease.

In 2009, New Mexico and Oregon became the first states to require licensing for diagnostic medical sonographers. Policies and procedures for licensure were being established at the time of this writing.

Several organizations certify diagnostic medical sonographers. The ARDMS awards the Registered Diagnostic Medical Sonographer (RDMS) credential. Candidates must pass two exams: a general Sonography Principles and Instrumentation exam and an exam in a specialty, such as breast scanning or fetal echocardiography. Certification must be renewed every three years, which requires continuing education.

The American Registry of Radiologic Technologists (ARRT) offers primary certification in sonography and post-primary certification in sonography and breast sonography. Those who meet the requirements are registered. Registration is renewed annually.

Work Responsibilities

A *sonogram*, or ultrasound, is a noninvasive procedure that does not require the use of radiation. It uses the echoes of sound waves, as submarines do in detecting undersea objects or as bats do in flying and finding prey.

To help conduct the sound waves, the sonographer spreads a gel on the patient's skin. Then the sonographer moves a transducer over the area to be scanned. A *transducer* is a device that emits sound and detects returning echoes. A computer in the ultrasound equipment analyzes the echoes and forms an image of the area being scanned.

During the scan, the sonographer looks carefully at the images for evidence of disease or other medical conditions. He or she decides which images the physician should see and stores them on a videotape, CD, or DVD. The sonographer analyzes the results of the scan and summarizes the preliminary findings for the physician, orally or in writing.

Diagnostic medical sonographers have several other duties. They keep patient records, and they adjust and maintain equipment. They also may prepare work schedules, evaluate equipment purchases, and have managerial or supervisory responsibilities.

Diagnostic medical sonographers can specialize in different systems or parts of the body. Two specialties, cardiac sonography and vascular sonography, were discussed earlier in the chapter. Four other specialties are common:

- **Obstetrics/gynecology**—imaging the female reproductive system. A familiar example is the ultrasound performed on a growing fetus during pregnancy.
- **Abdomen**—scanning the abdominal cavity, including the gallbladder, bile ducts, kidneys, liver, pancreas, spleen, and male reproductive system, as well as parts of the chest.
- **Neurosonography**—scanning the nervous system. In neonatal care, neurosonographers study and diagnose neurological and nervous system disorders in premature infants. They also may scan blood vessels to check for abnormalities in infants diagnosed with sickle-cell anemia.

- **Breast**—imaging the breasts for diseases, such as cancer. These sonograms are often performed as a follow-up to a routine or diagnostic mammogram that has indicated an abnormality and can distinguish a possible tumor from a benign cyst.

Typical Tasks of a Diagnostic Medical Sonographer

- Evaluate a requisition before a sonogram
- Set the Doppler parameters
- Select the proper transducer
- Apply sufficient coupling gel, eliminating air bubbles
- Perform an abdominal scan
- Identify artifacts (imaging errors)
- Prepare a written summary of findings
- Clean, check, and maintain equipment

Personal Characteristics of Diagnostic Medical Sonographers

Because diagnostic medical sonographers spend most of their time with patients, they need good people skills. They must be able to talk with patients to obtain a medical history, clearly explain procedures, direct patients during a scan, and calm and comfort them when needed.

SPOTLIGHT ON SKILLS Typical Task: Write a Preliminary Report

Position: Diagnostic Medical Sonographer

After completing a sonogram, the sonographer issues a preliminary report to quickly communicate the key sonographic findings, so that the physician does not have to wait for the official dictation to be typed. Promptness is important because the findings may indicate the need for immediate action. Sonographers entrusted with writing preliminary reports should confine themselves to describing the findings without offering a conclusion about pathology, unless they have prior approval from the physician.

Preliminary reports should be accurate, clear, complete, concise, and timely. This is a typical report on a normal study:

Liver No lesion seen; normal size.
Common bile duct 4 mm (normal for age).
Gallbladder No evidence of sludge or calculi. Normal wall thickness.
Pancreas No abnormality seen. No evidence of dilated ducts or focal lesions.
Spleen No focal lesions seen; normal size.

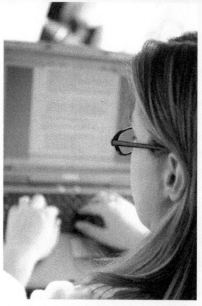

The sonographer must complete the preliminary report immediately after the procedure.

Patience and empathy are other personal characteristics of good sonographers.

Being a diagnostic medical sonographer requires an eye for detail. When performing a scan, sonographers must pay close attention to the images they see, and they must be able to detect signs of disease that can sometimes be very subtle. Since sonographers select the images that will be shown to the physician, this attention to detail is very important. This occupation also requires good judgment and a high degree of personal responsibility.

Sonographers do much of their work alone. They need to be self-motivated and comfortable working independently. At the same time, sonographers should be able to communicate and work well with others on the health care team, including technologists, supervisors, nurses, and physicians.

Employment Opportunities and Trends

In 2008, diagnostic medical sonographers held slightly more than 50,000 jobs, about 60 percent of which were in hospitals. Most of the remaining jobs were in physicians' offices, medical and diagnostic laboratories, and outpatient care centers.

From 2008 to 2018, the BLS projects employment of diagnostic medical sonographers to grow by about 18 percent. As with many medical occupations, this anticipated growth is due to the rising demand created by the needs of an aging population. Two other factors are the increasing use of sonography by health care practitioners as a safer, less expensive alternative to radiology and the development of new sonography procedures, so that more areas of the body may be scanned.

About 9,200 new jobs will be added between 2008 and 2018, with hospitals continuing to be the main employer. The BLS anticipates more rapid job growth in physicians' offices and medical and diagnostic laboratories, however, due to the increasing trend toward outpatient care.

Diagnostic medical sonographers can expect favorable job opportunities, with the number of job seekers roughly equal to the number of jobs available. Having more than one specialty or credential and being willing to relocate will provide the best job opportunities.

Professional Organization

The Society of Diagnostic Medical Sonography (SDMS, formerly the ASUTS) works to advance the profession and educate the medical community about diagnostic medical sonography. It advocates in state legislatures and Congress on issues affecting ultrasound, sonography careers, and patient interests.

The SDMS offers a variety of benefits to its 20,000 members. Its publications are the *Journal of Diagnostic Medical Sonography*, two newsletters, and examination guidelines. Online resources include free exams for continuing education credits; discussion groups for different specialties and areas of interest; and information regarding professional development, careers, and workplace issues. Members can purchase home-study courses, textbooks, national certification exam review materials, and admission to the annual conference at a discount.

The SMDS Educational Foundation awards scholarships to sonography students, grants to members to attend industry seminars, and research and grant monies to sonographers to recognize their research and contributions to the field.

✔ CHECK POINT

4 What education and training are needed to become a diagnostic medical sonographer?

RADIOLOGIC TECHNOLOGISTS/ RADIOGRAPHERS

Radiologic technologists perform diagnostic medical imaging tests and administer radiation therapy treatments for cancer and other diseases. They work in one of four practice areas: radiography, sonography (discussed in the previous section), nuclear medicine (profiled in the next section), and radiation therapy. This profile focuses on radiography.

Radiographers use x-rays to produce black-and-white images (*radiographs*) for the purpose of diagnosing an injury or illness. These images, which may be recorded on film, computer, or videotape, show the structure of organs, vessels, bones, and tissues. Radiographers x-ray the chest, bones, joints, GI tract, and other parts of the body. They may specialize in particular types of tests, such as computerized tomography (CT) scans or magnetic resonance imaging (MRI) scans. They work at the direction of a physician, and they do not make diagnoses.

History of the Profession

In 1895, German scientist William Conrad Roentgen made an accidental discovery: a previously unknown wavelength of energy that could penetrate materials that light could not, allowing the insides of objects, including the human body, to be "viewed" from the outside. Roentgen called his discovery *x-rays*.

Almost immediately, physicians began to experiment with medical uses of x-rays. X-ray equipment was costly, however, and difficult to operate. Companies sprang up to provide this service. Hospitals slowly began to add x-ray facilities. As x-ray equipment gradually improved, the medical specialty of radiology developed.

In the early 20th century, as x-ray equipment became more affordable and x-rays more widely used, physicians found that they didn't have enough time to take x-rays and develop the film, so they delegated those tasks to secretaries, receptionists, and nurses. These early technicians, nearly all of whom were women, were also responsible for repairing and maintaining the equipment.

In 1917, Ed Jerman, who had worked with x-ray technology for much of his career, convinced an x-ray equipment manufacturer to form an education department and hire him to head it. Jerman thought the company could sell its services teaching physicians and technicians to use the equipment, which would also increase equipment sales. Jerman's next step, in 1920, was to form a professional society of technicians, the American Association of Radiological Technicians (AART). This group later became the American Society of Radiographers and then the American Society of X Ray Technicians (ASXT).

The AART and the Radiological Society of America, a professional organization of radiologists, began collaborating on a means of certifying x-ray technicians. In 1922, the first certification exam was given, and the following year, the American Registry of X Ray Technicians (ARXT) was established. AART soon began to list approved schools for x-ray technicians. By 1940, there were 90 accredited training programs. The AMA Council on Medical Education and Hospitals assumed responsibility for accreditation in 1944.

During World War II, the army established training programs in 16 training centers that eventually graduated 9,000 technicians. In civilian hospitals, female x-ray technicians took many positions vacated by male technicians in radiology departments.

In the 1950s, rapid advances in technology prompted ASXT to develop a model standardized curriculum. It was submitted to the American College of Radiology in 1952 and approved the same year. By 1956, there were nearly 15,000 registered technicians.

Since then, the profession has continued to grow. Some hallmarks of its growth are higher educational standards, state licensing, and different practice areas and specialties.

Education, Training, and Legal Requirements

Most people wishing to become radiographers complete a two-year associate's degree program. Other options are a certificate program typically lasting 21 to 24 months or a four-year bachelor's degree program. Hospitals, colleges and universities, and some technical schools offer radiography training.

The Joint Review Committee on Education in Radiologic Technology accredits educational programs for radiographers and other radiologic technologists. As of 2009, there were 397 associate's degree programs, 213 certificate programs, and 35 bachelor's degree programs. Applicants to these programs should have a high school diploma or the equivalent; programs may impose additional standards. For students interested in a career in radiography, helpful classes are biology, chemistry, physics, algebra, geometry, photography, health sciences, psychology, and a second language.

Radiography programs provide classroom instruction and clinical practice in these subjects:
- Anatomy and physiology
- Patient care procedures
- Radiation physics
- Radiation safety and protection
- Principles of imaging
- Medical terminology
- Patient positioning
- Medical ethics
- *Radiobiology* (the effects of radiation on humans and other living organisms)
- Pathology

Radiographers can choose to specialize in other imaging procedures, including these:
- CT scans, which produce cross-sectional x-rays that are assembled into three-dimensional images
- MRIs, which are similar to CT scans, but use a magnetic field and radio waves
- Mammograms, which are breast x-rays

Federal law requires workers who operate radiologic equipment to be properly trained, but states handle the actual licensure. As of 2010, 38 states had licensure or certification laws for radiographers. Students interested in becoming radiographers should check with their state's health board to learn the requirements. Links to state licensing authorities and up-to-date information regarding licensure or certification are available at the web site of the American Society of Radiologic Technologists (ASRT), formerly the ASXT.

Radiographers can choose to be certified by the American Registry of Radiologic Technologists (ARRT), formerly the ARXT. As of 2010, 35 states used ARRT exams in licensing. Certification also gives an advantage in the job market. For certification, applicants must graduate from an ARRT-approved educational program, pass an exam, and meet a set of ethical standards. Recertification requires continuing education credits or passing an exam. ARRT also offers certification in a number of specialties, including mammography, computerized tomography, and magnetic resonance imaging.

Work Responsibilities

Before a patient arrives for an x-ray, the radiographer prepares the room and assembles all supplies and equipment that will be needed. He or she explains the procedure to the patient. For a fluoroscopy—a test that uses a continuous beam of x-rays to observe movement in the body—the radiographer may prepare a contrast medium for the patient to drink to help make soft tissues visible. The radiographer positions the patient and x-ray unit, measures the thickness of the area to be x-rayed, and sets the controls to yield images with the appropriate density, detail, and contrast. The radiographer then places the film beneath the area and takes the x-rays.

The radiographer takes precautions to avoid exposure to radiation and to prevent exposing the patient to more radiation than necessary. For example, he or she may place a lead shield over part of the patient's body or limit the size of the x-ray beam.

After making the exposure, the radiographer removes the film and develops it. He or she examines the x-rays to determine whether they're satisfactory for diagnosis or need to be retaken.

Not all radiographers work in radiography departments. Some operate mobile x-ray equipment, taking x-rays in emergency rooms, operating rooms, or patients' hospital rooms.

Radiographers have several other tasks. They keep patient records and adjust and maintain equipment. They may also escort patients to and from the x-ray room, take histories, educate patients, prepare work schedules,

Typical Tasks of a Radiographer

- Obtain and document the patient's history
- Provide a radiation protection shield for the patient
- Identify radiographs with appropriate lead markers
- Manipulate radiographic equipment with ease
- Expose film after telling the patient to hold still and giving breathing instructions
- Process film
- Evaluate images for appropriate positioning and quality

SPOTLIGHT ON SKILLS Typical Task: X-Ray a Patient with a Fracture

Position: Radiographer

Traumatic injuries are caused by external force or violence, the result of car accidents, falls, sports injuries, and other occurrences. Often, patients with traumatic injuries cannot be transported to the hospital's imaging department for x-rays they need. Therefore, many are imaged with mobile radiography equipment.

The radiographer's first task is to assess the situation and plan the imaging procedure. He or she determines the patient's mobility and the equipment and accessories needed and provides protective apparel for anyone who needs to be in the room.

The limb or body part with the fracture is kept immobilized. Any patient movement must be directed by the physician in charge of the patient. The radiographer informs the patient in advance of any moves that will be required and enlists the patient's support.

If the patient has an open fracture (where the bone protrudes through the skin), the radiographer wears gloves and uses standard precautions to protect against infection. The radiographer observes the patient for signs and symptoms of shock and must be prepared to act if such an emergency occurs.

The radiographer takes at least two radiographs for each injured body part, which must include all anatomy of interest.

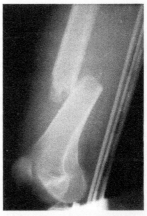

And x-ray is an important diagnostic tool.

evaluate equipment purchases, conduct quality assurance programs, and manage radiology departments.

Personal Characteristics of Radiographers

Radiographers typically work with many different patients in the course of a day. Some will be injured or ill, and some are facing difficult diagnoses. A positive attitude, empathy, and good human relations skills are valuable characteristics in this occupation.

Much of a radiographer's work is carried out with little supervision. Radiographers should be confident, self-motivated, and comfortable working independently. At the same time, they are part of the radiology team, so they need good teamwork skills. Radiographers must be able to follow instructions.

Several other personal characteristics are important. One is manual dexterity. Radiographers should be flexible and good at multitasking. They need to pay careful attention to detail. Finally, radiographers need good communication skills to communicate clearly with patients, physicians, and other health care professionals.

Employment Opportunities and Trends

The BLS projects that employment of radiographers and other radiologic technologists will increase by about 17 percent from 2008 to 2018. Growth of the population in general, and the population of older adults in particular, will create a need for more diagnostic imaging. Increased use of imaging to monitor the progress of treatment is also anticipated.

In 2008, radiographers and other radiologic technologists held about 196,000 jobs. Their main employer was hospitals, accounting for more than 60 percent of positions. Most of the remaining jobs were in physicians' offices; medical and diagnostic laboratories, including diagnostic imaging centers; and outpatient care centers. From 2008 to 2018, 37,000 new jobs will be added. Hospitals will continue to be the main employer, but physicians' offices and diagnostic imaging centers will also be hiring. Like diagnostic medical sonographers, radiographers will benefit from technological advances that make imaging equipment less expensive, allowing more procedures to be performed in physicians' offices.

Radiographers can enhance their job prospects in several ways. They can specialize in CT scans or MRIs, as the use of both types of scans is increasing. They can also learn more than one specialty, as health care facilities are trying to control costs by hiring employees who can do more than one type of scan.

Professional Organization

With more than 130,000 members, the American Society of Radiologic Technologists (ASRT) is the largest professional organization representing medical imaging technologists and radiation therapists. It is also the oldest, founded in 1920. The ASRT's mission includes fostering professional growth and developing the radiologic technology community. The ASRT represents radiologic technologists in government and education. It monitors state and federal legislation and works with accrediting and certifying agencies to develop and revise curriculums, set practice guidelines, and implement entry-level standards.

The ASRT offers members a number of ways to earn continuing education credits. These include directed reading programs through its two professional journals and an online learning center. Courses at its two annual meetings and state conferences, seminars, and symposiums provide additional opportunities for continuing education and for networking.

The organization actively promotes careers in radiologic technology. It offers students and educators a wealth of career-related materials. The ASRT Education and Research Foundation, the organization's philanthropic wing, awards scholarships and provides research grants to students and practicing technologists.

✓ CHECK POINT

5 What are the typical work responsibilities of a radiographer?

NUCLEAR MEDICINE TECHNOLOGISTS

Nuclear medicine is the use of radioactive materials inside the body to create diagnostic images or to treat cancer and other diseases. A radiologic technologist who specializes in nuclear medicine is called a *nuclear medicine technologist*. Some common diagnostic nuclear medicine procedures are bone scans for orthopedic injuries, lung scans for blood clots, and cardiac stress tests that gauge the heart's degree of function. (These are not the same tests that cardiographic technicians perform.) Like other imaging technologies, nuclear medicine imaging gives physicians a means of obtaining information about a patient's condition that might otherwise require surgery or not be obtainable at all. Unlike other imaging technologies, which show structures, nuclear medicine imaging actually shows the function of organs or tissues.

History of the Profession

Not long after the discovery of radioactivity by Henri Becquerel in 1896, scientists began to observe that it had medical uses. A key factor in the development of nuclear medicine was the work of Georg Von Hevesy, a Hungarian chemist, in the first part of the 20th century, in developing radioisotope tracers.

Radionuclides, or radioisotopes, are unstable atoms of an element that give off radiation. They behave chemically like that element, but they are radioactive. Because of that radioactivity, they can be traced. In diagnostic nuclear medicine imaging, many radionuclides are bound to a stable molecule or compound to make drugs known as radiopharmaceuticals. Radiopharmaceuticals are targeted to accumulate temporarily in specific tissues or organs. A higher or lower concentration of radioactivity than expected can indicate disease. Radionuclides are also used in treating diseases, particularly in killing cancer cells.

Although some radioisotopes occur naturally, trying to isolate them proved impractical. With the invention of the cyclotron by Ernest Lawrence in 1929, scientists began to make and discover artificial radionuclides, including iodine-131, used to treat thyroid disease, and technetium-99m, the most commonly used radionuclide in medicine. In the 1930s, physicians treated blood disorders with radioactive phosphorus produced in cyclotrons. The invention of the nuclear reactor in 1942 made producing radionuclides easier. An important event took place in 1946, when a patient with thyroid cancer was treated with radioactive iodine, which stopped the cancer from spreading.

The discipline of nuclear medicine took shape in the 1950s, with the development of the first imaging devices and the use of iodine-131 to diagnose and treat thyroid disease. From the mid-1960s forward, nuclear medicine grew rapidly, with the integration of computers into imaging devices and the development of new technology and instruments such as positron emission tomography (PET) scans. Physicians could now see the function, as well as the structure, of most organs in the body. In the 1980s, radiopharmaceuticals were developed to diagnose heart disease and other medical problems. Today, they're also used in treatment.

With widespread clinical applications and rapidly developing technology, the need for more technologists became pressing, and radiologic technologists began to specialize in nuclear medicine.

Education, Training, and Legal Requirements

People can enter the field by completing an associate's degree, bachelor's degree, or certificate program in nuclear medicine technology. Certificate programs, available at hospitals, are intended for health care professionals, such as diagnostic medical sonographers or registered nurses, who already hold an associate's or bachelor's degree but want to change fields or add a specialty.

The Joint Review Committee on Educational Programs in Nuclear Medicine Technology (JRCNMT) accredits formal educational programs in nuclear medicine technology. In 2010, 101 accredited programs were available. Programs must either include, or require as a prerequisite, college-level courses in human anatomy and physiology, physics, algebra, medical terminology, computer applications, oral and written communications, and general chemistry. Coursework covers at minimum the following areas:

- Patient care methods
- Nuclear medicine computer applications
- Nuclear medicine physics and radiation physics
- Diagnostic nuclear medicine procedures
- Immunology relating to nuclear medicine
- Radiation safety and protection
- Radionuclide therapy—the use of radiopharmaceuticals to treat diseases
- Radionuclide chemistry and radiopharmacy, which deals with radiopharmaceuticals
- Quality control and quality assurance
- Nuclear instrumentation
- Statistics

Accredited programs must also include a clinical component that covers patient care and recordkeeping, radiation safety, quality control, work with radiopharmaceuticals, performance of a sufficient number and variety of procedures to meet the program's stated competencies, and correlation of procedures.

More than half the states have licensure or certification laws for nuclear medicine technologists. Requirements differ from state to state. Certification is voluntary, but it is the standard for the field, and employers generally expect it—in part because many health insurers require it.

Both the ARRT and the Nuclear Medicine Technology Certification Board (NMTCB) certify nuclear medicine technologists. Technologists can qualify for certification by completing an educational program approved by the organization, such as a JRCNMT-accredited program. For the NMTCB, candidates can also qualify in a number of other ways, such as by holding a bachelor's or associate's degree in a biological science, gaining a set number of hours of clinical experience in nuclear medicine technology, and completing 15 hours of coursework in nuclear medicine topics. Both organizations require an exam, and they have additional criteria. The NMTCB also offers specialty certification in nuclear cardiology and PET scanning.

For both organizations, technologists must renew their certification annually and complete continuing education every two years. The ARRT offers the option of an exam in another ARRT-recognized discipline instead of continuing education.

Work Responsibilities

A major responsibility of nuclear medicine technologists is performing diagnostic scans. Some examples of nuclear medicine scans are PET scans, single photon emission computed tomography (SPECT) scans, bone scans, and cardiovascular imaging.

Before a scan, the nuclear medicine technologist gets the camera and computer system ready and prepares the radiopharmaceutical that the patient will receive. The amount of radiologic exposure for the patient is similar to that of an x-ray. The technologist explains the procedure to the patient and administers the radiopharmaceutical by mouth, injection, inhalation, or other means.

When it is time to begin a scan, the technologist positions the patient and starts the x-ray unit. The gamma camera or scanner picks up the gamma rays emitted by the radiopharmaceutical. A computer then builds an image of the area being scanned, showing where the radioactive material is distributed and its concentration.

The nuclear medicine technologist selects, processes, and enhances the images. He or she does preliminary

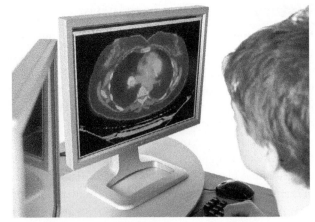

In addition to performing diagnostic scans, nuclear medicine technologists select and process the images.

analysis on the computer, sometimes using spreadsheets, and provides the results to the physician, along with images or film and patient information.

Nuclear medicine technologists also assist in radionuclide therapy. They ensure that the correct radiopharmaceuticals and dosages are prepared and perform other tasks, such as verifying patients' identities, preparing or coordinating the preparation of supplies, and observing radiation safety procedures.

Technologists have several additional duties. They record procedures in patients' records. They also document the amount and type of radionuclides that they receive, use, and dispose of. They maintain and run quality control checks on equipment. They may also supervise students, technologists, and other personnel; help schedule exams; purchase supplies and equipment;

SPOTLIGHT ON SKILLS Typical Task: Perform a Wipe Test

Position: Nuclear Medicine Technologist

A routine task in laboratories that work with radiation is conducting wipe tests to ensure that surfaces are not contaminated.

Before doing a wipe test, the nuclear medicine technologist washes his or her hands, gathers supplies, and puts on personal protective equipment, such as gloves and safety glasses. It is important not to touch anything but testing materials during the test. The technologist places a clean cotton swab, filter paper, or paper towel in a vial to serve as a background sample. Then he or she closes the vial.

A sample is taken by wiping a surface from side to side, using an S motion. The sample is placed in the appropri-

ate vial, which is then closed. These steps are repeated for each sample.

Next, the technologist adds LSC (liquid scintillation counter) cocktail to each vial, enough to cover the sample. This cocktail is a fluid that holds the sample while it is analyzed. After discarding gloves in a radioactive waste container, the technologist loads the rack of vials into the radiation counter, sets it, and runs the samples.

Each test must be documented on a record sheet. If a result is three times or more than the count for the background sample, the surface must be cleaned and retested.

> **Typical Tasks of a Nuclear Medicine Technologist**
>
> - Select and prepare prescribed dosages of radiopharmaceuticals
> - Verify the correct syringe and dose
> - Position the patient appropriately
> - Select images for processing
> - Record receipt of radioactive materials
> - Evaluate the performance of a scanner
> - Perform wipe tests for radiation
> - Collect blood samples by venipuncture
> - Conduct and document radiation surveys

and take part in inspections by external agencies and research activities.

Personal Characteristics of Nuclear Medicine Technologists

Nuclear medicine technologists work closely with patients, so they should have good interpersonal and communication skills. They should be able to help ease a patient's concerns before and during a procedure, gather relevant information about the patient's history, explain the procedure, and give clear directions. Technologists must also be able to communicate clearly with physicians regarding scan results.

Many tasks that nuclear medicine technologists perform require attention to detail. Working with radioactive materials demands careful adherence to safety procedures. In preparing radiopharmaceuticals, technologists must be meticulous and precise. Technologists must pay careful attention to a scan to distinguish abnormalities that may signal disease. Enhancing images and completing documentation also require sharp focus on detail.

Nuclear medicine technologists typically work independently, so they need to be self-motivated and comfortable working on their own. At the same time, they are usually part of a team that includes fellow technologists, physicians, support staff, and other personnel. As a result, teamwork skills are valuable.

Two additional personal characteristics that nuclear medicine technologists should have are flexibility and a willingness to learn. They need to be able to deal with shifts in schedules, shuffled priorities, unexpected exam results, and other changes, with ease. Nuclear medicine technology is constantly evolving, as new procedures and applications are added and existing procedures are improved. For this reason, people considering this occupation should enjoy learning.

Employment Opportunities and Trends

The BLS projects 16 percent job growth for nuclear medicine technologists from 2008 to 2018. It cites three reasons for this projected growth:
- Development and increased use of newer imaging technologies, such as PET and SPECT
- The development of new nuclear medicine treatments
- The rising share of the population that is middle-aged or older, which is likely to result in higher demand for diagnostic and treatment procedures

The cost of new imaging technologies will temper job growth, however. Although the new technologies will be used more often, they are likely to replace, rather than supplement, older technologies, which also will limit growth. The BLS predicts that there will be more qualified technologists than jobs available, which will make competition keen. Nuclear medicine technologists can increase their employability by cross-training in another type of imaging, such as radiography, diagnostic medical sonography, or nuclear cardiology.

In 2008, nuclear medicine technologists held nearly 22,000 jobs. Hospitals were the main employer, accounting for about two-thirds of jobs. Physicians' offices and medical and diagnostic laboratories, including diagnostic imaging centers, supplied most of the remaining jobs.

Professional Organization

The Society of Nuclear Medicine (SNM), founded in 1954, represents physicians, scientists, and technologists specializing in nuclear medicine. It publishes journals, newsletters, and books; sponsors international meetings and workshops; monitors congressional and regulatory activities; advocates for nuclear medicine science and research; and offers grants, awards, and scholarships. Membership benefits include a professional journal and newsletter; discounted admission to the organization's national meeting; courses and audiovisuals that earn continuing education credits; and free online exams and CE credits. The SNM provides an online resource center and job bank.

> **✓ CHECK POINT**
>
> **6** What education and training are needed to become a nuclear medicine technologist?

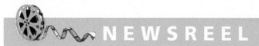

Imaging and Costs

The 64-slice CT scan is a powerful tool for identifying clogged arteries and diagnosing cardiovascular disease. High-resolution images can be obtained much more quickly than with older scanners, with far fewer flaws resulting from a patient's accidental movements. The entire heart can be imaged in less than 15 seconds. The scan is an alternative to invasive procedures, such as cardiac catheterization, and is increasingly being used for other applications.

Sophisticated CT scans, MRIs, and PET scans have transformed the diagnosis and treatment of a steadily expanding list of diseases—but at a price. A 64-slice CT scanner costs about $1 million. A scan costs from $500 to $1,500. Scans are typically covered by insurance if prescribed by a physician, but not if the patient opts to have them done as a preventive measure.

Both the number of scans performed and the cost of imaging in the U.S. have skyrocketed. An American College of Radiology blue-ribbon panel found that, over a 15-year period, the number of annual CT scans alone increased from 3 million to 60 million. A 2008 study by the U.S. Government Accountability Office (GAO) found that Medicare spending on imaging services had more than doubled from 2000 to 2006, from $6.89 billion to $14.11 billion, and spending on CT scans and other advanced types of imaging had risen much faster than spending on ultrasound, x-rays, and other more basic procedures. According to a 2008 report by America's Health Insurance Plans, a health insurance lobbying group, spending on imaging was nearing $100 billion a year and was expected to double in the next four years.

As a result, physicians, the federal government, insurance companies, and the press are debating the proper use of imaging scans.

Don't forget to visit thePoint* companion website for additional study resources!

CHAPTER HIGHLIGHTS

- Cardiographic technicians perform diagnostic tests to help determine the cause and extent of cardiovascular illnesses. They perform basic electrocardiograms (ECGs or EKGs), which record the electrical activity of the heart. With additional training, they may perform other types of tests.
- Cardiovascular technologists perform diagnostic tests on the heart and blood vessels and help treat patients with cardiac and vascular disease. They usually specialize in one or more of three areas: (1) invasive procedures, such as cardiac catheterization and balloon angioplasty, in which they assist a physician; (2) noninvasive cardiology, including echocardiography, the use of ultrasound to examine the heart and blood vessels; and (3) noninvasive peripheral vascular study, or ultrasound scans of the blood vessels.
- Phlebotomists are clinical laboratory technicians who collect blood samples for testing and draw blood for transfusions. They collect blood by a variety of methods, including venipuncture, or drawing blood from a vein, and capillary puncture, or finger stick.
- Diagnostic medical sonographers perform sonograms, or ultrasound scans, of various parts of the human body. They may specialize in different systems or parts of the body, including cardiac sonography, vascular sonography, neurosonography, obstetrics/gynecology, and abdomen and breast scans.
- Radiologic technologists perform diagnostic medical imaging tests and administer radiation therapy treatments for cancer and other diseases. They work in one of four practice areas: radiography, sonography, nuclear medicine, and radiation therapy. Radiographers take x-rays. They may specialize in CT scans, MRIs, or other imaging procedures.
- Nuclear medicine technologists perform diagnostic tests that use radioactive materials, such as positron emission tomography (PET) scans, single photon emission computed tomography (SPECT) scans, bone scans, and cardiovascular imaging, They also assist in the use of radiopharmaceuticals to treat diseases.

REVIEW QUESTIONS

Matching

1. _____ Venipuncture

2. _____ Mammography

3. _____ PET scan

4. _____ Holter monitor test

5. _____ Balloon angioplasty

    a. Cardiographic technician   **b.** Cardiovascular technologist   **c.** Phlebotomist
    d. Radiographer   e. Nuclear medicine technologist

Multiple Choice

6. Ultrasound scans of fetuses during pregnancy are performed by _____.

    a. radiographers   **c.** diagnostic medical sonographers
    b. phlebotomists   **d.** cardiographic technicians

7. Which procedure does a cardiographic technician typically perform?

   a. Echocardiography
   b. Stress test
   c. Noninvasive peripheral vascular study
   d. Electrophysiology testing

8. Which is NOT a job responsibility of nuclear medicine technologists?

   a. Prepare radiopharmaceuticals
   b. Perform wipe tests for radiation
   c. Select and enhance images
   d. Deliver radionuclide therapy

9. Which statement about phlebotomists is NOT true?

   a. Most states require phlebotomists to be licensed.
   b. Phlebotomists must be able to work with patients of all ages.
   c. The BLS predicts excellent job opportunities for phlebotomists from 2008 to 2018.
   d. Some phlebotomists are also laboratory assistants and EKG technicians.

10. Which type of educational program do most radiographers complete?

    a. On-the-job training
    b. Certificate
    c. Two-year associate's degree program
    d. Four-year bachelor's degree program

Completion

11. _____ is the use of radioactive materials inside the body to create diagnostic images or to treat cancer and other diseases.

12. The word _____ refers to procedures that don't involve entering the body or breaking the skin.

13. _____ is the use of high-frequency sound waves to construct images of organs and other structures in the body.

14. _____ means drawing blood from a vein.

15. The word _____ refers to the blood vessels.

Short Answer

16. Which of the occupations profiled in this chapter require good people skills? Why?

   _____

   _____

17. In terms of job responsibilities, what is the difference between a cardiographic technician and a cardiovascular technologist?

   _____

   _____

18. Describe the education or training options for becoming a phlebotomist.

   _____

   _____

19. What are some areas in which diagnostic medical sonographers can specialize?

   _____

   _____

20. Explain the tasks that a nuclear medicine technologist performs before, during, and after a diagnostic scan.

   _____

   _____

INVESTIGATE IT

1. Write a brief story describing a typical day on the job for someone in one of the occupations described in this chapter. To get the information you need, you can interview a person who works in the field, read interviews in print or online, watch online career videos, review the "Work Responsibilities" description in this chapter, or even draw on TV programs or movies (but make your description realistic!). Some web sites with interviews and videos are listed below.

    http://www.mayoclinic.org/careerawareness/ce-patientcare.html ("Career Exploration: Patient Care")

    https://www.asrt.org/content/RecruitmentRetention/RecruitmentTools/career_videos.aspx ("Career Encounters Video Kit")

    http://science.education.nih.gov/LifeWorks.nsf/Interviews ("LifeWorks: Explore Health and Medical Science Careers: Interviews")

2. This chapter's Newsreel feature describes the tremendous growth in the number and cost of imaging procedures performed in recent years. Why is this happening? What roles do the health care system, physicians, and patients play? What are some ways of controlling costs? Use the search term *imaging costs* in your Internet search.

RECOMMENDED READING

American Society for Clinical Pathology. The Laboratory Medicine Profession. Available at: http://www.ascp.org/MainMenu/laboratoryprofessionals/CareerCenter.aspx.

Association for Career and Technical Education. Career Curve: Nuclear Medicine Technologist. *Techniques: Connecting Education and Careers* [serial online]. February 2009;84(2):58. Available at: http://www.acteonline.org/uploadedFiles/Publications_and_E-Media/files/files-techniques-2009/career_curve%281%29.pdf.

Nobel Foundation. Electrocardiogram [game]. Available at: http://nobelprize.org/educational_games/medicine/ecg.

Public Broadcasting Service (PBS). The Mysterious Human Heart. Available at: http://www.pbs.org/wnet/heart/index.html.

Radiological Society of North America. Radiology in Motion. Available at: http://www.radiology-info.org/en/video/index.cfm.

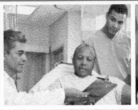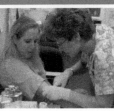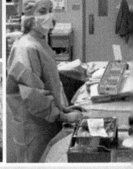

Therapy and Rehabilitation

CHAPTER OBJECTIVES

After careful study of this chapter, you should be able to:

⁕ State the education, training, and legal requirements for becoming a physical therapist, physical therapist assistant, occupational therapist, occupational therapy assistant, respiratory therapist, and massage therapist.

⁕ Describe the typical work responsibilities in each profession.

⁕ List desirable personal characteristics of physical therapists, physical therapist assistants, occupational therapists, occupational therapy assistants, respiratory therapists, and massage therapists.

⁕ Identify employment opportunities and key trends for these occupations.

KEY TERMS

bronchoscopy (brong KOS kŏ pē)

chest physiotherapy

holistic (hō LIS tik)

intervention

modality

polysomnography (POL ē som NOG rǎ fē)

rehabilitation

respiratory therapy

spirometry (spī ROM ě trē)

Rehabilitation is the restoration, after a disease or injury, of the ability to function in a normal or near-normal manner. The careers described in this chapter focus on helping people to develop or recover the ability to move without pain and to perform tasks of everyday life. From premature infants to older adults, many people use the services provided by these professionals at some time during their lives.

PHYSICAL THERAPISTS

Physical therapists help people who have been injured, are in pain, or suffer from some other disabling condition to recover or improve in their ability to carry out routine life activities. Their patients include people with low-back pain, arthritis, or cerebral palsy; people who've broken a leg in a car accident or torn a rotator cuff playing tennis; people who've had strokes or have suffered spinal cord injuries; soldiers who've lost arms or legs; and many others.

This high-growth occupation is also personally rewarding. *U.S. News and World Report* included physical therapy in its 50 Best Careers of 2010 (and 2009). The magazine noted that physical therapists ranked second only to clergy in job satisfaction in a recent survey.

History of the Profession

The physical therapy profession began during World War I, with the rehabilitation of wounded U.S. soldiers. In 1917, the surgeon general of the army established a program that trained 800 individuals, called *reconstruction aides*, in physical therapy. After the war, these aides continued to be in demand to work with veterans, either in the civilian sector or in veterans' hospitals. At the time, all of these workers were women.

In 1921, a group of reconstruction aides who had served in the war formed a professional association, the American Women's Physical Therapeutic Association. This organization eventually became the American Physical Therapy Association (APTA), the national association of physical therapists in the U.S. today.

In the 1940s and 1950s, the demand for therapists increased to meet the needs of servicemen injured in World War II and to care for victims of several polio epidemics. During the war, many people entered the profession through federally-funded programs that trained college graduates with degrees in physical education and other related areas. During the polio epidemics, the National Foundation for Infantile Paralysis (the March of Dimes) funded student recruitment drives, scholarships, salaries for new faculty, and faculty training programs.

In the 1960s, when polio had largely disappeared after the development of the Salk and Sabin vaccines, physical therapists shifted to the treatment of many other disabling conditions. In 1968, Congress authorized outpatient physical therapy services for the Medicare program, which boosted demand for these services.

State licensing for physical therapists, which had begun in the 1910s, intensified during the 1950s. By the end of that decade, 45 states had enacted physical therapy practice laws. In 1954, the APTA, working with the Professional Examination Service, developed a competency exam for entry-level physical therapists and made it available to state licensing boards. Over the following decades, the activities of noted physical therapists and physicians, the development of new technology, and federal legislation expanded the physical therapist's scope of practice.

Education, Training, and Legal Requirements

Becoming a physical therapist normally requires at least a master's degree from an accredited physical therapy pro-

gram and a state license. The profession is moving swiftly toward a doctoral degree as the entry-level educational requirement.

The Commission on Accreditation in Physical Therapy Education (CAPTE) accredits physical therapist educational programs. As of January 2010, there were 203 accredited programs leading to a doctoral degree and 19 accredited programs leading to a master's degree. Doctoral degree programs take three years; master's degree programs typically take two to two and a half years.

Accredited programs include academic classes, lab work, and clinical work. Programs cover these areas:

- Biological and physical sciences, such as anatomy/cellular biology, physiology, exercise physiology, neuroscience, and pharmacology
- Behavioral sciences, such as applied psychology, applied sociology, communication, clinical reasoning, and applied statistics

The clinical component, which makes up at least one-third of the curriculum, must include opportunities to manage patients whose conditions are representative of those that physical therapists commonly encounter; to work in typical practice settings; to interact with practicing therapists, who serve as role models; and to take part in interdisciplinary care.

Accredited programs must also prepare students to meet a lengthy set of professional practice expectations in areas such as professional duty, screening, examination, diagnosis, prognosis, plan of care development, management of care delivery, practice management, and consultation.

Generally, doctoral programs differ from master's degree programs in offering more content in areas such as diagnostics, pharmacology, and advanced practice skills, such as pediatrics and geriatrics. Doctoral programs also involve longer clinical rotations with more hours and more roles than master's programs. The educational approach focuses on *evidence-based practice*, which relies on the best clinical research currently available when making decisions about a patient's care. Programs focus on graduating students who can work autonomously, exhibit professionalism, and have high-level clinical decision-making and diagnostic skills.

Undergraduates considering becoming physical therapists should take science, math, and social science courses. Many physical therapist programs require applicants to have volunteer experience in the physical therapy department of a hospital or clinic.

All states require physical therapists to be licensed. Licensure requirements vary by state, but generally, applicants must have graduated from an accredited program, passed the National Physical Therapy Examination

(NPTE), and fulfilled other requirements of the state, such as a jurisprudence exam. The NPTE is administered by the Federation of State Boards of Physical Therapy (FSBPT), and requirements to sit for the exam vary by state. People interested in this occupation can learn state requirements by locating the state licensing authorities at the FSBPT web site. State renewal requirements may include continuing education.

The American Board of Physical Therapy Specialties awards specialist certification to licensed physical therapists who have been in practice for at least ten years. The specialties are cardiovascular and clinical electrophysiology, geriatrics, neurology, orthopedics, pediatrics, sports, and women's health. Requirements vary but generally include 2,000 hours of direct patient care in the specialty area, 25 percent of which must have been in the past three years. Recertification requirements also vary but generally include 200 hours per year of direct patient care in the specialty area in the previous two years.

Work Responsibilities

A physical therapist's work begins with a review of the patient's medical history. Based on that history, physical therapists select appropriate physical tests to use to evaluate the patient's abilities and condition. Therapists test and measure factors such as overall strength; aerobic capacity and endurance; range of motion; gait; locomotion; stability when walking; balance and coordination; posture; and muscle strength, endurance, tone, and reflexes. They may assess whether the patient needs devices like braces or prostheses and whether the patient is using them properly.

Once the examination is complete, physical therapists develop a treatment plan that addresses one or more of these goals:
- Restoring function
- Improving mobility
- Relieving pain
- Preventing or limiting permanent physical disabilities

Most treatment plans include exercises to increase flexibility and range of motion. More advanced exercises focus on improving strength, balance, coordination, and endurance. Treatment can include many different types of exercise, from those that people would typically do at a gym or outdoors to others that are especially designed for a particular therapy goal. Physical therapy often includes *manual therapy*, skilled hand movements performed by the therapist or therapist assistant. Goals of manual therapy may include increasing range of motion, easing pain, and reducing swelling.

A plan may include the use of modalities, or treatment tools, such as hot or cold packs, whirlpools, nerve stimulation, ultrasound, and traction. In addition, patients may need to be taught to use devices, such as crutches, prostheses, and wheelchairs. Physical therapists may instruct patients in biofeedback for pain management. They may also show patients and their families how to do exercises and carry out other treatment procedures at home.

Physical therapists may work directly with patients to carry out the treatment plans or delegate that work to physical therapist assistants. In either case, physical therapists monitor patients' progress during treatment. They reevaluate patients periodically and modify the plans when necessary. Physical therapists are sometimes asked to perform a systems review of all body systems to screen patients and determine whether they need physical therapy or should be referred to another health care professional.

Physical therapists often consult or work with other health care professionals, such as physical therapist assistants, physicians, nurses, social workers, occupational therapists, speech-language pathologists, and audiologists.

Some physical therapists specialize in certain areas, such as pediatrics, geriatrics, orthopedics, sports medicine, and cardiopulmonary physical therapy. Physical therapists also work to prevent injury or disability by developing health, fitness, and wellness programs. Some design conditioning programs to help athletes prepare for events.

Typical Tasks of a Physical Therapist

- Do a systems review
- Take a patient's medical history
- Conduct motor function tests
- Develop a treatment plan
- Perform gait and locomotion training
- Assess a patient's progress
- Educate patients about expected outcomes
- Coordinate with home care agencies

Personal Characteristics of Physical Therapists

When physical therapists are asked why they chose the field or what they find personally satisfying about their jobs, a frequent response is the opportunity to work intensively with patients. Physical therapists should have a caring, compassionate, and positive attitude and the ability to work well with others. Whether they do physical therapy themselves or design and supervise it, physical therapists need to be able to interact effectively with patients, their families, and other health care professionals.

SPOTLIGHT ON SKILLS Typical Task: Make a Proximal Interphalangeal Joint (PIP) or Distal Interphalangeal Joint (DIP) Mobilization Splint

Position: Physical Therapist

A mobilization splint helps patients regain range of motion by gently extending an injured joint over time. It might be used with a finger stiffened by arthritis, for example. Sometimes a prefabricated splint is suitable. In other instances, physical therapists make their own.

The first steps in making a splint are to cut and fit the straps. The therapist cuts a strip of elastic strapping of sufficient length and width and places the center of the strip along the back of the patient's distal phalanx. Then the therapist has the patient flex the PIP and DIP joints of the affected digit (in a claw position), while the strap ends are stretched to meet across the back of the proximal phalanx. The therapist holds the straps together, adjusts the tension, marks both pieces of elastic, and removes them slowly from the digit.

The next step is to sew or connect the straps together. A safety pin or staples may be used for a simple, quick closure technique. The corners of the straps are rounded, and a piece of soft foam is added under the portion that comes in contact with the nail.

After making the splint, the physical therapist gives the patient written materials describing the purpose, pre-

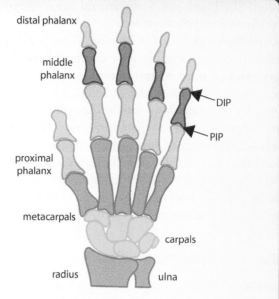

Bones of the hand and arm.

cautions, wearing schedule, and proper care of the splint. He or she schedules a follow-up visit to reevaluate and adjust the strap tension as range of motion increases.

Physical therapists need to be good observers and problem solvers. Physical therapists have to closely observe a patient's condition, find the cause of problems, and devise appropriate treatments. They need to carefully assess a patient's progress, determine why a treatment isn't working, and modify the treatment plan when needed.

Employment Opportunities and Trends

Physical therapists will enjoy strong employment growth of 30 percent from 2008 to 2018, according to the Bureau of Labor Statistics (BLS). Several factors are driving this growth:

- Easing of service restrictions by insurers
- The rising population of older adults, who are more likely to suffer chronic medical problems requiring therapy and rehabilitation
- The needs of trauma victims and infants with birth defects, who are surviving more often than in the past, due to improvements in medicine and technology

- Treatment of previously untreatable conditions, made possible by advances in technology and the use of evidence-based practices
- The influence of the Individuals with Disabilities Education Act, which guarantees physical therapy services for students who need them

In 2008, physical therapists held about 185,500 jobs. The actual number of practicing therapists could be smaller, however, as some held more than one job. About 35 percent worked in physicians' and physical therapists' offices and the offices of other health practitioners. Roughly 30 percent worked in hospitals, and about 10 percent worked in home care services. Approximately 8 percent were self-employed. Others worked in nursing care facilities and outpatient care centers. Some physical therapists did research and taught.

From 2008 to 2018, physical therapists will have good job prospects, especially in acute hospitals, skilled nursing facilities, and orthopedic settings, where older adults are most often treated. Physical therapists who are willing to work in rural areas should also have good job prospects, because many physical therapists work in urban and suburban areas.

Professional Organization

As noted earlier, the American Physical Therapy Association (APTA) is the national association of physical therapists in the U.S. The APTA is a 72,000-member organization with an overall goal of helping to advance physical therapy practice, research, and education. It monitors legislation and advocates for the profession before Congress, state legislatures, and other executive agencies. The APTA operates a political action committee and a grassroots campaign for members. It conducts research on the profession, certifies specialists in physical therapy, and credentials residency and fellowship programs.

The association offers a variety of ways for members to engage with one another. Besides the national conference, there are chapter meetings, sections devoted to staying current in different areas of expertise, and special interest groups within sections.

The APTA offers members continuing education opportunities through a national conference, meetings, workshops, seminars, home-study courses, audio conferences, and an online learning center. Other member benefits include an online career planning center, a professional journal and other publications, an honors and awards program, a mentoring program, and special initiatives for students, women, members of minority groups, and new professionals.

CHECK POINT

1 What are the typical work responsibilities of physical therapists?

PHYSICAL THERAPIST ASSISTANTS

When people need physical therapy services, the person who provides them is often a physical therapist assistant. Working under the direction of a physical therapist, physical therapist assistants carry out the treatment plan. Physical therapist assistant ranks seventeenth among the fastest-growing occupations in the nation, and *U.S. News and World Report* named it one of the 50 Best Careers of 2010.

History of the Profession

The profession of physical therapist assistant developed as a result of the expansion of the physical therapy profession after World War II and the increasing demand for

physical therapy treatments. The first assistants, informally trained, appeared in the 1950s. After studies found that physical therapists spent about a third of their time on tasks that could be delegated to workers with less training, the APTA formed a committee to develop a policy for using nonprofessional personnel. The first two physical therapist assistant education programs were approved in 1967. Soon afterward, CAPTE began setting program accreditation standards, and APTA developed guidelines for tasks that physical therapist assistants could perform.

From the 1970s through the 1990s, physical therapist assistant training programs grew rapidly, fueled by federal legislation supporting allied health programs and an increasing demand for physical therapy services.

Education, Training, and Legal Requirements

Most physical therapist assistants enter the occupation by earning an associate's degree from an accredited physical therapist assistant program. The accrediting organization is CAPTE. As of January 2010, there were 252 accredited physical therapist assistant programs in the U.S.

Accredited associate's degree programs are usually two years long. They include, or require as a prerequisite, general education classes in basic sciences, as well as in applied physical therapy science. The second component, technical education classes, prepares graduates to meet a set of performance expectations in physical therapy interventions (active treatment processes, such as exercises to improve muscle extension), communication, behavior and conduct, data collection, and other areas. The third component is 520 to 720 hours of clinical experience.

The AMA recommends that students interested in becoming physical therapist assistants take classes in biology, chemistry, math, physics, English, and social sciences. Program prerequisites vary, so students should check the requirements for the particular programs that interest them.

Most states require physical therapist assistants to be licensed, registered, or certified. In most states, physical therapist assistants must obtain at least an associate's degree from an accredited physical therapist assistant program and pass an NPTE exam. In some states, candidates must pass a state exam. State licensing authorities can be accessed through the FSBPT web site. In most states, continuing education is a requirement for license renewal.

The APTA's PTA Recognition Program recognizes physical therapist assistants with advanced proficiency in one or more work areas: musculoskeletal, neuromuscular, geriatric, pediatric, cardiovascular/pulmonary, and integumentary (skin). This distinction can be an asset in career advancement.

Work Responsibilities

Physical therapist assistants work one-on-one with patients to carry out a treatment plan. For example, a physical therapist assistant may help a patient do stretching exercises to increase muscle flexibility, monitoring the patient during the exercises and correcting any incorrect moves. Physical therapist assistants can assist patients with stretching and strengthening exercises, aerobic conditioning, and balance and coordination training. They may help patients learn to manage wheelchairs or crutches or to walk and run with prosthetic legs. Like physical therapists, physical therapist assistants may massage injured tissues, use interventions, or administer other therapies.

After each session with a patient, the physical therapist assistant writes notes on the patient's progress. Physical therapist assistants communicate regularly with physical therapists about patients' conditions, through progress notes or in person. They may work with the same patients from the beginning of their physical therapy to the end.

Physical therapist assistants work under the direction and supervision of a physical therapist. Although physical thera-pist assistants can perform many types of physical therapy, there are some procedures that only physical therapists can do or that a physical therapist assistant can perform only under a physical therapist's direct supervision. A physical therapist assistant's exact responsibilities vary by state.

Typical Tasks of a Physical Therapist Assistant
● Measure height, weight, length, and girth
● Use hip and knee flexion techniques
● Use static stretching techniques
● Conduct gait training
● Collect patient data
● Massage tissues to ease swelling
● Teach a patient to use a walker
● Update progress notes after a session

Personal Characteristics of Physical Therapist Assistants

Physical therapist assistants need empathy and good people skills. They may work with many different patients in

SPOTLIGHT ON SKILLS Typical Task: Use a Stretching Technique to Increase Flexibility

Position: Physical Therapist Assistant

Stretching exercises help increase muscle flexibility and improve range of motion. Some stretching exercises make use of the body's natural ability to relax muscles through the Golgi tendon organ, a set of nerve fibers between a muscle and a tendon. When a muscle is stretched for a prolonged period of time and tension builds in the tendon, the GTO fires and inhibits the tension, allowing the muscle to relax and elongate.

Before performing the stretch, the physical therapist assistant explains the procedure to the patient and has the patient assume the appropriate position.

First, the physical therapist assistant passively moves the limb to be stretched to the full range of motion. For example, if the hamstring muscles are to be stretched, the physical therapist assistant flexes the patient's leg to full hip flexion. *Flexion* is a bending motion that decreases the angle between bones.

Once the muscle's end range of motion is attained, the physical therapist assistant has the patient contract the hamstring muscles by extending the hip against the assistant, who holds the leg without allowing it to move. The contraction of the hamstring muscle increases tension in the muscle, which stimulates the GTO. The GTO causes the muscle to relax before it is moved to a new stretch position.

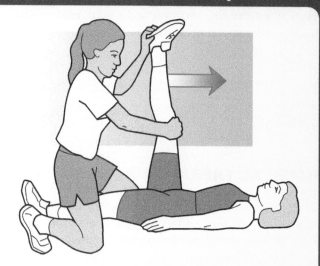

The PTA flexes the patient's leg to full hip flexion.

After the contraction, the physical therapist assistant instructs the patient to relax. Then he or she moves the limb to a new stretch point beyond the original starting point and holds the patient's leg in the new position for 10 to 15 seconds.

Without having the patient lower the leg, the process may be repeated three to five times. After the last sequence, the leg is lowered.

the course of a day and with the same patient for weeks or even months. Rehabilitation can be slow and challenging. The physical therapist assistant's ability to establish a rapport with patients; to understand their feelings; and to support, motivate, and encourage them can make a significant difference in their recovery.

People in this occupation should have good communication skills. They need to teach patients to do exercises and to use prostheses and other devices, and some of the instructions can be complicated. Physical therapist assistants also talk with patients about their condition and progress. In addition, they must be able to communicate clearly with physical therapists and other members of the health care team. In writing progress notes, physical therapist assistants must be clear and precise and include all necessary details.

Several other personal characteristics are important. Carrying out each patient's treatment plan and performing all the communication and documentation tasks associated with it require both good organizational skills and attention to detail. Finally, physical therapist assistants often work in a team environment, and therefore, they need good teamwork skills.

Employment Opportunities and Trends

In 2008, physical therapist assistants held nearly 63,800 jobs. Approximately 72 percent worked in hospitals or offices of other health practitioners. Others were in nursing care facilities, home health care services, and outpatient care centers.

The physical therapist assistant profession is a rapidly growing occupation. The BLS projects that employment will increase by 33 percent from 2008 to 2018, and 21,200 new jobs will be added. Reasons for growth are similar to those for physical therapists.

The BLS projects very good job opportunities for physical therapist assistants. As with physical therapists, physical therapist assistants will find especially good job prospects in acute hospitals, skilled nursing facilities, orthopedic settings, and rural areas.

Professional Organization

The APTA, described earlier in the chapter, represents physical therapist assistants, as well as physical therapists. Within the APTA, physical therapist assistants have their own representative organization, the National Assembly. Physical therapist assistants have continuing education opportunities, special interest groups, awards, a career planning center on the APTA web site, and other membership benefits.

✓ **CHECK POINT**

2 What personal characteristics should a physical therapist assistant have?

OCCUPATIONAL THERAPISTS

Occupational therapists help people to regain, develop, or master everyday skills so they can function better at work and in life. Their clients include people who have been injured, have a serious illness, have suffered a stroke, are depressed, have Alzheimer's disease, or have disabilities, such as cerebral palsy. Occupational therapists provide a wide range of treatments to help people be independent and to lead productive and satisfying lives. *U.S. News and World Report* included occupational therapy in its 50 Best Careers of 2010.

History of the Profession

Many people think that *occupational therapy* means "vocational training." However, occupational therapy is actually based on the idea that *purposeful activity* ("occupation") can help to protect and improve physical and mental health.

The foundation of early occupational therapy is *moral treatment*, an 18th- and 19th-century approach to treating mental illness. At that time, the common practice was to lock mental patients away, often in shackles and in isolation. Moral treatment focused on providing these patients with activities, exercise, and pleasant surroundings. In the late 19th and early 20th centuries, people in several different fields began to practice occupational therapy, not just for the mentally ill, but also for people who had disabilities or were recovering from illnesses. Among them was George Edward Barton, an architect who had been disabled and who had opened a school, workshop, and vocational bureau to help others recovering from injuries and illnesses.

In 1917, Barton invited five people who shared his ideas to form a professional association, the National Society for the Promotion of Occupational Therapy. These men and women all believed in the value of occupation, but they thought about it in different ways. Putting together their ideas, they defined *occupation* to include crafts, vocational work, healthful habits, and graded physical exercise. Four years later, the organization changed its name to the American Occupational Therapy Association (AOTA).

One of the AOTA's first actions was to convince the U.S. military to hire 5,000 reconstruction aides to provide occupational therapy for soldiers wounded in World War I. These women engaged their patients in metalworking, woodworking, and other crafts. While occupational therapists continued to work with patients with mental illness, they expanded the scope of their practice to include patients with physical disabilities and other medical conditions.

The growth of occupational therapy was strongly influenced by ties to organized medicine. Physicians, seeing the benefits of occupational therapy for their patients, provided support, and as early as 1935, the AMA joined the AOTA in accrediting occupational therapist training programs. During World War II, the profession grew rapidly, especially in physical rehabilitation of wounded soldiers. This emphasis on rehabilitation and the alignment to medical models continued after the war. Therapists began to specialize in certain areas, such as physical rehabilitation, mental health, or pediatric practice. Beginning in the 1960s, some leaders in the field called for the profession to return to its occupation-centered roots and a more holistic view of the patient. Opportunities arose with the Rehabilitation Act of 1973 and the independent living movement, which enabled people with disabilities to move more readily into the workplace, schools, and community life. At the same time, the creation of occupational science has resulted in a fuller definition of occupational therapy and given added credibility to occupation as a type of therapy. In 2002, the AOTA adopted a new practice framework that retains elements of medical models but puts occupation at the core of practice and asserts that the profession is continuing to evolve.

Education, Training, and Legal Requirements

Becoming an occupational therapist requires a minimum of a master's degree in occupational therapy from an accredited college or university. Programs are accredited by the Accreditation Council for Occupational Therapy Education (ACOTE). As of December 2009, 151 accredited institutions offered entry-level master's degree programs (including combined bachelor's and master's degree programs), and 4 offered entry-level doctoral programs. Combined programs, which accept students before they have finished their bachelor's degree, may be six-year programs or accelerated five-year (3 + 2) programs.

Although some schools offer undergraduate degrees in occupational therapy, students accepted into graduate OT programs may have had a variety of undergraduate majors, such as biology, psychology, sociology, anthropology, anatomy, and liberal arts. Educational programs have different prerequisites, so undergraduates should check the requirements for the particular programs that interest them. Paid or volunteer work in health care can help in gaining admission. Courses in biology, chemistry, physics, health, art, and the social sciences are also useful.

Students in an accredited master's degree program will take core classes in biological, physical, social, and behavioral sciences, either as prerequisites or as part of the program. Professional subjects include a general introduction to occupational therapy; skills in screening, evaluating, and referring clients; development of an intervention plan (a written treatment plan); interventions; accommodation to different work settings; management of occupational therapy services; research; and professional ethics, values, and responsibilities. Programs must also include at least 24 weeks of supervised fieldwork.

Compared to a master's degree program, doctoral programs offer additional instruction in a number of subjects, including clinical practice skills, administration, leadership, program and policy development, advocacy, education, and theory development.

Every state requires occupational therapists to be licensed. Applicants must graduate from an accredited program and pass a national certification exam administered by the National Board for Certification in Occupational Therapy (NBCOT). Specific licensing requirements vary by state and can be accessed through the AOTA web site. Generally, to sit for the national exam, a student must be a graduate of an accredited program. Upon passing the exam, the candidate is awarded the designation of Occupational Therapist Registered (OTR). Renewal, which can occur every three years, requires 36 Professional Development Units (PDUs), earned through continuing education, supervised fieldwork, or a variety of professional activities.

The AOTA offers board certification in several specific areas, including gerontology, mental health, pediatrics, and physical rehabilitation. It also gives specialty certification in driving and community mobility; environmental modification; feeding, eating, and swallowing; and low vision. Requirements include a professional degree or the equivalent; a set number of years of practice; and a certain number of hours working as an occupational therapist and performing occupational therapy services in the certification or specialty area. Certification must be renewed every five years.

Work Responsibilities

An occupational therapist's work typically begins with screening individuals to determine whether they need occupational therapy. For example, the therapist might test the motor skills and perceptual abilities of young children entering the school system to discover developmental delays or other problems that would affect learning.

Once a client has been identified as requiring therapy, the occupational therapist gathers and analyzes data about the client. These data may come from observation, the client's medical history, reports of past treatment, and interviews with clients and family members. The occupational therapist may administer tests to determine the client's abilities and identify areas needing improvement.

After analyzing the data, the occupational therapist develops an intervention plan. For clients with physical disabilities, the plan might begin with basic skills, such as bathing and dressing, and then progress to skills needed to be in school, find and keep a job, care for a home and children, and so forth. For clients with mental illness, skills might include budgeting, time management, shopping, doing housework, and using public transportation. Using a computer, working with a guide dog, making lists to aid recall, and exercising to improve coordination are a few examples of the many different types of activities occupational therapists teach. They also design, build, and modify equipment for clients, evaluate workplace areas, and plan job activities.

Once a plan is implemented, occupational therapists document the patient's progress and periodically reassess the plan and modify it if necessary. When treatment ends, occupational therapists prepare a written summary of the process and the outcomes, which may include recommendations for follow-up services.

Occupational therapists may focus their practice on particular age groups, such as children or older adults, or on a certain type of problem, such as mental illness. The AOTA has identified six broad areas of practice:
- Mental health
- Productive aging
- Children and youth
- Health and wellness
- Work and industry
- Rehabilitation, disability, and participation

Some newer specialties include teaching employees ergonomics, evaluating and training older drivers, and consulting on health and wellness.

Typical Tasks of an Occupational Therapist

- Screen for learning disabilities
- Perform muscle testing
- Test visual acuity
- Evaluate a home environment
- Develop an intervention plan
- Select assistive technology
- Teach a patient to dress
- Instruct in reading strategies
- Modify classroom equipment
- Write progress notes

Personal Characteristics of Occupational Therapists

In their interactions with clients, occupational therapists need good interpersonal skills, empathy, and patience. The ability to get along well with others will help them to establish positive working relationships with clients. Therapists can serve their clients better if they understand the challenges clients face and how difficult progress might be. Patience is another important quality because treatment can be a long process with improvements coming only in small increments.

Developing and managing intervention plans requires several other personal characteristics. Occupational therapists should be good observers to assess patients and environments accurately. Creativity is helpful in devising ways to adapt activities, equipment, and physical arrangements to a particular client's needs. Occupational therapists need strong organizational skills, and they must be detail-oriented. Working with clients and other health care professionals also calls for good communication skills.

Employment Opportunities and Trends

In 2008, occupational therapists held about 104,500 jobs. About 29 percent were in offices of health practitioners (including occupational therapists), 28 percent in hospitals, 13 percent in educational services, and 10 percent in nursing and residential care facilities. About 5 percent were in individual, family, community, and vocational rehabilitation services. Other employers included home health care services, outpatient care centers, community care facilities for senior citizens, and government agencies. A few occupational therapists were in private practice, treating clients referred by other health care professionals or providing contract or consulting services to nursing care facilities, schools, adult day care programs, and home health care agencies.

The BLS projects that employment of occupational therapists will increase by 26 percent between 2008 and 2018. As with physical therapists and physical therapist assistants, the needs of older adults will spur job growth. Another factor is medical advances that will enable more patients with critical problems to survive.

Occupational therapists will find good employment opportunities in many health care settings, particularly acute hospital, rehabilitation, and orthopedic settings, where older patients are most often treated. Hospitals will also hire them to work in outpatient rehabilitation programs. Schools will be a promising source of employment, as the school-age population increases and disabled

SPOTLIGHT ON SKILLS Typical Task: Perform a Functional Active Range-of-Motion Scan

Position: Occupational Therapist

A functional active range-of-motion scan is appropriate for patients who are wholly or partly unable to do activities important to them because of impairments in range of joint motion. For example, a person who cannot fully flex the elbow may have difficulty eating a meal independently. Measurement of joint range may be done actively or passively. *Active range of motion* is the amount of motion at a given joint achieved by a patient using his or her own strength.

First, the occupational therapist greets the patient and explains the procedure. To estimate the amount of active movement in certain motions, the therapist gives instructions to the patient, such as those in the table below. If the patient has a language barrier or cognitive problems, the therapist demonstrates the movements. The therapist observes for complete movements, symmetry of movements, and timing of movements.

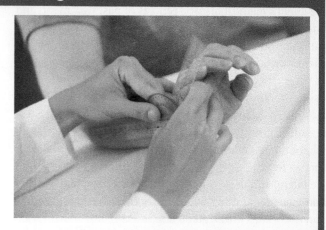

Therapist measuring wrist motion with goiniometer.

Motion*	Examples of Instruction
Shoulder flexion (sagittal plane)	Lift your arms straight up in front and reach toward the ceiling.
Shoulder abduction (frontal plane)	Move your arms out to the side. Now reach over your head.
Shoulder horizontal abduction and adduction (horizontal plane)	Raise your arms forward to shoulder height. Move each arm out to the side and then back again.
External rotation	Touch the back of your head with your hand.
Internal rotation	Touch the small of your back with your hand.
Elbow flexion and extension	Start with your arms straight down by your sides. Now bend your elbows so your hands touch your shoulders.
Forearm supination and pronation	With your arms at your sides and your elbows flexed to 90 degrees, rotate your forearms so the palms of your hands face the floor and then the ceiling.
Wrist flexion and extension	Move one of your wrists up and down. Now move the other one.
Finger flexion and extension	Make a fist; then spread your fingers out.
Finger opposition	Touch your thumb to the tip of each finger, one at a time.

students receive more services. Therapists with specialized knowledge in a treatment area will have better job prospects. Two newer practice areas are driver rehabilitation for older adults and ergonomic consulting.

Professional Organization

The AOTA is the professional organization for occupational therapists in the U.S. The organization has about 36,000 members, including occupational therapy assistants and students. Its goals are to represent the interests and concerns of its members and to improve the quality of occupational therapy services. The AOTA monitors legislation and regulations affecting the profession, working at both the federal and the state level. It advocates for the profession and operates a political action committee. In addition, it offers board and specialty certifications.

The AOTA provides a number of benefits for its members. Continuing education opportunities include online classes, self-paced clinical courses, articles, conference session webcasts, and audio conferences. The organization has several publications, including the *American Journal of Occupational Therapy*. The AOTA hosts an annual conference and has special interest sections in which members sharing professional interests can network. It also provides an online career center; professional development materials; and consumer education, awareness, and career materials.

The organization's philanthropic wing, the American Occupational Therapy Foundation, funds awards, honors, scholarships, and grants; operates Pi Theta Epsilon, a national honor society for occupational therapy students; and maintains the world's largest collection of occupational therapy literature.

✓ **CHECK POINT**

3 What are the typical work responsibilities of occupational therapists?

📷 **ZOOM IN**

Physical Therapy and Occupational Therapy

Physical therapy and occupational therapy sometimes overlap. For example, occupational therapists and physical therapists perform some of the same types of exercises, and both teach people to use wheelchairs and other assistive devices. However, the two fields are different in essential ways.

Physical therapy is the diagnosis and treatment of physical illnesses and injuries that limit people's ability to move and to perform activities in their daily lives. The goals of physical therapy are to restore function, improve mobility, relieve pain, and prevent or limit physical disabilities. Physical therapy focuses on regaining and improving movement and mobility.

The AOTA defines *occupational therapy* as "the therapeutic use of everyday life activities (occupations) . . . for the purpose of participation in roles and situations in home, school, workplace, community, and other settings." The goal of occupational therapy is to develop, regain, or improve the skills needed to live an independent, productive, and satisfying life. Occupational therapy focuses on acquiring and improving everyday life skills.

Physical therapists and occupational therapists frequently work together to achieve the best outcomes for their patients.

OCCUPATIONAL THERAPY ASSISTANTS

Occupational therapy assistants work under the direction of an occupational therapist to provide occupational therapy services. They perform many of the same tasks as occupational therapists. Their most common responsibility is working directly with clients, carrying out intervention plans.

History of the Profession

The occupational therapy assistant profession emerged in the 1950s. After World War II, there was a shortage of occupational therapists. At the same time, these professionals were taking on more rehabilitation work. In the early 1950s, the AOTA conducted a study to determine if support personnel could be trained to assist occupational therapists. The results showed that assistants could play a useful role, and in 1958, the AOTA began approving educational programs for assistants. Early programs were three months long and were often based in hospitals, but they later moved to community colleges and technical schools, and the period of study gradually lengthened.

The profession continues to develop. Occupational therapy assistants have moved from hospitals into other practice settings. More tasks and skills are demanded of them, and they've earned increased privileges and broader representation within AOTA.

Education, Training, and Legal Requirements

Occupational therapy assistants typically need a two-year associate's degree from an accredited occupational therapy assistant program. The ACOTE accredits these programs. As of 2009, there were 145 such programs in the U.S.

Students in an accredited occupational therapy assistant program will take core classes in biological, physical, social, and behavioral sciences, either as prerequisites or as part of the program. Professional subjects include a general introduction to occupational therapy; skills in screening and evaluation; assistance in the development of an intervention plan; occupational therapy skills; accommodation to different work settings; assistance in management of occupational therapy services; use of professional literature; and professional ethics, values, and responsibilities. Programs also must include at least 16 weeks of supervised fieldwork.

Students who are considering becoming occupational therapy assistants should take classes in biology and health and volunteer in nursing care facilities, occupational or physical therapists' offices, or other health care settings.

Forty states and the District of Columbia regulate occupational therapy assistants through licensure, certification, or registration. Requirements vary, so students interested in this occupation should check with the licensing board of the state where they would practice. In several states, continuing education is required for renewal.

Occupational therapy assistants can earn optional certification by passing a national exam administered by the NBCOT. The exam is required by some states, while others have their own exam. Generally, to sit for the national exam, a student must be a graduate of an accredited program. Upon passing the exam, a candidate is awarded the credential of Certified Occupational Therapy Assistant (COTA). Renewal, which can occur every three years, requires 36 PDUs earned through continuing education, supervised fieldwork, or a variety of professional activities.

The AOTA offers the same specialty certifications to occupational therapy assistants as to occupational therapists (driving and community mobility; environmental modification; feeding, eating, and swallowing; and low vision). Requirements include at least 2,000 hours of experience and at least 600 hours providing services to clients in the certification area. Certification must be renewed every five years.

Work Responsibilities

Occupational therapy assistants work under the supervision of an occupational therapist. Under state law, they can perform many of the same tasks as occupational therapists. When an occupational therapist delegates a task to an occupational therapy assistant, the expectation is that the same result will be obtained as if the occupational therapist were carrying out the task. The level of supervision varies from direct, daily contact to supervision on an as-needed basis. The occupational therapist is responsible for the overall safety and effectiveness of the service, however.

The most common role of occupational therapy assistants is carrying out intervention plans. For example, they may perform passive range of motion exercises on a patient recovering from a stroke, teach an older adult exercises for strengthening muscles, educate school personnel about the needs of a disabled student, convince a client with depression to participate in some social activity, or teach a patient with a spinal cord injury to do light meal preparation.

Occupational therapy assistants may be involved at every stage of occupational therapy service. They may administer tests during screening and assessment and help to evaluate client data. Occupational therapy assistants may also contribute ideas to intervention plans. In addition, they write progress notes and may handle periodic reassessments and final written summaries after treatment has ended.

Occupational therapy assistants can assume a wide variety of additional roles. For example, they may serve as directors of residential activities at nursing homes, group homes, or residential facilities. In these settings, they provide an ongoing program of activities intended to promote the health and well-being of residents. Occupational

---

SPOTLIGHT ON SKILLS Typical Task: Teach a Patient to Transfer into and out of a Bathtub After Hip Surgery

Position: Occupational Therapist Assistant

Following a hip fracture and surgery, patients have certain restrictions on weight bearing and hip movement. Occupational therapy assistants teach these patients to complete daily activities safely, in accordance with the physician's orders and the patient's physical therapy progress.

To Get into the Bathtub

The occupational therapy assistant begins with the patient standing with feet parallel to the tub, with the injured leg next to the bathtub. Body weight is shifted to the uninjured leg , and the patient holds a grab-assist rail for support. The assistant instructs the patient to raise the injured leg with the knee bent and then extend the hip forward to allow the leg to go over the edge of the bathtub.

Once the injured leg is over the tub edge, the assistant instructs the patient to extend that knee and place the foot on the non-skid bath mat inside the tub. When the patient's balance is secure, the patient transfers body weight to the injured leg, lifts the other leg over the edge of the tub, and places that foot on the bath mat.

To Get out of the Bathtub

The occupational therapy assistant instructs the patient to stand with feet parallel to the side of the tub. As with getting into the tub, the patient should move the injured leg first. The rest of the procedure is the same as the procedure used in getting into the tub.

therapy assistants may lead exercise and stress reduction programs, organize and manage adaptive driving programs for people with disabilities, and teach pain management techniques to groups of patients.

Typical Tasks of an Occupational Therapy Assistant

- Screen for visual perception
- Test touch awareness
- Evaluate client data
- Select therapy activities to fit a client's needs
- Develop energy-saving strategies for a client with multiple sclerosis
- Convince a patient with mental illness to try clay modeling
- Write progress notes
- Devise memory aids for a patient with dementia
- Teach a patient with arthritis to use assistive devices in dressing
- Play ball games with a child with Down syndrome to improve hand-eye coordination

Personal Characteristics of Occupational Therapy Assistants

Like occupational therapists, occupational therapy assistants need good people skills, empathy, and patience. They may see many patients in the course of a day. They need to be able to get along with different people, understand them as individuals, and appreciate the challenges they're facing. Occupational therapy assistants also need patience to work with clients through long courses of therapy, even when progress is slow.

Occupational therapists delegate important responsibilities to occupational therapy assistants, so assistants need to be responsible. They need to follow the intervention plans; work diligently with clients; and keep regular, accurate, detailed progress notes. If occupational therapy assistants have any concerns about a patient's progress or care, they need to tell the occupational therapist in a timely manner.

A good therapist-assistant relationship is a partnership, with both parties knowing and accepting their roles. Occupational therapy assistants need to be willing to take direction and should be comfortable working as part of a team.

Employment Opportunities and Trends

In 2008, occupational therapy assistants held about 26,600 jobs. Three-quarters were in hospitals, offices of other health practitioners, and nursing care facilities. Most of the rest were in community care facilities for older people, home health care services, individual and family services, and government agencies. From 2008 to 2018, nearly 8,000 new jobs will be available.

The BLS projects that employment of occupational therapy assistants will grow by 30 percent from 2009 to 2018. Some of the same factors that will spur growth in the occupations already described in this chapter will stimulate demand for occupational therapy assistants as well. In addition, occupational therapists will increasingly employ occupational therapy assistants to help control costs. Another source of jobs will be the growing school-age population and federal laws requiring funding for education for people with disabilities.

Job prospects for occupational therapy assistants will be very good from 2008 to 2018. Assistants with experience in an occupational therapy office or other health care facility will have the best job opportunities.

Professional Organization

The AOTA, which represents occupational therapists, also represents occupational therapy assistants. The organization offers many of the same benefits to occupational therapy assistants, including specialty certifications and continuing education opportunities. The AOTA web site has a page devoted to occupational therapy assistant resources. These include links to educational programs for occupational therapy assistants who want to become occupational therapists; an occupational therapy assistant listserv; leadership development tools; and awards.

 CHECK POINT

4 What education and training are needed to become an occupational therapy assistant?

RESPIRATORY THERAPISTS

Respiratory therapy is the treatment of patients with breathing and other cardiopulmonary disorders, and it is delivered by respiratory therapists. Respiratory therapists evaluate, treat, and manage these patients. They work with patients of all ages, from premature infants with congenital heart-valve defects to older adults with chronic lung disease. Working in all hospital areas, respiratory therapists assess patients with many different conditions and are a vital part of emergency response teams.

History of the Profession

The first widely successful efforts in using oxygen to treat patients with cardiopulmonary disorders occurred in the

20th century. This success was made possible by a succession of technological developments, including the oxygen tent, nasal catheter, oxygen mask, and ventilator. For many years, nurses administered oxygen therapy. After World War II, however, oxygen therapy equipment became increasingly complex, and orderlies who transported the heavy cylinders of oxygen were trained to give oxygen therapy. They came to be known as oxygen orderlies. These orderlies became skilled at operating and maintaining the equipment, and they developed specialized knowledge of gas therapy through their interactions with physicians.

When oxygen orderlies set out to establish themselves as a separate profession, they had strong support from physicians. In 1946, a group of oxygen orderlies, physicians, and nurses met in Chicago and formed the first professional respiratory care organization, the Inhalation Therapy Association. It eventually became a national organization, the American Association for Respiratory Care (AARC).

In 1954, the New York State Society of Anesthesiologists and the Medical Society of the State of New York formed a joint committee to set guidelines for schools of inhalation therapy. The AMA formally approved the guidelines in 1962. The guidelines have since been revised several times, most recently in 2009.

Education, Training, and Legal Requirements

At least an associate's degree is needed to be a respiratory therapist. A bachelor's or master's degree may help in advancement. Colleges and universities, medical schools, vocational-technical institutes, and the armed forces offer training programs. Most programs award an associate's or bachelor's degree and prepare students for jobs as advanced respiratory therapists. A few associate degree programs prepare students for entry-level jobs. As of November 2009, the Commission on Accreditation for Respiratory Care (CoARC) had accredited 378 advanced-level programs and 27 entry-level programs. Ten programs featured an added specialty of polysomnography, the diagnosis of sleep disorders, which often involve respiratory conditions.

Respiratory therapy programs include courses in these areas:
- General education, such as communication, social and behavioral sciences, math, and computer science
- Basic sciences related to respiratory care, such as cardiopulmonary anatomy and physiology, chemistry, microbiology, and pharmacology
- Specific respiratory care content areas, such as assessment of cardiopulmonary status, airway management, lung inflation therapy, and alternate site care (hospice, for example)

Students choosing to specialize in polysomnography must take additional classes in polysomnographic technology.

Students interested in becoming respiratory therapists should take classes in health, biology, chemistry, math, and physics.

In all states except Alaska and Hawaii, respiratory therapists must be licensed. Licenses must be renewed every one to three years, and renewal usually requires continuing education. Licensing generally follows the certification requirements of the National Board of Respiratory Care (NBRC).

The NBRC awards four respiratory therapist credentials. Each credential requires an exam, and an RRT credential requires two exams.
- **Certified Registered Therapist (CRT).** To take the exam, candidates must have graduated from an accredited entry-level or advanced program, be within 30 days of graduation, or be enrolled in an accredited program and have a special certificate of completion from their educational institution upon completion of specific coursework.
- **Registered Respiratory Therapist (RRT).** Candidates must have graduated from an accredited advanced program or be enrolled in such a program and have a special certificate of completion. Other requirements exist for practicing CRTs with clinical experience and graduates of bachelor's degree programs not in respiratory care. This credential is usually required for supervisory positions and intensive care specialties.
- **Neonatal/Pediatric Specialist (CRT-NPS or RRT-NPS).** Candidates must be RRTs, or they must be CRTs with one year of clinical experience caring for newborns or children.
- **Sleep Disorders Testing and Therapeutic Intervention Respiratory Care Specialist (CRT-SDS or RRT-SDS).** Candidates must have completed an accredited program with a sleep add-on track or be practicing with six months' (CRT) or three months' (RRT) full-time clinical experience following certification in a sleep diagnostics and treatment setting under a physician's supervision.

Respiratory therapists must renew their credentials annually and, within a five-year period, complete 30 hours of continuing education, retake and pass the credentialing exam, or pass another credentialing exam.

Work Responsibilities

Respiratory therapists provide respiratory care for patients with heart and lung disorders. They perform diagnostic tests and evaluate the results; help prepare and modify a patient's plan of care; administer oxygen, aerosol medications, and many other types of treatment; monitor the patient's responses; and manage the patient's overall respiratory care. While they work under a physician's direction, respiratory therapists are in charge of respiratory care diagnostic procedures and therapeutic treatments, and they exercise a high degree of independent judgment.

Respiratory therapists typically begin their careers in a hospital. In these settings, they practice their clinical skills, see patients of all ages with many different illnesses, and become adept at using many types of respiratory tools and equipment. They can specialize in a number of areas, including continuing and long-term care, critical care, diagnostics, disease management, home care, pediatrics, and pulmonary rehabilitation.

- In continuing and long-term care, respiratory therapists work with mostly older adults who have serious respiratory problems, including chronic diseases like emphysema. They continually assess their patients, modify the plan of care as needed, and work with other health care professionals.
- In critical care, respiratory therapists care for critically ill patients in an intensive care unit. They also work on surface and air transport teams or as part of rapid-response teams in hospitals. These therapists must be constantly alert to potentially life-threatening changes in a patient's condition.
- In diagnostics, respiratory therapists perform a wide range of tests to help in the diagnosis of symptoms,

such as shortness of breath. They begin by interviewing the patient and conducting an abbreviated physical exam. Tests include breathing tests, blood tests, and exercise tests. The most common test is spirometry, a test in which a patient breathes into a machine, the *spirometer*, to test lung function. Respiratory therapists may also assist in a bronchoscopy, in which a flexible tube is inserted into the nose or mouth and through the trachea (windpipe) to view the lungs. Polysomnography is one of the fastest-growing diagnostic specialties.

- In disease management, respiratory therapists help patients with chronic pulmonary conditions to live with their diseases and manage their care. Patient education is an important part of this specialty.
- In home care, respiratory therapists have a wide variety of responsibilities. Working with patients with chronic pulmonary conditions, they bring equipment to patients' homes, teach them and their families to use it, maintain the equipment, and make emergency visits if it breaks down. They also perform inhalation therapies, keep the primary care physician informed about the patient's condition, and coordinate with different agencies. Therapists working in this specialty have a good degree of independence.
- In pediatrics, respiratory therapists work with children of all ages, from newborns in a neonatal ICU to teenagers with asthma. They perform tests, provide treatment, and teach patients and their families how to use medicines and equipment.

SPOTLIGHT ON SKILLS Typical Task: Perform Closed Tracheal Suction

Position: Respiratory Therapist

Patients having difficulty breathing may be on a *ventilator*, a machine that helps them breathe. Air from the ventilator flows through a tube inserted into the trachea through the nose or mouth (an endotracheal tube) or through a hole made in the neck (a tracheostomy tube). A common task of respiratory therapists is to clear a patient's airways of secretions that interfere with breathing. A closed tracheal suction system (see photo) can make this process easier and reduce patient complications. With this system, the patient can stay connected to the ventilator during suctioning.

First, the respiratory therapist greets and identifies the patient and explains the procedure. After putting on gloves, the therapist attaches the control valve of the suction system to the connection tubing. He or she presses

the suction control valve while setting the suction pressure to the desired level.

Next, the therapist connects the suction system's T-piece to the ventilator breathing circuit and the patient's endotracheal or tracheostomy tube. The therapist advances the catheter through the tube and into the patient's windpipe and the passageways connecting it to the lungs. If necessary, the therapist gently retracts the catheter sleeve as he or she advances the catheter.

While continuing to hold the T-piece and control valve, the respiratory therapist applies intermittent suction and withdraws the catheter until it reaches its fully extended length in the sleeve.

The closed suction system is changed every 24 hours to minimize the risk of infection.

- In pulmonary rehabilitation, respiratory therapists help patients learn to live with chronic respiratory diseases. They teach special breathing techniques, relaxation techniques, and stress management; instruct patients about medication use; and develop exercise routines that patients can use at home.

Respiratory therapists work in several other areas, including smoking cessation counseling, disease prevention, case management, education, and research.

Typical Tasks of a Respiratory Therapist

- Do a pulmonary function test
- Set up a mechanical ventilator
- Monitor arterial blood gases
- Insert an airway tube
- Obtain and analyze oxygenation level of arterial blood
- Administer aerosol medications
- Perform chest physiotherapy, a variety of techniques used to eliminate secretions, re-expand lung tissue, and promote efficient use of respiratory muscles
- Check lung sounds

Personal Characteristics of Respiratory Therapists

Difficulty breathing can be frightening for patients. Respiratory therapists should have a calm, reassuring manner and should be sensitive to their patients' needs.

Good communication and teamwork skills are also important. People in this occupation spend a lot of time educating patients and their families. Respiratory therapists need to be able to explain procedures and the use of medicines and equipment. Since they work as members of a health care team, they must be able to communicate clearly (and know when to communicate) with other health care professionals and work effectively on teams.

Flexibility is essential. For example, if a treatment isn't working, respiratory therapists need to be ready to try other treatments. In the case of life-threatening situations, they must adapt quickly and efficiently.

The equipment and procedures used in respiratory therapy change constantly. Respiratory therapists should enjoy learning and should be committed to keeping up with the latest information in their field.

Employment Opportunities and Trends

In 2008, respiratory therapists held nearly 106,000 jobs. About 81 percent were in hospitals, mostly in the respiratory care, anesthesiology, and pulmonary medicine departments. Most other jobs were in the offices of physicians or other health care practitioners, companies that rent respiratory equipment to consumers, nursing care facilities, temporary employment agencies, and home health care services.

According to the BLS, employment in this occupation will grow by 21 percent from 2008 to 2018. The BLS identifies three factors driving this demand. One is the increasing number of middle-aged and older adults, who are more prone to respiratory illnesses and cardiopulmonary diseases. A second is advances in inhalable medications and treatment for premature babies, lung transplant patients, and accident and heart attack victims. A third factor is the movement of respiratory therapists into case management, prevention, emergency care, and early detection of pulmonary disorders.

Job prospects will be very good, especially for therapists with a bachelor's degree and certification, skills in cardiopulmonary care, or experience working with infants.

Professional Organization

Founded in 1947, the American Association for Respiratory Care (AARC) is dedicated to the professional development of respiratory therapists, the science and practice of respiratory care, and the promotion of good lung health. The organization works with federal, state, and local government on legislative and regulatory issues and sends representatives to various agencies, including accrediting, credentialing, and medical agencies.

The AARC accredits continuing education programs and offers members several means of earning continuing education credits. The organization also provides a number of ways for its more than 47,000 members to associate professionally. It sponsors an annual congress and a three-day summer meeting, as well as meetings, workshops, and seminars. Specialty sections and roundtables allow members to network with others who share their professional interests.

Additional benefits include a variety of print publications and online resources, including a professional journal; an online career section; discounts on credentialing exams; and a message board for urgent professional questions. The American Respiratory Care Foundation funds awards, fellowships, research grants, publications, and educational activities and also sponsors conferences.

CHECK POINT

5 What are the typical work responsibilities of respiratory therapists?

MASSAGE THERAPISTS

Massage therapy is the manipulation of muscles and other soft tissues to maintain or improve health. According to the AMA, massage has been proven to help lower blood pressure, relax muscles, and improve range of motion, among other benefits. Massage can speed recovery after an injury and can lead to more complete recovery. It is also used to reduce stress and promote general health. The following statistics are from the American Massage Therapy Association (AMTA):

- According to consumer surveys, more than one in five adult Americans have at least one massage each year.
- Nearly one in four has used massage therapy at least once for pain relief.
- Some 69 percent of massage therapists receive referrals from health care professionals.

History of the Profession

Massage dates to ancient cultures around the world, where it was a means of healing and maintaining and improving health. It was practiced in China, India, Egypt, and many other societies. In Greece, where the Olympic Games started, athletes received massages before and after competitions. Hippocrates used massage to treat sprains, dislocations, and other medical problems and recommended that all physicians be trained in it. In Greek and Roman society, where many people went to public baths, massage was part of the bathing process.

In the U.S., massage gained popularity in the mid-1800s, when Dr. George H. Taylor incorporated it into his natural approach to health care. Taylor promoted Swedish massage, a method of massage developed by Per Henrik Ling. A physical educator, Ling developed a system of exercise that included massage to promote health and treat joint and muscle problems. Massage was also popularized by 19th-century physician John Harvey Kellogg, who started the health food movement.

In the first half of the 20th century, massage in the U.S. declined, due in part to scientific and technological advances in medical treatment. However, people continued to practice massage, and the first professional organization in the U.S. was founded in 1927.

Massage regained popularity in the U.S. in the 1960s and 1970s, especially among athletes and members of the counterculture movement, which sought holistic approaches to health that treated both mind and body. It also began to gain acceptance in the medical community as clinical studies proved its effectiveness. Today, massage in the U.S. includes methods from both Eastern traditions—Indian Aryuvedic massage, for example—and Western traditions, such as Swedish massage.

Massage therapy is a developing profession. The AMA recognizes it as a health care career, and it is profiled at the National Center for Complementary and Alternative Medicine of the National Institutes of Health. Several agencies accredit massage training programs, and most states regulate the practice. There are nationally recognized exams, and therapists can earn a nationally recognized credential from the AMTA.

Education, Training, and Legal Requirements

Most massage therapists complete a formal training program. These programs comprise both academic classes and hands-on practice. Coursework typically includes anatomy, physiology, the study of organs and tissues, *kinesiology* (the study of human movement in terms of anatomy and mechanics), pathology, massage theory and application, business, and ethics. Some programs focus on particular modalities, such as Swedish massage. In massage, a *modality* is a set of therapies that tend to use similar movements or strokes to reach a similar goal.

Massage therapy programs are generally approved by a state board and sometimes by an independent accrediting agency, such as the Commission on Massage Therapy Accreditation (COMTA). Programs are typically offered by private and public postsecondary schools and take 500 hours or more to complete. Applicants generally need a high school diploma or the equivalent. The AMTA suggests that students considering this occupation take classes in science, especially anatomy and physiology; psychology; business; and the humanities.

According to the AMTA, 44 states and the District of Columbia had laws regulating massage therapy as of May 2009, and four additional states had introduced or were drafting legislation. Idaho and Wyoming were the exceptions. Most regulating states require therapists to complete a state-approved formal education program and pass a national certification exam or a state exam. Some also require continuing education. People interested in becoming massage therapists should check information on licensing, required exams, certification, and accreditation in their state.

After training, many massage therapists choose to take one of two national certification exams administered by the National Certification Board for Therapeutic Massage and Bodywork (NCBTMB). To sit for an exam, candidates must have completed or, in some circumstances, be enrolled in a formal NCBTMB-approved training program or submit a portfolio of training experience for review. Certification must be renewed every four years. For renewal, applicants must have completed 200 hours of work experience and 48 hours of continuing education during the four-year period. The Federation of State Massage Therapy Boards (FSMTB) also offers a national licensing exam, with no eligibility requirements. Both organizations' exams are used by many states for licensure.

Work Responsibilities

Massage therapists press, rub, or otherwise manipulate the muscles and other soft tissues of the body. They usually use their hands and fingers but may use their forearms, elbows, and feet. Goals of massage therapy are usually to relax the soft tissues, increase circulation in the massaged areas, warm those tissues, and reduce pain.

In performing their work, massage therapists use different strokes that vary in direction, length of skin covered, rate, rhythm, and pressure. They can draw on a number of different modalities, such as deep-tissue or trigger point/neuromuscular massage, and many types of massage within those modalities, such as acupressure, Shiatsu, and sports massage. Acupressure, for example, requires the use of firm fingertip pressure at certain points in the body. Most massage therapists are skilled at several types of massage.

Massage therapists usually work by appointment. A session can last from five or ten minutes to two hours, depending on the client's needs and physical condition. It usually begins with an interview or client history. The therapist needs to ensure that the client's medical condition warrants massage and that the client's needs match the type of massage the therapist offers.

A massage is performed with the client lying on a massage table or sitting on a chair or stool. To help create a relaxed atmosphere, massage therapists often use dim lighting, fragrances, or soft music. Frequently, lotions or oils are used, and therapists may also apply ice or compresses, use an infrared lamp or whirlpool bath, or employ other tools. A massage therapist observes a client's responses during the massage, listens to any feedback; and then adjusts the actions appropriately. A session can include recommendations for self-care, such as stretches, heat applications, and rest.

Other duties of massage therapists include scheduling sessions, developing treatment plans, and maintaining client records. Therapists who own their own businesses perform business-related tasks, such as marketing, ordering supplies and equipment, billing, and maintaining financial records. Massage therapists often work independently, but they may also be part of a health care team,

SPOTLIGHT ON SKILLS Typical Task: Perform Skin Rolling

Position: Massage Therapist

Skin rolling is a common massage technique used to treat restrictions in the *fascia*—fibrous tissue that underlies the skin—or muscle. A *restriction*, sometimes called an adhesion, can form as a result of injury or chronic patterns of muscular tension. Adhesions can limit movement and create pain. Massage therapists try to break up the adhesions and restore space to the tissues.

The massage therapist begins by determining the direction of the restriction, or the direction in which tissues do not move easily. To do so, he or she pushes the tissue forward and backward and to the left and right.

Next, the therapist grasps the tissue in a roll, pulling it slightly in the direction of ease, toward the client's spine. Then, gently changing direction, he or she pulls the rolled tissue into the direction of restriction.

The massage therapist slowly transports the rolled tissue in the direction of restriction by gathering the tissue between fingers and thumbs, keeping the roll of tissue elevated. The skin roll continues for several inches or until the restriction diminishes.

The therapist releases the roll of tissue carefully. Next, he or she applies a resting stroke, lightly resting relaxed hands on the area for several seconds without moving. This stroke allows tissues to reorganize. Then the therapist returns to the original contact area and reevaluates the tissue for restriction.

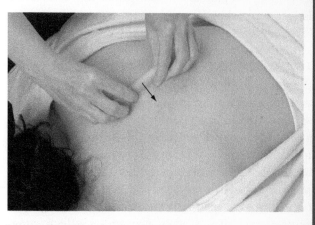

Massage therapist performing skin rolling.

working with chiropractors, physical therapists, physicians, and others.

> **Typical Tasks of a Massage Therapist**
>
> ● Do a client assessment
> ● Prepare an initial treatment plan
> ● Position the client's body
> ● Use a relaxation technique
> ● Give a simple chair massage
> ● Assist a draped client off the table
> ● Provide a contrast foot bath (using hot and cold water)
> ● Provide a pre-event massage for a long-distance runner

Personal Characteristics of Massage Therapists

Two important personal characteristics for massage therapists are sociability and empathy. For many massage therapists, building a solid, loyal client base is essential for success. A friendly, outgoing personality and the ability to get along well with different people will help a therapist gain and keep clients and get referrals. As in many health care occupations, being able to understand a client's feelings and the pain a client may be experiencing helps a massage therapist to deliver better care.

Massage therapists also need good communication skills. They need to be able to explain treatment plans or techniques to clients, give them directions, and discuss methods of self-care. Massage therapists may also need to communicate with physical therapists and other health care professionals regarding a patient's condition and needs. Self-employed therapists need good verbal and writing skills to promote their businesses.

Employment Opportunities and Trends

In 2008, massage therapists held about 122,400 jobs. About 57 percent were self-employed, most owning their own businesses and the rest working as independent contractors. For many more therapists, massage therapy is a secondary source of income. Some massage therapists worked in salons, spas, and other businesses offering personal care services. Others worked in physicians' and chiropractors' offices; fitness and recreational sports centers; and hotels. Jobs were available throughout the country, but cities, resorts, and upscale tourist areas had the most opportunities.

The BLS predicts that from 2008 to 2018, employment of message therapists will increase by 19 percent, with 23,200 new jobs added. Job growth will result from more people learning about the benefits of massage therapy; the formation of more spas and massage clinic franchises; and companies adopting seated massage as a workplace benefit. Two other factors that should lead to job growth are the growing number of older adults in nursing homes or assisted living facilities, many of whom can benefit from massage, and the increasing demand for massage therapy among young adults.

In states that regulate massage therapists, graduates of formal training programs who pass a national exam will have an edge in securing employment. Most new therapists should expect to work part-time in spas, hotels, hospitals, physical therapy centers, and other businesses until they build a pool of clients. Because referrals are an important source of work, networking increases job opportunities. State and local chapters of professional associations provide opportunities for networking and making job contacts.

Professional Organizations

The massage therapy profession has two major professional associations. Formed in 1943, the AMTA represents more than 58,000 massage therapists. Its goals include advancing the profession and establishing massage therapy as essential to good health and a complement to other types of therapy. The AMTA monitors state and federal legislation, maintains guidelines for practice standards, and operates the COMTA. The organization's national convention and its national and state conferences and workshops offer opportunities for continuing education and networking. Online training is available at the AMTA web site, and members can also order home study courses and DVDs. Other benefits include a job bank, enrollment in a national massage therapist locator service, liability coverage, and a professional journal. The AMTA Foundation funds massage therapy research, community service, and scholarships.

Founded in 1987, Associated Bodyworks & Massage Professionals (ABMP) is the largest massage therapy association in the U.S., with more than 70,000 members. The ABMP seeks to advance its members' professional interests in many ways. These include providing advice about career paths and starting and building a practice; advocating on professional regulation; and keeping members informed about major issues and educational developments. It offers members a wide variety of benefits related to professional development and business growth. These include professional publications, free and discounted continuing education courses, an online referral service, liability insurance, and a database of educational articles.

CHECK POINT

6 What are the typical work responsibilities of massage therapists?

Chapter Wrap-Up

Don't forget to visit thePoint companion website for additional study resources!

CHAPTER HIGHLIGHTS

- Physical therapists help people who have been injured, are in pain, or suffer from some other disabling condition. They develop treatment plans to restore function, improve mobility, relieve pain, or prevent or limit permanent physical disabilities. They may work directly with patients to carry out the treatment plans or delegate that work to physical therapist assistants. In either case, they monitor patients' progress during treatment.
- Working under the direction of a physical therapist, physical therapist assistants carry out treatment plans, working individually with patients. They may assist patients with stretching and strengthening exercises, aerobic conditioning, and balance and coordination training. They may also help patients learn to manage wheelchairs or crutches or to walk and run with prosthetic legs.
- Occupational therapists help people to regain, develop, or master everyday skills so they can function better at work and in life. Their clients include people who have been injured, have a serious illness, have suffered a stroke, are depressed, have Alzheimer's disease, or have disabilities, such as cerebral palsy. Occupational therapy is based on the idea that purposeful activity ("occupation") can help to protect and improve physical and mental health. Occupational therapists screen individuals to determine whether they need occupational therapy and then develop intervention plans for those who do.
- Occupational therapy assistants work under the direction of an occupational therapist, performing many of the same tasks as occupational therapists. Their most common responsibility is working directly with clients, carrying out intervention plans.
- Respiratory therapists evaluate, treat, and manage patients with breathing and other cardiopulmonary disorders. They are often among the first workers to assess a patient and are a vital part of emergency response teams. While they work under a physician's direction, respiratory therapists are in charge of respiratory care diagnostic procedures and therapeutic treatments, and they exercise a high degree of independent judgment.
- Massage therapists manipulate muscles and other soft tissues to maintain or improve health. The goals of massage therapy are to relax the soft tissues, increase circulation in the massaged areas, warm those tissues, and reduce pain. Massage can speed recovery after an injury and is also used to reduce stress and promote general health.

REVIEW QUESTIONS

Matching

1. _____ Develop an intervention plan to improve everyday life skills
2. _____ Perform a pulmonary function test
3. _____ Teach a patient to walk with a prosthetic leg
4. _____ Use acupressure
5. _____ Develop a treatment plan to restore function

   a. Physical therapist   **b.** Physical therapist assistant   **c.** Occupational therapist
   d. Respiratory therapist   **e.** Massage therapist

Multiple Choice

6. The entry-level educational requirement for physical therapists will probably soon be _____.
   - **a.** an associate's degree
   - **b.** a bachelor's degree
   - **c.** a master's degree
   - **d.** a doctoral degree

7. Physical therapist assistants _____.
   - **a.** carry out treatment plans
   - **b.** can perform all physical therapy procedures
   - **c.** usually work without supervision
   - **d.** develop intervention plans

8. Which person is *least* likely to be an occupational therapist's client?
   - **a.** An older adult driver
   - **b.** A teenager with asthma
   - **c.** A man who lost a hand in a car accident
   - **d.** A woman who's depressed

9. Which statement about occupational therapy assistants is NOT true?
   - **a.** They typically have an associate's degree.
   - **b.** They can perform many of the same tasks as occupational therapists.
   - **c.** Their most common role is to gather client data.
   - **d.** They are represented by the American Occupational Therapy Association.

10. Which is NOT a typical job responsibility of respiratory therapists?
    - **a.** Perform range-of-motion exercises on a patient
    - **b.** Monitor patients in an ICU
    - **c.** Educate patients and families
    - **d.** Be part of a rapid-response team

Completion

11. _____ is the restoration, after a disease or injury, of the ability to function in a normal or near-normal manner.

12. In occupational therapy, another term for *occupation* is _____ activity.

13. The most common type of test performed by a respiratory therapist is _____, a test in which a patient breathes into a machine to test lung function.

14. _____ is the manipulation of muscles and other soft tissues to maintain or improve health.

15. _____, the diagnosis of sleep disorders, is one of the fastest-growing specialties in respiratory therapy.

Short Answer

16. Compare and contrast the work of physical therapists and occupational therapists.

    _____

    _____

17. Compare and contrast the typical job responsibilities of physical therapist assistants and occupational therapy assistants.

    _____

    _____

18. Describe three areas in which respiratory therapists can specialize.

    _____

    _____

19. What kind of preparation is needed to become a massage therapist?

_____

_____

20. All the occupations described in this chapter are growing rapidly. What is a common factor driving demand for these occupations?

_____

_____

INVESTIGATE IT

1. During the 1940s and 1950s, physical therapists were in demand to care for victims of polio epidemics. These polio epidemics changed many facets of American society. Research one of these topics about the epidemics and their legacy:
   - Public perceptions about polio
   - How patients were rehabilitated
   - Living with polio, including the use of assistive devices
   - The iron lung
   - The March of Dimes
   - The Salk and Sabin vaccines

   The following web site will be a useful starting point:
   http://americanhistory.si.edu/polio/index.htm ("Whatever Happened to Polio?")

2. Respiratory therapists may specialize in sleep disorders testing. What happens during a sleep study? Why do physicians order it? What types of disorders do sleep studies reveal? This web site may be a good place to start:
   http://www.nhlbi.nih.gov/health/dci/Diseases/slpst/slpst_whatis.html ("What are Sleep Studies?")

3. Nintendo's Wii video game system has become a useful and popular physical therapy tool. Find a newspaper or magazine article about "Wiihab." Use the search term _Wii physical therapy_ to find helpful Internet resources.

RECOMMENDED READING

American Association for Respiratory Care. Career: Resources to help you begin or further your career in respiratory care. Available at: http://www.aarc.org/career. (Good career videos)

A Career in Massage Therapy: Healthcare Specialty. Chicago: Institute for Career Research; 2007.

Get Physical. _Career World._ April/May 2009;37(6):26–29.

Lais T. _Career Diary of a Physical Therapist._ Washington: Garth Gardner; 2008.

Precin P, ed. _Surviving 9/11: Impact and Experiences of Occupational Therapy Practitioners._ New York: Routledge; 2004.

U.S. News Staff. Occupational Therapist. In: The 50 Best Careers of 2010. _U.S. News & World Report_ [serial online]. Posted December 28, 2009. Available at: http://www.usnews.com/money/careers/articles/2009/12/28/occupational-therapist-2.html.

U.S. News Staff. Physical Therapist. In: The 50 Best Careers of 2010. _U.S. News & World Report_ [serial online]. Posted December 28, 2009. Available at: http://www.usnews.com/money/careers/articles/2009/12/28/physical-therapist.html.

U.S. News Staff. Physical Therapist Assistant. In: The 50 Best Careers of 2010. _U.S. News & World Report_ [serial online]. Posted December 28, 2009. Available at: http://www.usnews.com/money/careers/articles/2009/12/28/physical-therapist-assistant.html.

Weeks Z. _Opportunities in Occupational Therapy Careers._ New York: McGraw-Hill; 2006.

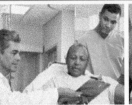
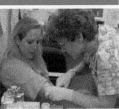

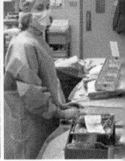

Health Information and Administration

CHAPTER OBJECTIVES

After careful study of this chapter, you should be able to:

* State the education, training, and legal requirements for becoming a health information technician, health information coder, and medical transcriptionist.

* Describe the typical work responsibilities in each profession.

* List desirable personal characteristics of health information technicians, health information coders, and medical transcriptionists.

* Identify employment opportunities and key trends for these occupations.

KEY TERMS

morbidity   mortality

People in health information careers don't work directly with patients. Instead, they work with documentation of client care. Health information technicians, health information coders, and medical transcriptionists provide accurate, timely patient documents in an easy-to-use form. Health care providers use that data in caring for patients, and insurers use it in evaluating claims for coverage.

HEALTH INFORMATION TECHNICIANS

Even the most routine physical exam generates paperwork regarding a patient's health—a history, a summary of the visit, and possibly lab test results. Health information technicians gather these and the many other documents that chronicle a patient's health, ensure they're complete, and assemble them into well-organized medical records that can be located and read easily.

History of the Profession

The occupation of health information technician evolved from that of medical record administrator. The first medical record administrator was Grace Whiting Myers, appointed in 1897 at Massachusetts General Hospital to organize patient care records from the preceding 80 years. Soon other hospitals began hiring such workers.

In 1928, the American College of Surgeons established an organization to improve the standards for medical records kept in hospitals and other health care institutions. Myers was its founder and president. This organization, the Association of Record Librarians of North America, went through several name changes that reflected the evolution of medical records occupations. In 1991, it became the American Health Information Management Association (AHIMA).

In 1934, the association set the first official standards for training programs, and at its request, the AMA began approving programs in 1942. This responsibility later shifted to the Commission on Accreditation for Health Informatics and Information Management Education (CAHIIM). The number of approved programs grew slowly, however. In 1953, partly to get more qualified personnel into the workforce, standards were established for programs to train a lower-level worker, the medical record technician. The first technician training programs were based in hospitals.

Medical record technicians have evolved into health information technicians. According to the AHIMA, the terminology change from *medical record* to *health information* reflects the expansion of this occupation's role from dealing with a single hospital medical record to managing health information that represents all of a patient's care.

Education, Training, and Legal Requirements

Most entry-level health information technicians have an associate's degree. Previous classes in biology, health, chemistry, math, and computer science help improve students' chances of admission into a program.

As of January 2010, there were 225 CAHIIM-accredited associate's degree programs in health information technology. The curriculum of an accredited program must meet or exceed the course content described in a set of entry-level competencies and knowledge clusters developed by the AHIMA. The program must include general education courses, professional education courses, and practicum experiences.

Students complete general education courses in these areas:
- Oral and written communication skills
- Social and behavioral sciences
- Humanities
- General sciences
- Math
- Computer literacy (hardware, software, operating systems, and file structure)
- Microcomputer applications (word processing, spreadsheet, database, and graphics and presentation)

Professional education courses cover the following areas:
- Biomedical sciences (anatomy, physiology, medical terminology, pathophysiology, and pharmacotherapy)
- Health data structure, content, and standards
- Health care information requirements and standards (for example, types and content of health records and documentation requirements)
- Clinical classification systems (coding)
- Reimbursement (billing)
- Health care statistics and research
- Quality management and performance improvement
- Health care delivery systems
- Privacy, confidentiality, legal issues, and ethical issues
- Information and communication technologies
- Data storage and retrieval
- Data security and health care information systems
- Organizational resources (such as teams and committees)

Technicians may seek the Registered Health Information Technician (RHIT) credential awarded by the AHIMA. This credential confers a strong advantage in the job market and typically leads to a higher salary. Candidates must complete a two-year associate's degree program accredited by the CAHIIM and pass a written exam. Several categories of students can take their certifying exam while still enrolled in school. To maintain their certification, RHITs must complete 20 continuing education units every two years, 80 percent of which must be in health information management.

Work Responsibilities

Health information technicians are responsible for ensuring that medical charts are complete, well-organized, and easily located. They gather patient notes, test results, consultation reports, diagnoses, treatment plans, and other documents related to patient care. If a document hasn't been received or information is missing, the technician contacts the appropriate health care provider for it. The health information technician also checks that the appropriate information from these documents is entered into the computer. For a new patient, the technician sets up a chart and organizes the contents so that information can be found quickly. For a returning patient, the technician puts new documents in the proper place in the file and places the file in the appropriate location so that it can be retrieved when needed. In carrying out these responsibilities, the health care technician follows the rules and procedures of the health care facility to ensure that records are consistent.

Health information technicians follow the law to ensure that patient information remains confidential and is released only to persons and agencies authorized to have it. The files they work with may be paper or electronic ones. Health information technicians may also process business and government forms and prepare admission and discharge documents.

When medical staff and administrators need patient data to evaluate care, help control costs, or do research studies, they often turn to health information technicians. Because of their familiarity with chart organization and contents and computer functions, health information technicians can readily assemble the data. They may also perform some data analysis.

The duties of health information technicians vary with the size of the facility. In small facilities, experienced workers may be charged with managing the department. In medium-size or large facilities, workers might specialize in a certain aspect of health care information or supervise health information clerks and transcriptionists. In large facilities, information departments are managed by a health information administrator.

Health information technicians can specialize in two areas: coding, discussed in the next section of this chapter, and cancer registry. Cancer registrars maintain databases of cancer patients. They review patient records and assign codes for the diagnosis and treatment of different types of cancer and some benign tumors. They also follow up with patients yearly, tracking their treatment, survival, and recovery. Physicians and public health administrators use this data to determine survival rates, assess treatments, and identify candidates for clinical trials.

Typical Tasks of a Health Information Technician

- Create a paper or electronic chart
- Add documents to a patient's chart
- Make written entries in a chart
- File and retrieve charts according to facility rules
- Release authorized data from a chart
- Compute health care statistics

Personal Characteristics of Health Information Technicians

Health information technicians need good organizational skills. They must file items in the correct place in patients' charts in a timely manner, because another professional could need the same records at any time. Especially in an emergency, any member of the health care team must be able to find a patient's file immediately.

SPOTLIGHT ON SKILLS Typical Task: Create a Patient's Electronic Chart

Position: Health Information Technician

A medical record, or chart, must be created for each new patient. Increasingly, electronic medical records are replacing paper charts.

To create an electronic medical record, a health information technician enters the patient's information into a computer using the facility's electronic charting software. Then the technician scans any existing paper records into the patient's computer file. These may include personal information and medical history forms that the patient completed, test results, past medical records, and a copy of the patient's living will or power of attorney for health care (if any). The technician then disposes of the scanned paper records according to the facility's policy.

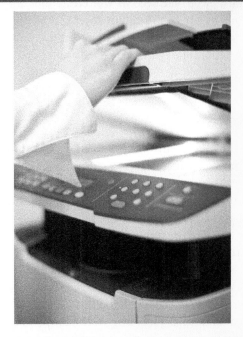

One step in creating an electronic medical record is scanning any existing paper records.

Being detail-oriented is another important quality. Health information technicians should be skilled at scanning test results, patient information sheets, and other documents and be able to note when information is misfiled, incomplete, or missing. Technicians must also be careful about entering the appropriate patient data into the computer. Accuracy in entering patient data into a computer and in filing is vital.

Finally, health information technicians need good communication skills. They communicate with other health care professionals and facilities and with insurance companies to obtain and send patient information. For this reason, they need to be able to speak clearly and directly and listen carefully.

Employment Opportunities and Trends

In 2008, health information technicians held about 172,500 jobs, nearly 40 percent of which were in hospitals. About 26 percent were in physicians' offices. Other significant sources of jobs were nursing care facilities, government agencies, outpatient care centers, home health care services, and administrative support services.

The BLS projects that jobs for health information technicians will increase by 20 percent from 2008 to 2018. More medical tests, treatments, and procedures will be performed. As the older population grows, the demand for medical services will increase. In addition, the shift toward electronic records will create jobs and new responsibilities for health information technicians. The BLS predicts especially good job prospects for technicians who have a thorough knowledge of technology and computer software.

Professional Organization

The AHIMA represents more than 53,000 health information professionals, including managers, technicians, and coders. Its services to the profession include accreditation; professional development of members through certification, continuing education, and other means; and advocacy before Congress, federal agencies, and other organizations.

The association offers members a number of benefits. State organizations provide opportunities for continuing education and networking. The AHIMA hosts a national convention and holds meetings, workshops, and conferences. Members receive a professional journal and other publications. Student members have access to a mentoring program. The AHIMA maintains a fellowship program

to recognize members who have made important contributions to the profession and a foundation that funds research and scholarships.

The organization offers a variety of online services, including training through quizzes, courses, webinars, audio seminars, and remote conferences. Members also have access to a career center and career counseling. They can join communities of practice, communicating with other members on topics of mutual interest via chat, email, and threaded discussions. Other online features include a library and an advocacy tool that facilitates member participation. Students can find general information about health information professions, including career paths, on the AHIMA's web site.

CHECK POINT

1 What personal characteristics should a health information technician have?

HEALTH INFORMATION CODERS

Health information coders assign numerical codes to identify patients' diseases, injuries, and conditions and the services they receive. These codes are used by insurance companies to determine whether, and how much, to pay for these services. They're also used by government agencies and the World Health Organization to gather data about common diseases, causes of death, and epidemic diseases.

History of the Profession

Medical coding dates to 17th-century London, when a wave of the bubonic plague, or black death, spread through the city. The city began to publish the London Bills of Mortality, listing the number of plague deaths and their locations. (In this usage, mortality refers to the incidence of death in a population.) The city continued to publish the bills of mortality, listing numbers of deaths, their causes, and age groups, until the early 19th century.

The recording of mortality data advanced significantly with the work of William Farr, a British medical statistician of the 1800s. Among other accomplishments, Farr worked actively for a uniform system of classification to be used by all nations. In 1855, the second International Statistical Conference adopted a classification system based partly on Farr's work. The system was the basis of the International List of Causes of Death adopted by the conference's successor, the International Statistical Institute, in 1893 and updated periodically afterwards.

Over time, it became apparent that the system for classifying diseases needed to be revised to meet the needs of many different organizations, including insurance companies, hospitals, and the military. Countries also needed morbidity statistics, not just mortality statistics. Morbidity—the incidence of disease in a population—includes all diseases, not just those that are fatal. Morbidity statistics allow countries to assess their progress in health care and the control of disease. At its creation in 1948, the World Health Organization (WHO) assumed responsibility for a revised list of diseases that incorporated both mortality and morbidity. WHO produces a manual generally known as the International Classification of Diseases (ICD), which is updated regularly. The U.S. has been using a clinical modification (CM) of the ninth revision, known as ICD-9-CM, for medical coding for insurance and other purposes. In 2013, it is switching to ICD-10 standards.

Education, Training, and Legal Requirements

Most coders learn their skills on the job. A few schools offer associate's degree programs in coding, but these programs are not accredited. Coding is included in an accredited health information technician associate's degree program. Certificate programs are also available. As of January 2010, the AHIMA had approved 36 coding certificate programs.

An approved coding program includes coursework in biomedical sciences, information technology, health information management, and clinical classification systems. Classes must cover a set of knowledge clusters and prepare students to perform a set of job competencies. Students take classes in anatomy and physiology, medical terminology, computer software applications in health care, health information management, coding, and other topics. They also receive at least 40 hours of practical coding experience.

Coders with certification earn more—according to a 2009 survey, an average of $7,000 more—than coders without it. The American Academy of Professional Coders (AAPC) awards five general credentials and 19 specialty credentials in areas like dermatology or pediatrics. For all credentials, candidates must pass an exam. The Certified Professional Coder (CPC), Certified Professional Coder–Hospital (CPC-H), and Certified Professional Coder–Payer (CPC-P) credentials also require two years of medical coding experience. Candidates who pass the exam for one of these three credentials, but who do not yet have the coding experience, earn apprentice status. Renewal requires various numbers of hours of continuing education.

The AHIMA offers entry-level coders the Certified Coding Associate (CCA) credential. Candidates must have a high school diploma or the equivalent and pass an exam. The AHIMA suggests, but does not require, that candidates have at least six months' experience in coding or have graduated from an AHIMA-approved coding certificate program or another formal coding training program. For renewal, candidates must complete ten continuing education units and two annual coding self-reviews every two years.

A number of other certifications are available. The AHIMA awards two advanced credentials. The Board of Medical Specialty Coding and the Professional Association of Healthcare Coding Specialists (PAHCS) also offer certification in specialty areas.

Codes are updated every year. In addition, the change from the ICD-9 coding system to the ICD-10 coding system in 2013 will introduce many more codes and will make coding more complex (see the "Newsreel" feature later in this chapter). It's easy to see why health information coders need continuing professional education.

Work Responsibilities

In the simplest terms, medical coding is assigning a number to a patient's medical problem or treatment. In practice, this process is anything but simple. This complex process requires accuracy, medical knowledge, and careful attention to detail. There are more than 10,000 codes, and codes are added, deleted, and revised each year. Accurate coding is essential to ensure that medical conditions are reported properly and that health care providers are properly compensated for their services.

Health information coders work with two types of codes:

- **Diagnostic codes.** There is a diagnostic code for nearly every illness, injury, or condition a patient may have.
- **Procedure codes.** The main source of these codes is the fourth edition of *Current Procedural Terminology*, or CPT-4 for short, produced by the AMA. This book and its annual updates provide codes for nearly every treatment, test, and service a patient might receive. For patients on Medicare, there's another set of codes called the Healthcare Common Procedure Coding System, or HCPCS.

The combination of diagnostic and procedure codes tells the insurance company what the patient's medical problem was and what type of care the patient received.

Coding typically involves combing through a patient's medical record, carefully reading documents to determine what the diagnosis was and which services were rendered, and using code books to select the right codes. According to a 2009 AAPC survey, the majority of coders worked from paper medical records and the next biggest group from paper billing forms. Just eight percent used an electronic medical records program.

A new trend in coding is computer-assisted coding, or CAC. CAC software scans transcription files and other electronic health care documents for key words and phrases and their locations and uses this information to predict the appropriate codes. This software has proven useful for routine coding and performing simple and repetitive coding tasks, relieving coders of these duties. Even with CAC systems, however, a coder is needed to check the software's work and do more advanced coding.

Codes can be very detailed. For example, for a patient who has broken a leg in a fall, the ICD-9-CM lists more than two dozen codes for describing how the fall occurred. The "Spotlight on Skills" describes what coding is like and how complicated it can be.

Typical Tasks of a Health Information Coder

- Assign diagnostic codes using ICD-9-CM or ICD-10 (after 2013)
- Assign procedure codes using CPT or HCPCS
- Monitor patient records for changes and update codes appropriately
- Investigate health plan payment denials
- Assist in using coded data for reporting
- Coordinate coding information with other health care professionals

SPOTLIGHT ON SKILLS Typical Task: Use the ICD-9-CM to Code Patient Diagnoses (Physician's Office)

Position: Health Information Coder

In assigning diagnostic codes, health information coders use the ICD-9-CM, which comes in three volumes. Volumes 1 and 2 contain the diagnosis codes that identify the reasons for physicians' services. These services will be billed by the physician's office, no matter where the services took place. Hospitals use Volume 3 to bill for the services and care they provide.

The health information coder begins by choosing the main term (the main diagnosis) in the diagnostic statement. Then he or she locates this main term in the alphabetic index of Volume 2. The term will be followed by a diagnostic code. An example is shown below:

Bleeding (see also Hemorrhage) 459.0

The coder carefully reads all of the information under the main term and follows appropriate references to other parts of the volume (such as the reference in the example above to *hemorrhage*). The coder reviews the list of indented terms—called *subterms*—that appear under the main term and selects the appropriate one. Use of subterms, which have codes of their own, helps to make the diagnosis more precise. For example, a few of the subterms under the main term *bleeding* are *anal* (code 569.3), *capillary* (code 448.9), and *ear* (code 388.69).

Next, the coder confirms the code selected from the index by looking it up in Volume 1, where he or she also looks to see if it is necessary to add any fourth or fifth digits. These digits, which follow the decimal point, make a diagnosis more specific. For example, fourth digits divide

the diagnosis of herpes simplex (054) into genital herpes (054.1), herpetic gingivostomatitis (cold sore on mouth) (054.2), and other categories. Fifth digits make diagnoses even more precise, allowing for the coding of such conditions as herpetic ulceration of vulva (054.12) or herpes simplex dermatitis of eyelid (054.41).

Once the code is complete, the coder places it on the claim form. He or she codes the reason for the visit first and then codes any other conditions that affect the patient's treatment for that visit. The coder must make sure that an ICD-9 code is linked to each service or procedure provided to the patient. Services for situations other than disease or injury, such as follow-up care, are identified with a distinct set of codes, called V-codes, also listed in Volume 1.

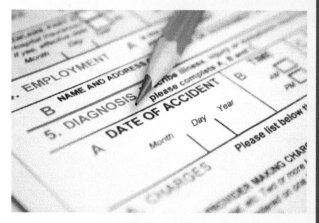

Medical coders assign diagnostic codes and are a key part of the health insurance claims process.

Personal Characteristics of Health Information Coders

Like health information technicians, health information coders must be detail-oriented and accurate. Determining the correct codes can take time and effort, and the stakes are high. If a code is incorrect or incomplete, a patient's insurance coverage may be affected, and payment may be reduced, delayed, or denied. Health information coders need persistence and diligence to work carefully through code books and different sources of patient information to determine the proper code. They also need to enjoy working alone and must be able to work without constant supervision.

Health information coders need to be good learners. Medical codes are updated constantly, so it is essential that coders keep abreast of changes.

Employment Opportunities and Trends

The BLS includes coders in the category of medical records and health information technicians, who held about 172,500 jobs in 2008. Hospitals employed nearly 40 percent of these workers, and physicians' offices about 26 percent. Nursing care facilities, government agencies, outpatient care centers, home health care services, and administrative support services were the other main sources of jobs. The 2009 AAPC survey found that coders who worked for physicians, groups, ambulatory surgery centers, outpatient departments, and payers enjoy especially good careers.

The Bureau projects that job growth for this group will be 20 percent from 2008 to 2018. Coders will benefit from rapid growth in the number of medical tests, treatments, and procedures that will be performed.

Professional Organizations

Health information coders are represented by a number of professional organizations. Three of these are the AHIMA (described earlier in the chapter), the AAPC, and the Professional Association of Healthcare Coding Specialists (PAHCS).

Founded in 1988, the AAPC has more than 86,000 members. Its goals are to provide education and certification for physician-based medical coders and to raise medical coding standards through certification, continuing education, and other means. Local chapters, national and regional conferences, and private online forums provide networking opportunities. To assist with professional development, the organization offers job tools and listings, résumé postings, and externship and consulting opportunities. Continuing education is available through local chapter seminars and meetings, workshops, audio conferences, national and regional conferences, and association publications. The group also offers its members extensive resources on coding, both in print and online.

The PAHCS strives to improve coders' professional capabilities, mainly through specialty certification. Members can attend a national conference, receive a quarterly newsletter, and have scholarship opportunities available to them. Through a members-only online network, they can share information and solve coding problems.

CHECK POINT

2 What education and training are needed to become a health information coder?

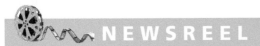

NEWSREEL

The Switch to ICD-10

On October 1, 2013, the U.S. Centers for Medicare and Medicaid Services (CMS)—and, in effect, the entire U.S. health care industry—is switching from the ICD-9 coding system, in use since 1979, to ICD-10. ICD-10 has been in use in WHO member states since 1994. It has been used in the U.S. to classify mortality data from death certificates since 1999.

ICD-10 has a number of advantages over ICD-9. With the newer system, diseases can be described in greater detail and with greater specificity. ICD-10 has more than 155,000 codes, in comparison with ICD-9's 17,000. ICD-10 also has room for growth. Its codes can contain 3–7 characters, whereas ICD-9 codes can contain just 3–5.

In addition, ICD-10 allows for combined diagnosis and symptom codes, reducing the number of codes needed to fully describe a condition.

The WHO approves all changes to the ICD. Such changes must conform to ICD code conventions so that data can be shared meaningfully across countries. The U.S. version of ICD-10 has two parts: ICD-10-CM, the clinical modification of WHO's ICD-10 diagnostic coding system, and ICD-10-PCS (for *Procedure Coding System*), a system for coding procedures. ICD-10-CM was developed through the work of a technical advisory panel and consultation with physician groups, clinical coders, and others and was field-tested in 2003. ICD-10-PCS was developed for inpatient hospital procedures.

MEDICAL TRANSCRIPTIONISTS

Medical transcriptionists transcribe recordings dictated by physicians and other health care professionals into medical reports and other documents. By producing accurate, readable documents in a timely manner, medical transcriptionists play an important role in ensuring that patients receive the proper care.

History of the Profession

Medical transcription dates almost to the beginning of medicine. The earliest physicians began the practice of recording information about their patients. Until the beginning of the 20th century, physicians made their own notes, for the most part. As medical research increasingly required that medical data be standardized, physicians began dictating their notes to medical stenographers, who would record them in shorthand and type them later.

As dictation equipment was developed, physicians began to dictate into recorders. Tapes went to secretaries for transcription or, increasingly, to specialized medical transcriptionists. By the 1960s, hospitals were staffing transcribing departments with large numbers of medical transcriptionists. Since then, to control costs, transcribing has been increasingly outsourced to medical transcription services in the U.S. and, more recently, overseas.

In 1978, the Association for Healthcare Documentation Integrity (AHDI) was formed to represent the growing profession. The AHDI has contributed strongly to the development of medical transcription as a profession by creating and maintaining a model curriculum, accrediting educational programs, and establishing a voluntary certification system. In 1999, the U.S. Department of Labor granted medical transcriptionists their own job classification.

Over time, the medical transcriptionist's role has evolved. As medical specialties become more complex and new tests and procedures are developed, medical transcriptionists need an increasingly stronger background in medical terminology and concepts to do their work accurately. Medical transcriptionists have always checked, corrected, and formatted their work. With speech recognition technology (which directly translates speech into a word-processed document) and overseas outsourcing, the demand for their editing services is stronger than ever.

Education, Training, and Legal Requirements

While formal education isn't always required, employers prefer to hire transcriptionists with postsecondary training in medical transcription. Medical transcriptionists can complete a two-year associate's degree or a one-year certificate program. Some transcriptionists, especially those already familiar with medical terminology from another job, need only refresher courses and training.

The Approval Committee for Certificate Programs, a joint committee of the AHDI and the AHIMA, offers optional approval for medical transcription programs. As of January 2010, 22 programs had been approved. Many are online or self-study programs. Students in an accredited program will take classes in these content areas and meet a set of competencies for each class:

- Medical style and grammar
- Medical knowledge (medical terminology, anatomy and physiology, concepts of disease, and pharmacology and laboratory medicine)
- Medical transcription technology
- Medicolegal aspects of the health care record
- Medical transcription practice

Students must also transcribe 2,400 minutes of actual health care provider-generated dictation.

The AHDI awards two credentials and a designation for medical transcriptionists:

- Registered Medical Transcriptionist (RMT)
- Certified Medical Transcriptionist (CMT)
- AHDI Fellow (AHDI-F)

The RMT and the CMT credentials are awarded based on a set of AHDI-established job skills, with the CMT indicating a higher level of skills. For both credentials, candidates must pass an exam. For the CMT, the candidate must have at least two years of work experience as a transcriptionist in an acute care setting before taking the exam. Both credentials are valid for three years. To renew, applicants must complete an online course and take an exam (RMT) or earn 30 hours of continuing education credit (CMT).

To become an AHDI Fellow, applicants must earn at least 50 points in the five years before applying. These points must be earned in at least five of eight categories: membership, professional meeting attendance, leadership, publications and presentations, mentorship, civic activities, awards, and credentials.

Graduates of an AHDI-approved program who earn the RMT credential can apply to the Registered Apprenticeship Program. This program offers entry-level medical transcriptionists on-the-job training and technical instruction.

Work Responsibilities

Medical transcriptionists listen to dictated recordings and interpret and transcribe them into medical reports and other documents. Consultation notes, patient histories, discharge summaries, diagnostic imaging studies, emergency room notes, correspondence, and autopsy reports are examples of the many types of documents that medical transcriptionists produce.

Typically, medical transcriptionists use special transcribing equipment and word processing software. In addition to traditional cassette tapes and digital recordings, many transcriptionists now receive transcriptions over the Internet. In medical transcription departments, transcriptions may be streamed over a network to handheld personal computers or PDAs.

Medical transcriptionists must be fast and accurate typists. More important, though, is a good working knowledge of anatomy, physiology, medical terms, diagnostic procedures, pharmacology, and treatments. This knowledge helps transcriptionists detect errors and inconsistencies and bring them to the dictator's attention. As they type, medical transcriptionists check the spelling and meaning of any medical terms they don't know, using standard print and online reference sources. They edit the text to turn incomplete sentences into sentences, and they replace abbreviations with full forms of words or phrases so that the document will be easier to read.

After typing documents, transcriptionists proofread, edit, and format them. When a document is properly formatted and error-free, the transcriptionist sends it to the health care professional who dictated it for a final check. That professional signs the document or sends it back for correction. Finished documents become part of a patient's permanent medical file.

Two trends in medical transcription are the outsourcing of transcription to foreign countries and the use of speech recognition technology. Both trends have generated jobs for medical transcriptionists in proofreading, editing, and formatting documents.

Typical Tasks of a Medical Transcriptionist

- Download and send files
- Transcribe a medical report
- Use references to check medical terms
- Edit, proofread, and format a transcription
- Query the professional who dictated a document
- Make corrections marked by the professional who dictated a document

Personal Characteristics of Medical Transcriptionists

Medical transcriptionists need good listening skills in order to transcribe dictation accurately and at a reasonable

---

 SPOTLIGHT ON SKILLS Typical Task: Proofread and Edit a Transcription

Position: Medical Transcriptionist

After transcribing a document, the medical transcriptionist proofreads and edits it. A few steps taken during the transcription process can help prevent errors and make proofreading and editing easier. For instance, the speed on the transcribing equipment should be set so that the transcriptionist can type at a comfortable pace, since typing rapidly can result in more errors. It is also good to stop when encountering an unfamiliar word and consult a reference source.

After transcribing, the transcriptionist allows a little time to pass before proofreading and editing, if possible. Having a break makes it more likely that errors will be caught.

When ready to edit, the transcriptionist begins by running a spell checker. Then he or she proofreads carefully, checking and editing for sense, clarity, grammar, punctuation, missing words, and mistyped words that get past the spell checker (*car* instead of *care*, for example). If the transcriptionist is unsure about an item, he or she doesn't guess, but flags it for the person who dictated the document to check. When a transcript has a lot of corrections, the transcriptionist may run the spell checker again and then proofread again, if needed.

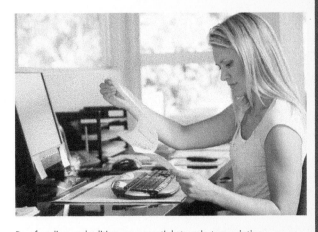

Proofreading and editing are essential steps in transcription.

pace and to understand dictation that's rushed, garbled, or spoken by someone with an accent. Several other personal characteristics are also desirable. The ability to focus closely on their work is helpful. Medical transcriptionists should also have a commitment to accuracy. Written communication skills, attention to detail, and analytical skills are important. Transcriptionists also need to enjoy working alone and must be able to work without constant supervision.

Employment Opportunities and Trends

In 2008, medical transcriptionists held about 105,200 jobs. About a third worked in hospitals, and nearly a quarter worked in physicians' offices. Other employers included business support services, medical and diagnostic laboratories, outpatient care centers, and offices of physical, occupational, and speech therapists and audiologists.

The BLS projects that employment of medical transcriptionists will grow by 11 percent from 2008 to 2018. The increasing number of older adults, who generally require more physicians' visits, tests, treatments, and procedures, increases documentation. As well, during the coming transition to electronic documentation, more medical transcriptionists will be needed to modify patient records, edit documents from speech recognition systems, and identify discrepancies in records.

Two alternatives to using in-house medical transcriptionists are outsourcing medical transcription to other countries, such as India and Pakistan, and using speech recognition systems. The BLS does not predict that these resources will replace well-trained U.S. transcriptionists. In fact, medical transcriptionists will continue to be needed to edit reports from both of these sources for accuracy.

Medical transcriptionists can expect good job opportunities, especially if they're certified. From 2008 to 2018, about 12,000 new jobs will be created. Hospitals will continue to be the main employer, but the BLS projects rapid job growth in physicians' offices, especially large group practices, because of the increasing demand for standardized records.

Professional Organization

The AHDI sets standards for the education and practice of medical transcriptionists, represents the profession before legislative and regulatory agencies, and seeks to educate these agencies and the public about the role of medical transcriptionists in patient safety and risk management. As noted earlier, the organization also awards professional certifications and a fellowship designation.

The AHDI offers members a number of benefits. These include a professional journal and several other publications. Its web site provides a job bank and other career resources, an online mentoring program for student or postgraduate members, and continuing education opportunities through online courses, webinars, and audio seminars. Members can also earn continuing education credits by reading articles, some with quizzes, in AHDI publications.

The group's annual convention and state chapter meetings provide networking opportunities. Members can also interact through an online professional practices network, introducing topics and posting and discussing questions, ideas, and concerns.

✓ **CHECK POINT**

3 What are the typical work responsibilities of medical transcriptionists?

Don't forget to visit thePoint. companion website for additional study resources!

CHAPTER HIGHLIGHTS

- Health information technicians gather and organize patient notes, test results, consultation reports, diagnoses, treatment plans, and other documents related to patient care. They are responsible for ensuring that paper or electronic documents are complete, well-organized, and easily located. Health information technicians may specialize in coding or cancer registry.
- Health information coders assign numerical codes to describe patients' medical problems and the services they receive. These codes are used by insurance companies to determine whether, and how much, to pay for these services. They're also used by government agencies and the World Health Organization to gather data about common diseases, causes of death, and epidemic diseases.
- Medical transcriptionists listen to dictated recordings made by health care professionals and transcribe them into medical reports and other documents. Finished documents become part of a patient's permanent medical file.

REVIEW QUESTIONS

Matching

1. _____ CAC software
2. _____ Speech recognition software
3. _____ ICD-9-CM
4. _____ Medical dictionary
5. _____ CPT-4

   a. Coding injuries, illnesses, or conditions   **b.** Coding treatments, tests, and services
   c. Suggesting codes   **d.** Proofreading dictation   **e.** Transcribing dictation

Multiple Choice

6. For which occupation is a background in anatomy, physiology, and medical terminology needed?
   - **a.** health information technician
   - **b.** health information coder
   - **c.** medical transcriptionist
   - **d.** all of the above

7. Which occupation requires proofreading and editing skills?
   - **a.** health information technician
   - **b.** health information coder
   - **c.** medical transcriptionist
   - **d.** all of the above

8. Which occupation requires good listening skills?
   - **a.** health information technician
   - **b.** health information coder
   - **c.** medical transcriptionist
   - **d.** all of the above

9. Which occupation checks patient documents for completeness?
   - **a.** health information technician
   - **b.** health information coder
   - **c.** medical transcriptionist
   - **d.** all of the above

10. Which occupation will see a significant change in 2013 when a new rule goes into effect?
    - **a.** health information technician
    - **b.** health information coder
    - **c.** medical transcriptionist
    - **d.** all of the above

Completion

11. Health information technicians can specialize in two areas: _____ and _____.

12. _____ means the incidence of death in a population.

13. _____ is the incidence of disease in a population.

14. Health information coders work with two types of codes: _____ codes and _____ codes.

15. The _____ approves all changes to the International Classification of Diseases (ICD).

Short Answer

16. Compare and contrast the typical education requirements for the occupations described in this chapter.

    _____

    _____

17. Why do health information coders need continuing education?

    _____

    _____

18. How has the trend toward outsourcing medical transcription to foreign countries affected the employment of medical transcriptionists? What effect may this trend have in the future?

    _____

    _____

19. What are the typical work responsibilities of health information technicians?

    _____

    _____

20. What are the primary uses of medical coding?

    _____

    _____

INVESTIGATE IT

1. Collecting morbidity and mortality statistics is part of the field of public health. Visit the "What Is Public Health?" web site at http://www.whatispublichealth.org and answer these questions:
   a. What is public health?
   b. What impact has it had?
   c. How do public health professionals use disease statistics?

2. Presidents George W. Bush and Barack Obama both made the switch to electronic health records a priority. Yet the majority of physicians' offices don't use them, and few hospitals do. Why is it taking so long for medical records in the U.S. to go electronic? What are the pros and cons of this change? Do an online search for "*electronic medical records*" to find a discussion of this issue.

3. Think about the health care careers you have learned about in the last seven chapters. Choose one that especially appeals to you. Write a paragraph explaining why. Then find ten facts about workers in this career. Make use of the lists of professional associations and

"Recommended Reading" resources at the end of each chapter and do some research of your own, through personal contact or on the Internet.

RECOMMENDED READING

Burns S. *You're a Medical What!?! A Lighthearted Peek into the World of a Medical Transcriptionist.* Bandon, OR: Robert Reed; 2008.

Mason PD. Medical Transcriptionist. [Health Professions Network website]. Last updated March 2005. Available at: http://www.healthpronet.org/ahp_month/03_05.html.

Morton G. *How to Become a Medical Transcriptionist.* Spring Valley, CA: Teresa Castaldi; 2006.

Wolgemuth L. Beyond Nursing: Hot Healthcare Jobs. *U.S. News & World Report.* July 1, 2009:45.

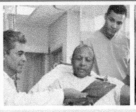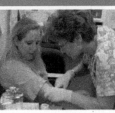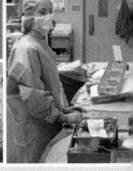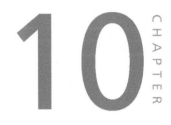

Personal Qualities and Professional Skills for Success

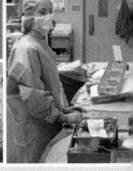

10 CHAPTER

CHAPTER OBJECTIVES

After careful study of this chapter, you should be able to:

✳ Recognize personal qualities and skills that are important for health care providers.

✳ List professional attributes that benefit all health care workers.

✳ Describe values and how they are developed.

✳ Identify important values in health care.

✳ Detect stress producers.

✳ Use strategies to cope with stress.

✳ Explain the role of nutrition, exercise, and sleep in maintaining a healthy body.

✳ Recognize the importance of good health behaviors, personal hygiene, and grooming for the health care professional.

KEY TERMS

altruism (AL-true-i-zəm)
autonomy (aw-TON-ă-mē)

competence
human dignity
initiative

public service
stress
time management

value
value system

To find success in any given career, you must possess the qualities essential to your chosen vocation. Professions in health care demand a unique combination of personal and professional qualities. Your attitude and integrity directly affect your ability to perform your work. And while medical skills are central to a majority of health-related jobs, other skills, like time management, are often just as important. Health care professionals should possess certain values, such as a respect for human dignity. They also need to take care of their own health and learn effective ways to cope with stress.

PERSONAL ATTRIBUTES

Most people begin to develop their personality early in life. This includes their interests, behavioral patterns, emotional responses, and attitudes. People's personalities affect how they cope with different situations, both at home and at work. Personal qualities and skills that are important for any successful health care professional include:

- **Enthusiasm.** When you're enthusiastic about your career, it shows in everything that you do. Professionals who are passionate about their work take an active interest in their duties and strive to do the best job possible. Enthusiasm for the care of others is essential in any health care career. Health care professionals with enthusiasm are more likely to do a better job.

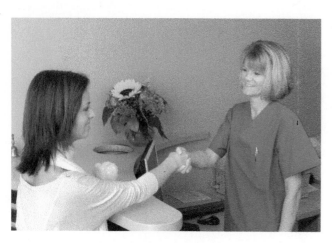

Enthusiasm is one of many important personal attributes for health care workers.

- **Optimism.** A positive attitude shapes a person's outlook on different situations and affects job performance. When your attitude remains bright, cheerful, and hopeful, you're more likely to focus on the positive aspects of a given situation. And a positive attitude is contagious: It can help encourage patients to remain focused on the positive aspects of their conditions.
- **Self-esteem.** High self-esteem leads to confidence in one's skills. Health care professionals who project confidence in their own abilities help their patients feel more secure. Coworkers generally develop a greater respect for individuals who are confident in their own abilities. A provider who is self-assured wins the confidence of patients and associates more easily than someone who is insecure and indecisive.
- **Honesty.** Health care professionals must earn the trust of those they serve and those they work with. Providers should always be truthful. This establishes trust in any relationship. The characteristics you display as a

student are predictors of those you will project as a health care professional. You can make a commitment to honesty by always doing your own work, avoiding plagiarism, and owning up when you're unprepared or your work isn't completed.

- **Patience.** Another fundamental trait for any health care professional is the ability to remain calm in the midst of difficulties. Complex and stressful situations are a normal part of the health care professional's day. Providers need to demonstrate patience when interacting with both patients and coworkers. Regardless of the circumstances, care workers need to take the time necessary to understand all aspects of a patient's situation. This will help patients feel that their well-being is a top priority.

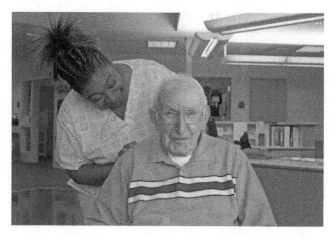

As a health care professional, it's important to be patient and sociable.

- **Cooperation.** An important personal skill for any health care professional is the ability to interact well with other health care team members. A patient's well-being and care are the most important objective, and all team members should work together toward this same goal. Through teamwork and cooperation, professionals can promote more effective and efficient methods of health care. When it comes to a health care team, all of the team members are important—from the professional handling the medical billing to the member providing direct patient care. To provide the best overall care, workers should show sensitivity to the needs, feelings, and ideas of other team members.
- **Organization.** Being organized is a key to success in almost any career. As a student, you learn early on that organization involves making a place for everything so that items can be easily accessed. The organizational skills you learn as a student and bring to your health care career will be a major professional asset. Materials, supplies, notes, charts, reports, schedules, and

contacts are just some of the many items health care workers reference and work with on a regular basis. Since time is valuable for you, your coworkers, and your patients, the more emphasis you place on getting and staying organized, the more effective you will be in your job and your interactions with others.

- **Responsibility.** Personal responsibility is important in school, work, and life. While in school, you know that you need to complete assignments and turn them in on time, without having to be reminded. This same sense of responsibility should carry over into your health care career. A person's willingness to fulfill obligations and accept responsibility for his or her own actions is extremely important in any health care career. Professionals must be counted on to complete their work in a timely, correct manner, always doing their best.

- **Flexibility.** Most health care positions require workers who are flexible with both their time and talent. Illnesses, emergencies, and other health-related issues don't keep to a regular 9-to-5 work schedule, and neither do those who deal with them. Laboratory and diagnostic tests can vary greatly in the amount of time they require to complete, and workers are often expected to run tests or perform procedures with very little advance notice. New and improved methods of care bring about frequent changes in health-related procedures, and professionals must be willing to acquire and perfect new skills as needed.

- **Sociability.** Since health care professionals interact with a wide range of people every day, sociability is an important interpersonal skill for those in health care professions. Whether providing care to a patient, overseeing office administrative tasks, or assisting a colleague, health care workers should be personable and at ease in work-related social situations. As a health care professional, your ability to interact well with others on a daily basis will directly impact your work, your patients, and other professionals working around you.

CHECK POINT

1 Why is a health care worker's personality important?

2 What are some personal attributes a health care professional should possess?

PROFESSIONAL ATTRIBUTES

Professionals are expected to behave in a manner consistent with the standards, views, and behaviors of their profession. Students often begin developing professional

qualities and skills while interacting with faculty members, administrators, and other students. These attributes continue to develop as students begin their health care careers and interact with patients, health care team members, and others in a professional environment.

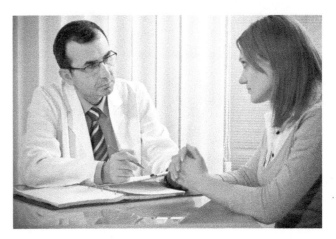

Your professional qualities will be critical beginning in school and carrying through to your first job interview and throughout your career.

Professional Qualities and Skills

For those who wish to become competent health care professionals, the right personal and professional characteristics are crucial. Like other professionals, health care workers must balance their personal and professional lives. Their personality traits don't affect just one aspect of their lives, but serve them on both a personal and a professional level.

Several qualities and skills are both personal and professional. For example, compassion, empathy, sympathy, honesty, integrity, and accountability are all traits that most people (including health care professionals) use in their personal lives. However, for health care professionals, these traits are also important career tools. Several of these characteristics were described as personal attributes earlier in the chapter, but they also affect a person's professional behavior.

Although different positions demand different qualities and skills, some professional attributes benefit all health care workers. These include:

- **Dedication to public service.** Health care professionals perform a type of public service, contributing to the good of society through their work with others. Those professionals who recognize and believe in the value of their work to society likely view their occupations as a calling, or their "life's work." They're attracted to their career because of the importance of the work itself, rather than what they stand to gain personally from the career.

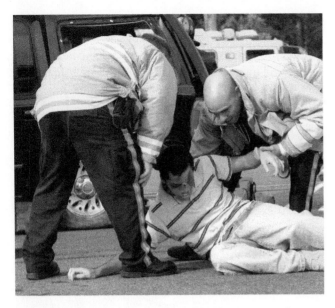

Motivation to help others and dedication to public service can offer health care workers true professional fulfillment.

A person's ability to act selflessly for the well-being of others is an essential attribute for health care workers. Professionals who are dedicated to public service consistently demonstrate attitudes of service to others; perform the duties of their work out of a desire to help, rather than merely an obligation; reap satisfaction from their work; and support and participate in professionally-related activities and groups, such as professional organizations.

- **Being motivated by job fulfillment.** A health care career provides many different rewards. Independence, continuing professional development, and economic security are attractive personal benefits for those in health-related careers. Professionals who choose this type of work because they enjoy it, however, gain a sense of satisfaction and contentment that can't be gained through an attractive salary alone. Those with a true passion, enthusiasm, and strong personal desire to help others are more likely to find fulfillment in a health-related career.
- **Trustworthiness.** Patients, coworkers, and supervisors need to know that they can trust a health care professional. Patients place their most precious possession, their lives, in the hands of their caregivers. Building trust requires dependability. This means that others can count on the person to follow through on promises, live up to agreements, and always be honest. Trustworthiness and dependability begin with regularly attending and being on time for school. Your attendance record is an important reflection of your dependability.
- **Competence.** People exhibit competence when they're proficient in what they've learned and are capable of performing related tasks. Competent people are able to follow steps and procedures accurately and in a timely manner. Competence involves a willingness to:
  - *Learn.* To be competent in any health care profession, you must be self-motivated and have a desire to learn. Because new techniques and health care technologies are developed frequently, a commitment to continuing education is necessary in order to maintain your competency.
  - *Change.* New technologies and innovations bring constant change to the field of health care. For the good of patients, health care professionals must be willing to change the way they perform their duties or administer treatments. Professionals shouldn't be resistant to change but should have a desire and enthusiasm for learning new techniques and better ways of doing their jobs.
  - *Admit mistakes.* Competent people willingly accept evaluation of their performance from managers, colleagues, and other professionals. They know that they need to keep the lines of communication open, even if at first they may not like what they hear. Whether in school, at home, or in the workplace, everyone makes mistakes. Mistakes aren't necessarily failures, so accepting and learning from those mistakes is an important trait.
  - *Accept criticism.* Constructive criticism from coworkers, teachers, friends, or patients can help a health care professional improve and become more successful on the job. Professionals should avoid negative reactions to criticism. Anger, excuses, laying the blame elsewhere, or walking away aren't acceptable, or professional, reactions to criticism.
- **Good time management.** People who are able to complete their work in a timely manner, while skillfully handling any tasks, concerns, or issues that arise, are using time management skills. A familiar saying in the business world is "time is money." In a health care setting, time may be even more valuable, because a patient's health and well-being may be at risk. Most health care professionals find themselves working on multiple issues at the same time, and these may involve numerous patients, tests, and documents. As you prepare for a health care career, it's imperative that you learn to deal with more than one task at a given time by setting priorities, staying focused on the task at hand, and avoiding procrastination. You can work to improve your time management skills while you are still a student by learning to balance your many different responsibilities.

- **Initiative, problem solving, and critical thinking**. Health care professionals often find themselves in situations that call for quick and decisive action. They need confidence in their own ability to make important decisions, because input from others isn't always immediately available. The ability to act and make decisions without the help or advice of others is known as *initiative*. For example, a care worker takes the initiative when realizing that a patient will need something even before the patient asks. Health care professionals also use initiative when they employ problem solving and critical thinking skills, both of which require independent and logical reasoning. Common sense and sound judgment gained through experience are also valuable assets for health care professionals.
- **Good communication skills.** As an allied health professional, you will frequently interact with other members of the health care team and—depending on the health care profession you choose—you may also interact with patients. Clearly and accurately conveying information in both verbal and written forms will be crucial to your professional success. Communication skills are discussed more fully in Chapter 16, "Health Care Communication."

Professional Attitude and Behavior

Your attitude and behavior in the workplace—with patients, coworkers, and administrators—are the outward display of your personal and professional qualities and skills. Whether treating a patient or consulting with another health professional, it is important to look and behave professionally.

Professional behavior involves not only appropriate use of language, manners, and dress, but also the outward expression of qualities and skills, such as integrity, honesty, and dependability. For example, how you handle mistakes is a reflection of your integrity. The mark of a true professional is the ability to admit mistakes and take full responsibility for all actions. Otherwise, patients and colleagues are likely to lose confidence in your abilities and judgment.

How and what you communicate with your patients and coworkers is a reflection of your honesty. Always present facts in a straightforward manner. It is never acceptable to mislead patients or health care associates.

Being dependable is another outward sign of your personal and professional qualities and skills. In most health care settings, you will work and interact with other members of a health care team, and your colleagues need to be able to depend on you to fulfill your duties and obligations and follow through in a timely manner.

VALUES

Personal qualities and professional behavior are often a reflection of a person's values. A *value* is a belief about the worth or importance of something that acts as a standard to guide one's behavior. The amount of time and money you devote to relationships, work, study, fitness, leisure, and other activities reveals something about the importance, or value, you attach to them.

Value System

A *value system* is a person's ranked personal principles, which often lead to a personal code of conduct. Your values influence your beliefs about human needs, health, and illness. They also impact how you practice health care and respond to illness. For example, individuals who place a high value on health and personal responsibility often work hard to reach their fitness goals. Individuals who value high-risk leisure activities may attach less value to life and health. Certain values, such as a concern for others and respect for human dignity, are essential for health care workers.

Development of Values

An individual isn't born with values. They're formed throughout one's lifetime from experiences combined with family, cultural, and environmental influences. Values are often formed by observing and modeling the behavior of parents, peers, colleagues, or others. They also may be acquired through instruction from parents or an institution, such as a church or school.

Important Values in Health Care

Values shape decisions in everyday life and are often echoed in one's behavior. These values are also the foundation for personal and professional qualities and skills.

Values supply a framework for a health care professional's career. Examine your personal values to ensure that they match up with the values regarded as essential by others in the profession. For example, health care workers should display tactfulness and discretion when dealing with patients' private medical information and should always value their patients' right to confidentiality. Sensitivity to a patient's situation, condition, and needs is another important value, and this extends to a patient's family as well. Other values that are essential in health care careers are:

- altruism
- respect for patient autonomy
- respect for human dignity

Altruism

A concern for the welfare and well-being of others is known as altruism. In health care, altruism is reflected in the provider's concern for the welfare of patients and other health care providers. Professional behaviors that display altruism include:

- demonstrating an understanding of the cultures, beliefs, and perspectives of others
- advocating for patients, particularly the most vulnerable
- taking risks on behalf of patients and colleagues
- mentoring other professionals

Respect for Patient Autonomy

Respect for the right to self-determination, or autonomy, is another important value in health care. Providers who value patient autonomy respect patients' rights to make decisions about their health care. Professional behaviors that display respect for patient autonomy include:

- planning a patient's care in partnership with the patient
- honoring the right of patients and their families to make decisions about health care
- providing information so patients can make informed choices

Respect for Human Dignity

To value human dignity is to respect the inherent worth and uniqueness of all individuals. Professional behaviors that demonstrate respect for human dignity include:

- providing culturally sensitive care
- protecting the patient's privacy
- preserving the confidentiality of patient and health care provider information
- designing care with sensitivity to individual patient needs

✓ CHECK POINT

5 What is a value system, and how does it impact a person's life?

6 What are some values that are essential in health care careers?

STRESS MANAGEMENT

Everyone feels stress, but professionals must manage it so that it doesn't affect their work. This is especially true for health care professionals. Stress is brought on by any number of physical, chemical, or emotional factors. It can produce both physical and emotional tension and has been linked to illnesses and disease. There are different types of stress and different reactions to stress.

📷 ZOOM IN

CPR: A Stress Inducer

Performing cardiopulmonary resuscitation (CPR) on a real person for the first time can be a very stressful situation for any health care provider. Just knowing that a person's life is in your hands is enough to raise your stress level. Health care professionals, however, must find ways to cope with this stress while still functioning, because others count on their skills and professionalism in the most difficult of situations.

When performing CPR, several different actions must be coordinated and recalled in an instant. Emergency situations often can be complicated by additional factors, such as:

- panicky family members
- language barriers
- unknown health conditions

The most important thing to remember when preparing to perform CPR is to stay calm, no matter what happens. This helps reduce any stressful feelings, which will allow you to focus on the patient. With proper training and practice, CPR skills can become almost second nature. In emergency situations, trained health professionals should be able to rely on that training to take over.

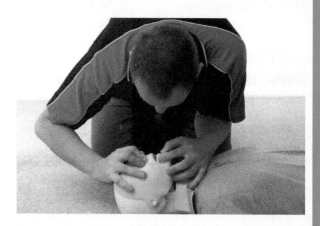

If you are called upon to perform CPR in a real emergency, stay calm and remember your training.

How people manage stress determines whether they react positively or negatively in stressful situations.

Types of Stress

There are two main types of stress—"good" stress and 'bad" stress. "Good" stress, called eustress (yōō-stres), leads to positive reactions. Low levels of stress often motivate people to complete tasks, meet deadlines, and solve problems. Many people experience this type of stress every day. Eustress can be helpful when it motivates a person to accomplish necessary tasks. "Bad" stress, also known as distress, causes negative reactions. High levels of stress often cause people to feel nervous and unfocused or to overeat or not be able to eat at all. Distress can hinder a person's ability to participate in and enjoy normal activities.

Stress Producers

Causes of stress typically depend on each individual's personality. What may be an extremely stressful situation for one person may produce little or no stress for someone else. However, there are some common stress producers that people struggle with every day:
- living a chaotic or disorderly lifestyle
- lacking the ability to say "no"

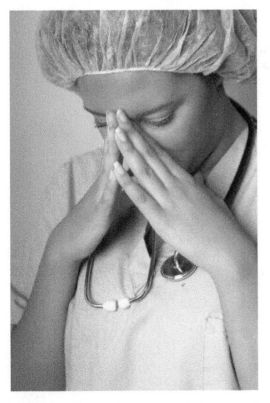

Even the best health care providers can begin to feel the strain when dealing with life and death situations on a regular basis.

- taking problems and criticism personally
- maintaining unrealistic expectations
- dealing with excessive demands
- remaining inflexible
- suffering self-doubt

For health care workers, excessive demands on their time and talent are often the rule rather than the exception. For some health care workers, handling emergencies is a normal occurrence. However, dealing with life and death situations on a regular basis puts strains and pressures on even the best providers. All of these factors are significant producers of stress.

A person feeling stress generally shows physical signs, such as increased anxiety, agitation, or depression. These signs often are easily detected by others. When a health care worker's attitude turns negative due to stress, it has a harmful effect on both the worker and his or her coworkers.

Strategies for Coping with Stress

Health care providers who are dealing with stress can have a difficult time focusing on the needs of others. It is vital that they develop methods and strategies for coping with stress before it has a chance to get in the way of the main goal—providing the best possible care for each patient.

Stress should be dealt with before it has a chance to lead to overload or burnout. Since stress producers vary from one person to another, individuals must first identify the specific situations, activities, and relationships that bring about stress in their lives. Only they can determine how they will respond to or manage their stress. Some people try to handle their stress by overeating, drinking, or using drugs. However, these strategies eventually produce more stress. Positive strategies that health care professionals can use to handle stress include the following:
- set priorities
- keep life and work simple
- identify and reduce stress producers
- shift thinking
- enlist social support
- relax and renew

Set Priorities

Oftentimes you can become stressed because you feel overwhelmed—too much to do and not enough time to do it. One way to reduce this stress is to set priorities and stick with them; as discussed earlier, this is a key aspect of time management. As you look at each task or commitment on your daily to-do list, determine which are necessary and which are not. Ask yourself, "Is it absolutely necessary that I get this task done today, or would it just be nice to get it done today?" Then move the absolutely necessary tasks to the top of the list. After—and only after—the most important tasks have been accomplished should you consider tackling the other items on the list.

Keep Life and Work Simple

A complicated schedule often produces stress. This is true in personal life, as well as professional life. Basic time management practices can help health care providers avoid this common stress producer. Once you've set priorities, avoid procrastination. Errands and tasks should be combined whenever possible. This not only saves time, it also reduces stress.

You shouldn't feel obligated to participate in optional activities that don't hold any professional or personal value to you. These activities consume time that could be used to complete necessary tasks. Also, remember that it's okay to say "no" to additional projects, responsibilities, or demands when accepting them would over-commit your time. Complaining, though, isn't the same as saying "no." Complaining doesn't relieve stress—it simply reinforces it.

Identify and Reduce Stress Producers

Once you have identified the main stressors in your life, you can stop them from getting out of control. A simple yet effective method anyone can employ is to write down tasks or situations that produce stress. Doing this often leads to new ideas for eliminating the stress. For example, suppose weekday morning activities—getting ready for school or work (showering, dressing, eating breakfast, packing a lunch, driving in rush-hour traffic, and so forth) causes stress for you each day. Writing down each of those stressors may help you think of ways to eliminate some or all of the stress, such as laying out your clothes the night before or beginning your morning routine 15 minutes earlier so that you beat the rush-hour traffic. Keep in mind, however, that there will always be new and changing situations that might cause stress.

Shift Thinking

Health care providers can cope with stress by changing how they think about stressful circumstances, activities, or relationships. They can greatly reduce stress by learning to look at problems or stressful situations as opportunities. Accepting a difficult task as a normal part of the job, rather than complaining about it, can reduce stress.

Enlist Social Support

The poet John Donne wrote, "No man is an island." There are times when everyone needs to depend on others for support. Having a network of supportive friends, family members, or colleagues helps individuals deal with stress. People in your support network may include:

- family members
- friends
- coworkers
- students or classmates
- members of religious groups
- people who share common interests or hobbies

When you discuss your problems or frustrations with others, this can help alleviate stress. And the people in your support network may be able to give advice or offer new perspectives.

Relax and Renew

When stress threatens to get the better of you, it's time to take a break and relax. By pausing the daily routine and engaging in enjoyable activities, you can reduce stress and help yourself cope with the stressful situations in your life.

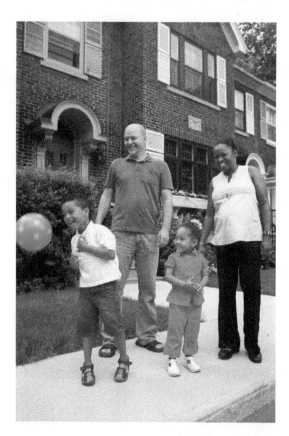

One way to cope with work stress is spending time with your family.

There are a number of ways to relax, but not everyone finds the same activities relaxing. For some, listening to relaxing music brings relief in a stressful situation. The aroma of a scented candle might bring relief to others. Time spent with family or friends can also help alleviate stress—as long as there are no ongoing conflicts that may surface and bring on additional stress.

A good laugh is a sure way to relieve any stressful situation. Professionals should ensure that they're sensitive to the opinions and feelings of others, however. What is funny to one person may be offensive to another.

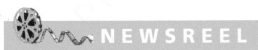

CHECK POINT

7 What is the difference between eustress and distress?

8 Why is it important for health care workers to develop methods and strategies for dealing with stress?

PERSONAL HEALTH

Since stress can take a physical toll on your body, taking proper care of your health helps prepare you to manage stressful situations. As a health care professional, you must take good care of yourself so that you will be able to provide proper care to others. You also need to be a good role model for others, including patients, friends, and family. With proper nutrition, exercise, and sleep, you stay on a healthy path to success.

Nutrition

Food can be thought of as fuel for the body. A proper breakfast prepares a person's body for the day ahead. You can give your body the energy it needs by eating healthy food. This also helps your body deal with stress, helps maintain a healthy body weight, and promotes good health generally. A wealth of information about nutrition and healthy eating can be found at MyPyramid.gov, a web site of the U.S. Department of Agriculture.

Exercise

Exercising is an important way to keep your energy level up, and it can help you feel good about yourself. Aerobic activities, such as running, swimming, or cycling, strengthen your heart and offer other benefits as well. People who exercise aerobically:

● have more energy.

● are less stressed and tense.

NEWSREEL

Disease Prevention through Diet and Exercise

Using data collected in Brazil, China, Britain, and the U.S., researchers have found that healthy living brings about a reduction in cancer rates. Findings suggest that a healthier diet, regular exercise, and maintaining a healthy weight could prevent nearly 34 percent of all cancer cases in the U.S. alone.

In the study, conducted by the American Institute for Cancer Research (AICR), along with the U.K.-based World Cancer Research Fund (WCRF), 12 common types of cancers were assessed against diet, exercise, and weight. Researchers wanted to find out how these factors contribute to the different types of cancer. Their conclusion is that, generally, cancer is preventable.

In their report, researchers recommend the development of a public health policy aimed at preventing, not just treating, cancer. They believe that this strategy would be a better way of treating cancer and that it also would reduce the amount of public health funds spent annually. Nutrition experts agreed that prevention is the clear winner in the contest of treatment versus preven-

tion. In addition to cancer, nutrition and exercise also help prevent cardiovascular and other diseases, such as diabetes.

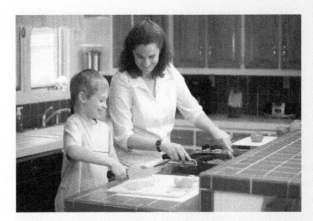

A healthy diet is important for cancer prevention.

World Cancer Research Fund. *Policy and Action for Cancer Prevention.* Available at http://www.dietandcancer report.org/?p=home.

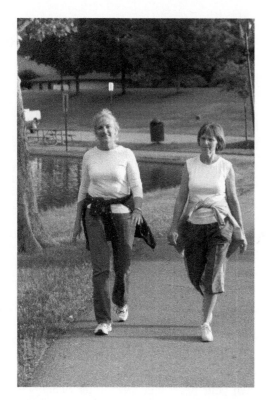

Walking with a friend is one way to relieve stress and preserve your own health.

- maintain an appropriate weight more easily.
- have improved self-esteem.

Choose an activity you truly enjoy. If you try to force yourself to do something you dislike, you won't be motivated to exercise on a regular basis. Another way to stay motivated is to exercise with a friend or in a group.

To receive the full benefits of exercise, work out at least three times a week for 20 to 30 minutes at a time. For even greater health, you can work your way up to exercising four to six times per week. However, it is important to allow at least one day of rest each week.

Sleep

Rest is also important for maintaining a healthy body. When you're well rested, you're able to complete tasks more efficiently. In contrast, feeling tired can increase the amount of stress you feel, which can wear you down even more. Take cues from your body: When you feel tired, give yourself time to rest.

According to the National Institutes of Health, most adults need eight hours of sleep each night. Going to bed at a reasonable hour aids in getting a good night's sleep. However, some people are unable to get a good night's rest, even after going to bed at a reasonable hour. Possible factors that can interfere with a good night's rest include:

- **Caffeine.** Drinking caffeinated beverages in the afternoon or evening can affect your ability to rest at the end of the day. Caffeine is a stimulant that can stay in your system for 6–12 hours. You may not be able to wind down properly in the evenings if caffeine is still affecting your system.
- **Nicotine.** Nicotine is another stimulant. Heavy smokers may experience nicotine withdrawal during the night, which can disrupt their sleep. Waking up multiple times can affect the quality of a person's sleep.
- **Alcohol.** While having a glass of wine or two with dinner makes some people feel drowsy, it can lead to sleep disruptions later on in the night. As a result, individuals may wake up the next morning feeling like they didn't get enough rest.
- **Food.** Eating foods that cause heartburn can interfere with sleep. Heartburn becomes worse after lying down. The amount of food you eat before falling asleep also may affect the quality of your rest.

On a positive note, a healthy diet and regular exercise can greatly improve one's ability to get a good night's sleep. Making changes in those two areas alone may be enough to promote quality sleep. However, when people still have trouble sleeping, they should discuss the problem with their physician. Good rest not only helps a person manage stress, it is also extremely important to physical, emotional, and mental health.

Personal Hygiene and Grooming

First impressions are often based on the image a person projects. As a health care professional, personal hygiene and grooming can set the tone for a patient visit or a meeting with colleagues. Your attire is also important. When your wardrobe consists of appropriate and professional attire, you're perceived as qualified and capable. Most workplaces have some form of a dress code, but general guidelines for professional dress include wearing:

- clean, pressed, and tear-free clothing
- polished, unsoiled, and professionally appropriate shoes
- plain and simple jewelry

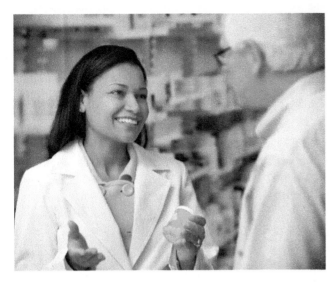

This pharmacy worker's hair is neat, her clothing is appropriate, and her make-up and jewelry are unobtrusive.

ZOOM IN

Hygiene and Grooming

Health care professionals should pay particular attention to their personal hygiene and grooming. People who are ill are often sensitive to odors and extremely susceptible to germs. Keep these things in mind if you come into regular contact with others:

- Daily showers or baths are important.
- Use unscented deodorant.
- Avoid perfume, cologne, fragrant lotion, and scented hair spray.
- Avoid foods that produce offensive odors, such as garlic or onions.
- Hair should be clean and pulled back.
- Fingernails should be trimmed and clean.
- Makeup should be natural, unscented, and lightly applied.

CHECK POINT

9 Why is it important to eat a healthy diet?

10 What influence does a healthy diet and regular exercise have on sleep?

Chapter Wrap-Up

Don't forget to visit thePoint* companion website for additional study resources!

CHAPTER HIGHLIGHTS

- Personal qualities and skills that are important for any successful health care professional include enthusiasm, optimism, self-esteem, honesty, patience, cooperation, organization, responsibility, flexibility, and sociability.
- A number of qualities and skills are both personal and professional, such as compassion, empathy, sympathy, honesty, integrity, and accountability.
- Professional attributes that benefit all health care workers include dedication to public service; being motivated by job fulfillment; trustworthiness; competence; good time management; initiative, problem solving, and critical thinking; and good communication skills.
- Your values influence your beliefs about human needs, health, and illness, and they impact how you practice health care and respond to illness.
- Stress can result from physical, chemical, and emotional factors. It can produce both physical and emotional tension and has been linked to illnesses and disease.
- Stress can be minimized by setting priorities; keeping life and work simple; identifying and reducing stress producers; shifting thinking; enlisting social support; and taking time to relax and renew.
- Proper nutrition, exercise, and sleep help health care professionals reduce stress and provide better patient care.
- Health care professionals should pay particular attention to personal hygiene and grooming, because people who are ill are often sensitive to odors and susceptible to germs.

REVIEW QUESTIONS

Matching

1. _____ A belief about the worth or importance of something that acts as a standard to guide one's behavior.

2. _____ Ability to act and make decisions without the help or advice of others.

3. _____ The right to self-determination, including the right to make decisions about one's own health care.

4. _____ Contributing to the good of society through one's work with others.

5. _____ Ability to set priorities and complete work in a timely manner.

   a. autonomy **b.** public service **c.** initiative **d.** time management **e.** value

Multiple Choice

6. Important personal skills for those entering a health care profession include
   - **a.** organization
   - **b.** flexibility
   - **c.** sociability
   - **d.** all of the above

7. One personal quality that is NOT important for health care professionals is
   - **a.** enthusiasm
   - **b.** self-esteem
   - **c.** honesty
   - **d.** none of the above

8. Health care professionals should possess a desire for
   - **a.** recognition
   - **b.** a regular work schedule
   - **c.** public service
   - **d.** all of the above

9. A person's ranking of personal principles, which often lead to a personal code of conduct, is known as
   - **a.** altruism
   - **b.** a value system
   - **c.** human dignity
   - **d.** initiative

10. A concern for the welfare and well-being of others is known as
    - **a.** optimism
    - **b.** altruism
    - **c.** autonomy
    - **d.** human dignity

Completion

11. _____ may be caused by any number of physical, chemical, or emotional factors and can produce both physical and emotional tension.

12. A common stimulant that can stay in a person's system from 6–12 hours is _____.

13. _____ involves a willingness to learn, change, admit mistakes, and accept criticism.

14. Health care professionals value _____ when they respect the inherent worth and uniqueness of all individuals and protect patients' privacy and confidentiality.

15. The two main types of stress are eustress and _____.

Short Answer

16. Why are enthusiasm and optimism important qualities for health care workers?

   _____

   _____

17. What are some ways health care workers can show patience and demonstrate that a patient's well-being is the top priority?

   _____

   _____

18. How do a person's values develop?

   _____

   _____

19. Briefly describe five common stress producers.

   _____

   _____

   _____

   _____

   _____

20. What are some positive strategies that health care professionals can use to handle stress?

   _____

   _____

INVESTIGATE IT

1. What are your strongest personal qualities? Which qualities do you feel are your weakest? Use the Internet to search for information on personality assessment resources, such as the Myers-Briggs Type Indicator and StrengthsFinder. In addition, you can also assess your learning style (visual, auditory, or kinesthetic) by using the *MyPowerLearning* diagnostic tool provided with this text. See the inside front cover for details on how to access all the student resources that accompany this text.

2. Playing games can actually be a great way to manage stress. Search the Internet and other available resources to locate stress management games. Use the search phrase *stress management games* to begin your Internet search.

RECOMMENDED READING

Eade, Diane M. *Motivational Management; Developing Leadership Skills.* Available at: http://www.adv-leadership-grp.com/Motivational_Article.html.

Heroux, Neomi. *Nutrition and Diet; Clean Living Could Reduce Your Cancer Risk.* Available at: http://www.healthnews.com/nutrition-diet/clean-living-could-reduce-your-cancer-risk-2706.html.

Medical Library Association. *Competencies for Lifelong Learning and Professional Success: The Educational Policy Statement of the Medical Library Association. Personal Attributes That Contribute to Success.* Available at http://www.mlanet.org/education/policy/success.html.

Quan, Kathy. *Skills for Health Care Workers; Beyond a Desire to Help is a Need for Talents and Abilities.* Available at http://healthfieldmedicare.suite101.com/article.cfm/skills_for_health_care_workers.

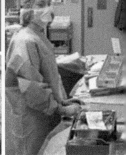
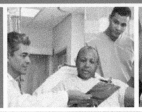
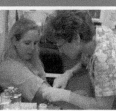

Law, Ethics, and Professionalism in Health Care

CHAPTER OBJECTIVES

After careful study of this chapter, you should be able to:

* Understand health care-related laws.
* Realize the difference between intentional and unintentional torts.
* Explain the importance of protecting patients' rights.
* Identify ethical principles.
* Understand ethical decision making.
* Recognize ethical dilemmas.
* Define characteristics of a professional attitude and behavior.
* Discuss the ethical code for health care professionals.
* Describe the importance of professional associations.

KEY TERMS

assault
battery
civil law
civil rights
common law
constitutional rights
defamation of character
durable power of attorney for health care

ethics
false imprisonment
Health Insurance Portability and Accountability Act (HIPAA)
human rights
implied consent
incapacitated (in-kə-PA-sə-tāt-ĕd)

informed consent
intentional torts
invasion of privacy
legal guardian
libel (LĬ-bəl)
litigation
living will
malpractice
negligence

professionalism
public law
restitution
slander
statutory law
tort
unintentional torts
ward

L egal, ethical, and professional responsibilities are an important part of any career, and this is especially true for health care professionals. The actions and decisions of health care providers have a direct impact on the lives of those they treat. All health care workers have a duty to provide the best possible care for every patient.

At the same time, they are obligated to protect each patient's civil, constitutional, and human rights.

- Civil rights are the basic legal rights held by all U.S. citizens.
- Constitutional rights are the rights afforded to all citizens through the U.S. Constitution.
- Human rights are the fundamental rights of all people regardless of citizenship status.

LAW

Citizens depend on the legal system to protect them from the wrongdoings of others. The American legal system ensures the rights of all citizens. Guidelines in the legal system protect health care workers, patients, and employers.

All health care professionals must understand the legal nature of the health care provider-patient relationship and their roles and responsibilities as the patient's advocate. Patients sometimes file lawsuits if they are unhappy after receiving health care treatment. Often, medical lawsuits prove to be unwarranted and never make it into the court system. But even in the best health care provider-patient relationships, litigation between patients and health care providers may occur. Litigation is a legal proceeding in a court. Litigation, or a lawsuit, may result from an unintentional medical error that has little or no consequences or from a life-ending mistake. A basic understanding of the legal system is important for all health care professionals.

Types of Law

Laws are rules of conduct that are enforced by government authorities. The two main branches of the legal system are public law and civil law. Public law focuses on issues between a government and its citizens and involves three main categories: criminal law, constitutional law, and administrative law. Civil law, sometimes referred to as private law, focuses on issues between private citizens, such as medical malpractice. Health care issues may involve either public law or civil law, depending on the circumstance (Figure 11-1).

The rights outlined in the U.S. Constitution and the laws established by the Founding Fathers make up the foundation of the U.S. legal system. Common law is a traditional civil law of an area or region resulting from rulings by judges on individual disputes or cases. Laws that are enacted by federal, state, and local legislators and enforced by the court system are known as statutory law.

Most legal issues in health care do not involve *criminal law*, or law concerned with punishing those whose conduct is so harmful or threatening to society that it is prohibited by governmental statute. Instead, most legal issues in health care involve tort law. A tort is any wrongful act that results in harm, for which restitution, or compensation,

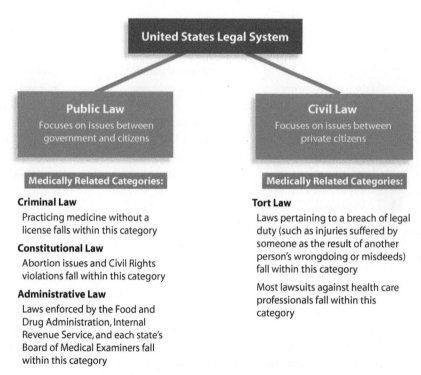

United States Legal System

Public Law
Focuses on issues between government and citizens

Civil Law
Focuses on issues between private citizens

Medically Related Categories:

Criminal Law
Practicing medicine without a license falls within this category

Constitutional Law
Abortion issues and Civil Rights violations fall within this category

Administrative Law
Laws enforced by the Food and Drug Administration, Internal Revenue Service, and each state's Board of Medical Examiners fall within this category

Medically Related Categories:

Tort Law
Laws pertaining to a breach of legal duty (such as injuries suffered by someone as the result of another person's wrongdoing or misdeeds) fall within this category

Most lawsuits against health care professionals fall within this category

Figure 11-1 Litigation of health care issues may involve either public law or civil law, depending on the circumstance.

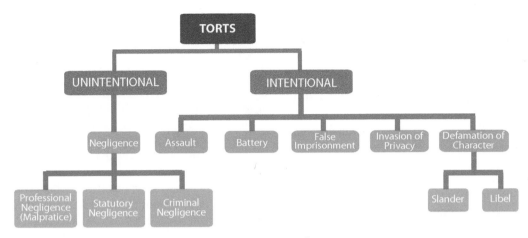

Figure 11-2 Health care professionals need an understanding of the different kinds of torts.

must be made. Penalties for torts are payments, not prison sentences as in criminal law. If a patient or other accuser believes a health care provider has done something wrong, the resulting lawsuit is usually based on a tort.

Torts may be unintentional or intentional. Unintentional torts are accidents or mistakes that result in harm. A prescription dosage error or inaccurate information entered in a patient's file is an unintentional tort. Intentional torts are deliberate acts intended to cause harm. This type of tort is far less common and involves deliberate and willful action. Health care professionals should be aware of the different kinds of torts, which are shown in Figure 11-2 and described below.

Assault and Battery

An assault happens when a threat or attempt is made to touch a patient without his or her permission. By law, a competent adult has the right to refuse medical care. For example, if a patient refuses to take medication, a health care provider can't threaten to put a tube down the patient's nose, as this would be assault.

A charge often associated with assault is battery. Battery occurs when a non-consenting patient is actually touched. Assault and/or battery charges may result when a caregiver improperly or aggressively touches a patient, threatens a patient, or forcefully performs a procedure without the patient's permission. For example, if the provider forcefully gives a patient medication that he or she has already refused, this is battery.

Invasion of Privacy

Patients have a right to privacy when receiving medical care. A provider who intentionally and unreasonably exposes a patient's body or reveals a patient's personal information without consent commits invasion of privacy.

Inadequately covering a patient's body during treatment and, therefore, exposing the patient's body to others is an example of invasion of privacy. Communicating patient information to an insurance company or any other entity without the patient's written permission is also invasion of privacy. The protection of medical information is detailed later in this chapter.

False Imprisonment

Patients must agree to medical treatment, unless they are minors or declared mentally incompetent. Any attempt to restrain an individual or restrict his or her freedom is false imprisonment. A health care provider who refuses to allow a competent person to go home, even if this is against medical advice, would be committing false imprisonment.

Defamation of Character

Making false or malicious statements that do harm to a person's reputation is called defamation of character. Attacks on a person's professional character or claims that a person has done something immoral are examples of defamation of character. When the information is written, it is called libel. When the information is spoken, it is called slander.

Liability and Negligence

Litigation often results when a health care professional fails to take reasonable precautions against harm to a patient. Careless or senseless behavior by a health care practitioner that results in harm is called negligence. When a health care worker is accused of negligence, a charge of malpractice is made. The term malpractice involves any illegal, unethical, negligent, or immoral behavior that

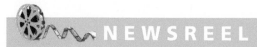

NEWSREEL

Legal and Ethical Dilemma Surrounding Results of Genetic Testing

According to the National Cancer Institute (NCI), of the more than 192,000 American women diagnosed with breast cancer each year, 5 to 10 percent will learn that they have a hereditary form of the disease. Genetic research has shown that women with inherited alterations in certain genes, known as the BRCA genes, are more likely to develop this hereditary form of breast cancer.

Scientists have developed genetic testing to look for alterations in these genes. With this test, women with a family history of breast cancer can choose to find out whether or not they carry altered BRCA genes. Positive or negative, the results of this test allow women and their doctors to make informed health care decisions.

This test also has raised a legal and ethical debate concerning genetic testing results and health insurance providers. The question in this debate is whether or not insurers can deny coverage to at-risk patients on the basis of genetic tests.

Although insurance companies don't presently require genetic testing, the American Society of Human Genetics (ASHG) is concerned about the potential use of genetic test results by health insurance companies. Could those whose test results show a genetic predisposition to a disease be required to pay higher premiums?

The ASHG also expresses concerns that health care professionals may be legally forced to share genetic test results with insurers. If an insurance applicant has signed a statement authorizing the insurer to collect all "pertinent information," is a physician required to send genetic information?

The AMA's Code of Ethics states that physicians shouldn't provide health insurance companies with the results of a patient's genetic tests. They recommend physicians maintain separate patient files for genetic testing results. This may help ensure that test results aren't accidentally sent to insurance companies with a patient's medical records. They also recommend that, when sending medical records, all physicians should make a sweeping statement that genetic testing results are purposely not included, whether the patient underwent testing or not.

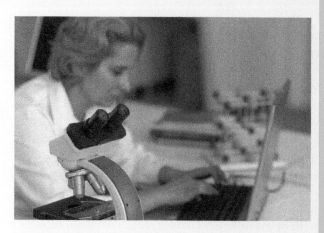

Genetic testing is now contributing to patients' ability to make informed decisions about their health care. However, there is some concern that insurance companies will use genetic information to deny coverage.

ZOOM IN

Good Samaritan Laws

Each state has a Good Samaritan Act. These laws are designed to encourage people to give emergency medical care without fear of being sued if something goes wrong. The laws vary from state to state, but generally, the person giving care is protected from litigation when the following conditions are met:

- The victim, if conscious, seeks or is willing to accept aid.
- The care provider behaves in a way that any reasonable person would in the same situation.
- The care provider doesn't act recklessly and doesn't intentionally do anything wrong.
- The care provider doesn't expect or receive payment for administering aid.

results in a failure of duties or responsibilities on the part of a health care professional. Examples of behaviors that can prompt a charge of malpractice include medication errors, improper assessment, improper use of equipment, and failure to properly communicate a patient's condition to a physician.

Reporting Abuse

One of the most important legal and ethical duties of any health care provider is guarding their patients' well-being. Individual states enforce laws that protect people from abuse, neglect, and other mistreatment. Generally, any mistreatment of people who are unable to protect themselves must be reported by health care providers.

Federal law requires health care workers to report threats to a child's physical or mental well-being. The law shields health care workers, teachers, and social workers who report suspected child abuse. They aren't identified to parents, and they are protected from being sued for reporting their suspicions. Many states also have laws that safeguard older adults and the mentally incompetent. Health care professionals should be familiar with these and other laws relating to their field.

Protecting Patients' Rights

The health care provider-patient relationship entails clear rights for each patient, such as the right to choose his or her own provider, the right to decide when to begin or end treatment, and the right to understand expectations about the treatment. The role of the health care professional is to maintain patient autonomy, maintain and/or improve health, promote good, do no evil, and create a relationship based on trust.

Physicians also retain certain rights in this relationship, such as the right to limit their practice to a certain specialty or location, the right to refuse to serve new patients, and the right to change policies after giving fair notice of change.

Advocacy

A primary responsibility of any health care professional is to be a patient advocate. An advocate always supports the best interests of all patients and helps them secure quality care. To deal objectively with each situation, a caregiver must be willing and able to put aside personal opinions, beliefs, and biases. In their role as advocates, many health care professionals work with insurance companies to help

---

ZOOM IN

Patient's Bill of Rights

In 1998, the Advisory Commission on Consumer Protection and Quality in the Health Care Industry developed the Consumer Bill of Rights and Responsibilities in health care, often referred to as the Patient's Bill of Rights. These rights have been adopted by most health care professionals, health care facilities, and health insurance providers, but they are not federal law. As of this writing, the health care reforms proposed by President Barack Obama include a patient's bill of rights that would apply to all Americans. The Patient's Bill of Rights has three goals: to strengthen consumer confidence that the health care system is fair and responsive to consumer needs; to re-affirm the importance of a strong relationship between patients and their health care providers; and to reaffirm the critical role consumers play in safeguarding their own health. The Commission proposed seven sets of rights and one set of responsibilities:

- **The Right to Information.** Patients have the right to receive accurate, easily understood information to help them make informed decisions about their health plans, facilities, and professionals.
- **The Right to Choose.** Patients have the right to a choice of health care providers so that they have access to appropriate high-quality health care. This includes giving women access to qualified specialists such as obstetrician-gynecologists and giving patients with serious medical conditions and chronic illnesses access to specialists.
- **Access to Emergency Services.** Patients have the right to access emergency health services when and where the need arises. Health plans should provide payment when a patient goes to any emergency department

with acute symptoms, such as severe pain or impairment of bodily functions.
- **Being a Full Partner in Health Care Decisions.** Patients have the right to participate fully in all decisions related to their health care. Consumers who are unable to participate fully in treatment decisions have the right to be represented by parents, guardians, family members, or others. Contracts with providers should not contain any so-called "gag clauses" that restrict the provider's ability to discuss and advise patients on medically necessary treatment options.
- **Care Without Discrimination.** Patients have the right to considerate, respectful care from all members of the health care industry at all times and under all circumstances. Patients must not be discriminated against based on race, ethnicity, national origin, religion, sex, age, current or anticipated mental or physical disability, sexual orientation, genetic information, or source of payment.
- **The Right to Privacy.** Patients have the right to communicate with health care providers in confidence and to have the confidentiality of their individually-identifiable health care information protected. Patients also have the right to review and copy their own medical records and request amendments to their records.
- **The Right to Speedy Complaint Resolution.** Patients have the right to a fair and efficient process for resolving differences with their health plans, health care providers, and the institutions that serve them, including a system of internal review and independent external review.
- **Taking on New Responsibilities.** In a health care system that affords patients rights and protections, patients must also take greater responsibility for maintaining their own good health.

ensure patients receive the best possible care based on their coverage and benefits.

Consent

When people give consent, they are agreeing with, or giving approval to, someone or something. When patients are given information about their care and voluntarily consent to particular treatments or procedures, this is referred to as informed consent. Health care professionals must obtain a patient's written, informed consent for most medical procedures, including:

• an invasive procedure, such as surgery
• the use of experimental drugs
• possibly dangerous procedures, such as stress tests
• any procedure that poses significant risk to the patient

Care is typically not provided until a patient gives informed consent. This verifies that the patient is aware of the benefits and risks associated with a procedure and its alternatives and voluntarily agrees to be treated. Informed consent is generally given through a signed consent form stating that the patient understands all of the issues and options related to the specific procedure or treatment.

Another form of consent occurs when a patient does not sign a written statement but gives permission for care to be provided, or is assumed to have given permission if unconscious. This is called implied consent. For example, if you are in an accident and call 911, you are giving implied consent to the paramedics to treat your injuries when they arrive.

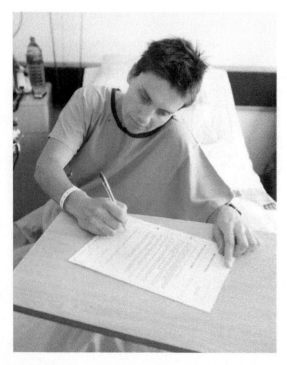

Health care professionals must obtain a patient's written, informed consent for most medical procedures.

ZOOM IN

Signing Consent Forms

A person shouldn't be asked to sign a consent form in the following situations:

- The patient doesn't understand the treatment.
- The patient has unanswered questions about the treatment.
- The patient is unable to read the consent form.
- The patient is a minor.
- The patient isn't mentally competent or is under the influence of drugs or alcohol.

Health care professionals should never try to force or convince patients to sign a consent form if they don't want to. Patients should never feel pressured to sign the form.

A legal guardian is someone appointed by a judge to act for another person, such as a minor or mentally incompetent adult. A legal guardian may sign consent forms on behalf of the ward, the person who is under legal guardianship.

Confidentiality and the Health Insurance Portability and Accountability Act (HIPAA)

One of the most important responsibilities of any health care professional is ensuring confidentiality and privacy when providing care. A patient's right to privacy is a basic civil right protected under the Health Insurance Portability and Accountability Act (HIPAA). Enacted in 1996, HIPAA contains regulations often referred to as the Privacy Rule. These regulations protect a patient's personal health information from being used or shared without the patient's written consent. This consent is obtained in the form of a signed authorization form.

Professionals working in all health care fields and facilities, including hospitals, providers, and insurers, are required to follow HIPAA privacy mandates. These mandates state that all patient information is protected. This includes information found in medical records, billing records, and health insurance computer systems.

HIPAA's main focus is to safeguard each patient's individual health information and protect patient privacy. Therefore, providers must not leave any paperwork containing patient information where it can be seen by others. HIPAA does allow some basic patient information to be displayed for identification purposes.

For example, a patient's name can appear on a sign-in sheet in the waiting room and outside the door where they are to receive care.

Releasing Confidential Information. Providers can't share information about patient care with anyone without written authorization from the patient except:

- The patient's legal guardian, a person with the patient's durable power of attorney for health care, or next of kin (if the patient is incapacitated). More information on the durable power of attorney for health care is provided under "Right to Die" later in this chapter.
- For operations of the hospital (for example, quality assurance, incident reports, teaching and education of residents and students).
- To allow the facility to be paid for services rendered.
- When there's a legal duty to report (such as child abuse, domestic violence, or gunshot or stab wounds).
- To another health care provider treating the same patient and seeking payment for services rendered.

What is Confidential Information? Confidential information includes a patient's:

- name
- age
- e-mail address
- social security number
- address
- phone number
- medical history
- medications
- diagnosis
- observations on health
- medical record number

ZOOM IN

HIPAA Do's and Don'ts

- *Do* keep all information you hear about a patient to yourself.
- *Do* dispose of written patient information by placing it in properly designated shredder bins for destruction.
- *Don't* tell anyone what you may overhear regarding a patient.
- *Don't* discuss a patient in public areas such as elevators, hallways, or cafeterias.
- *Don't* look at information about a patient unless you need to as part of your job.
- *Don't* look up information about friends or relatives unless required to perform your work.

- any unique identifier
- the fact that the patient is in the hospital

Right to Die

Health care providers have a professional and ethical duty to protect life. On occasion, this responsibility can conflict with a patient's wishes. Patients have the right to make decisions affecting their own health care, including the right to refuse or discontinue treatments that can sustain their lives.

In the event that a patient is unable to communicate his or her wishes, care providers must follow any specific instructions the patient previously outlined in an advance care directive. There are several different types of advance care directives.

One form of advance directive is a living will. A living will documents what steps, if any, are to be taken in order to save or prolong a person's life. A living will goes into effect when a person becomes incapacitated, or unable to make his or her own medical decisions.

Another type of advance directive is a durable power of attorney for health care, which designates a person to make health care decisions on behalf of the patient in the event the patient becomes incapacitated. Like a living will, a durable power of attorney for health care goes into effect when a person becomes incapacitated.

CHECK POINT

1 What are some health care-related laws that all health care providers should know?

2 When is a consent form required? Who is able to sign a consent form, and who shouldn't sign a consent form?

ETHICS

The laws described earlier in this chapter were established to differentiate between right and wrong behavior. Another set of guidelines that help determine right or wrong behavior in health care is called ethics. Laws reflect the values of an entire society, while ethics reflect the values of a certain group—in this case, those who practice health care.

Ethical Principles

Ethical principles are standards of conduct based on moral judgment. Morality involves traditions of belief about right and wrong human conduct. The principles listed in Table 11-1 are basic truths that guide conduct in health care, based on ethical and philosophical traditions. They are reference points for ethical decision making.

Table 11-1 Ethical Principles for the Health Care Professional

Autonomy	One should respect the capacity and right of rational people to self-determination. In health care settings, the patient has the capacity to act intentionally, with understanding, and without controlling influences. This is the basis for the practice of informed consent.
Justice	One should treat others fairly and equitably.
Nonmaleficence (do no harm)	One should never cause needless harm and injury to a patient. Health care professionals should act according to acceptable standards of practice. For example, if a health care worker fails to employ proper safety precautions, a patient may fall from an x-ray table—in an incident of professional negligence.
Beneficence (do good)	One should perform actions that are of benefit to others, weighing the good of actions against the risks. For example, in emergency medicine when a patient is incapacitated by accident or illness, the health care professional assumes that the person would want to be treated.
Veracity (honesty)	The patient has a right to know the truth, and one should be honest and forthcoming and interact with patients without deceit. An example of a lack of veracity is a physician who decides not to tell a patient that he or she is terminally ill.
Fidelity (keep promises)	One should keep promises regardless of payment, expectations for payment, or the personal characteristics of the patient. Health care professionals must be committed to providing quality health care to all patients.
Confidentiality	Medical and personal information obtained during health care must remain private. Sharing patient information outside the confines of direct patient service is never appropriate.

Health care providers must always follow ethical standards when performing duties. They must show all patients the same kindness and respect at all times. Their most important responsibility is to place the patient's best interests first, even if this goes against their own personal beliefs.

Joint Commission

Previously known as the Joint Commission on Accreditation of Hospital Organizations (JACHO), the Joint Commission's mission is to improve the safety and quality of care provided to the public by accrediting health care facilities and supporting performance improvement in health care organizations. The Joint Commission also establishes standards of care related to ethics. These standards are a defined way to address ethical issues in patient care. The Joint Commission's code of ethics is as follows:

- You are guided by your profession's code.
- You maintain patient confidentiality.
- You need to be a patient advocate. Advocacy means seeing that the patient's rights are maintained and speaking for people who are unable to so.
- You give care in a nonjudgmental and nondiscriminatory manner that is sensitive to patient diversity.
- You give care in a manner that preserves and protects the patient's autonomy, dignity, and rights.
- You seek available resources to help formulate ethical decisions.

Ethics Committees

The Joint Commission requires health care institutions to establish mechanisms for addressing ethical issues related to patient care. Generally, ethics committees consist of individuals from diverse professional backgrounds who use a multidisciplinary team approach for ethical decision-making. Goals of ethics committees may vary, but often include:

- Promoting patient rights
- Promoting shared decision making between health care providers and patients (or significant others if the patient is incapacitated)
- Assisting institutions in the development and review of policies related to ethical responsibilities
- Ensuring that policies are implemented and understood by changing groups of health care providers
- Serving as resource persons or consultants for specific situations with ethical dimensions

Health care professionals can and should consult ethics committees anytime they encounter an ethical dilemma in the care of a patient.

Professional Codes of Ethics

Most professional codes of ethics are similar in that they promote ethical behavior. Professional codes in health care have these common factors:

- *Quality of care*—Health care professionals evaluate the quality and effectiveness of their practices.
- *Primary commitment to patient*—Health care professionals respect human dignity, worth, and the rights of human beings regardless of the nature of their health problems.
- *Education*—Health care professionals acquire and maintain current knowledge in their practices.
- *Collegiality*—Health care professionals contribute to the professional development of peers, colleagues, and others. For example, when someone new joins the health care profession, other professionals help the new professional in learning the new job. If health professionals attend an educational seminar, they share their new knowledge with others.
- *Ethics*—Health care professionals make decisions and act on behalf of patients in an ethical manner.
- *Collaboration*—Health care professionals collaborate with patients, significant others, family, and other health care providers in providing appropriate patient care. Health care professionals don't make all the decisions for the patient.
- *Research*—Health care professionals advance the profession through scholarly inquiry to identify, evaluate, refine, and expand their profession's body of knowledge.
- *Resource utilization*—Health care professionals consider factors related to safety, effectiveness, and cost in planning and delivering patient care.

- *Confidentiality*—Health care professionals respect the patient's right to privacy and reveal confidential information only as required by law or to protect the welfare of the individual or the community.

Health care employers expect their employees to honor their professional code of ethics. They also develop and implement policies, standards, and procedures related to legal and ethical issues for the health care practice, institution, or agency. For example, institutional policies may be established for living wills and other forms of advance directives, for child and elder abuse, for reportable conditions such as gunshot wounds, and for organ donations. Often developed jointly by ethics committees and legal counsel, agency policies have ethical and legal implications for the health care provider.

Ethical Decision Making

Ethical decision making is rational and systematic. It is based on ethical principles and codes rather than on emotions or intuition. Figure 11-3 provides a systematic approach for ethical decision making. A good decision is one that is made in the patient's best interest and that also preserves the integrity of all involved. All health professionals have ethical obligations to patients, to their employing agency, and to other health care professionals.

Ethical Dilemmas

Codes of ethics generally state that health professionals must recognize and accept their responsibilities to both

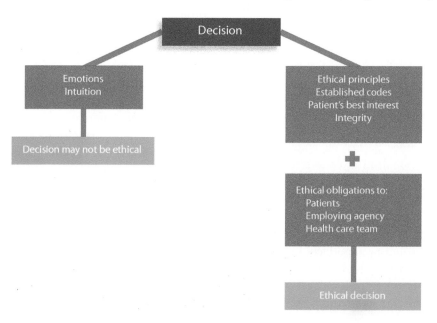

Figure 11-3 When faced with a difficult decision, use a systematic approach to ensure your decision is ethical.

ON LOCATION

Ethical Dilemma

How would you handle the following hypothetical situation?

You are a certified nursing assistant in a hospital, and one of the physicians with whom you work has diagnosed a female patient on your floor with cancer. The physician informs the patient's husband of the diagnosis, but does not plan to tell the patient that she has cancer or that she has six months to live. The husband agrees with the doctor's decision not to tell the patient because he believes his wife will become depressed or hysterical. Do you think the doctor acted ethically? How do the doctor's actions affect your and other health care workers' abilities to care for the patient?

patients and society. However, opposing ethical positions often arise as a result of modern medical advances. Genetic testing, stem cell research, cloning, and physician-assisted suicide are just a few of the medical issues that spark ethical debates.

In addition to the ethics of these situations, there are also many state and federal laws to consider. While there are no easy ways to reconcile opposing ethical positions, health care providers must strive to make the best decision for each situation—keeping in mind that the right decision for one set of circumstances may be wrong for another.

✔ CHECK POINT

3 How do medical ethics differ from laws?

4 What are the basic ethical principles that all health care professionals should follow?

PROFESSIONALISM

Professionalism is another quality all employers seek. In health care, professionalism involves a set of values, behaviors, and relationships that form a foundation on which patient and colleague trust is formed. Health-related careers are often prestigious and exciting, but they also require a responsibility to the patients being served. This requires professionalism and a commitment to excellence.

Health care careers are self-regulated in many ways. Professionals are expected to follow legal and ethical guidelines without constant supervision. With ongoing

medical advances, health care professionals have an obligation to remain lifelong learners in their fields.

Competence

Before beginning a new career in health care, a professional's initial formal health care training has likely concluded, but one's education is never complete. Professionals must commit themselves to continued learning in their health field in order to remain competent. In fact, many health care careers require continuing education credits.

Gaining information concerning new technologies, procedures, and legal issues is vital in any health-related career. Membership in a peer association or professional organization provides ongoing educational resources. Books, web sites, and seminars are good sources of information for health-related advances.

The humble and grateful acceptance of constructive criticism from a coworker or peer is another characteristic of a true professional. On the same note, the ability to offer constructive criticism to others in a positive manner is just as important. Regardless of a one's level of education or expertise, there's always room for improvement in any career.

Professional Associations

Professional associations provide many advantages in one's career. There are professional associations for almost all health care careers, such as the Association of Health Care Office Management and the American Association of Medical Assistants. Membership provides health care professionals with support and assistance throughout their careers. These professional associations offer members a wide range of benefits, including:

- Continuing education classes
- Subscriptions to professional publications
- Access to online resources
- Professional conferences, conventions, and workshops
- Networking opportunities
- Information on new technologies
- Management tools
- Ethics guidelines
- Patient educational materials
- News on emerging technologies

✔ CHECK POINT

5 How does membership in a professional association benefit health-related careers?

Don't forget to visit thePoint₊ companion website for additional study resources!

CHAPTER HIGHLIGHTS

- Health care professionals have a duty to protect patients' civil rights, constitutional rights, and human rights.
- Laws are rules of conduct enacted and enforced by government authorities. All health care professionals must understand the legal nature of the health care provider-patient relationship.
- Health care professionals are generally required to report the mistreatment of people who are unable to protect themselves.
- A health care professional's key responsibility is being a patient advocate.
- A health care provider must obtain a patient's written, informed consent for most medical procedures, including an invasive procedure like surgery, the use of experimental drugs, and potentially dangerous or risky procedures.
- A patient's right to privacy is a basic civil right protected under the Health Insurance Portability and Accountability Act (HIPAA).
- Ethical principles are standards of conduct based on moral judgment. While laws reflect the values of an entire society, ethics reflect the values of a certain group, such as those who practice health care.
- Ethical decision making is rational and systematic and is based on ethical principles and codes, rather than on emotions or intuition. A good decision is one that is made in the patient's best interest and preserves the integrity of all involved.
- Professional associations are a good source for educational materials, networking opportunities, and management tools.

REVIEW QUESTIONS

Matching

1. _____ Basic rights held by all citizens
2. _____ Laws that protect people who give emergency medical care from being sued if something goes wrong
3. _____ False or malicious written statements that do harm to a person's reputation
4. _____ False or malicious spoken statements that do harm to a person's reputation
5. _____ A threat or attempt to touch a patient without the patient's permission

   a. Good Samaritan Acts   **b.** libel   **c.** civil rights   **d.** assault   **e.** slander

Multiple Choice

6. Laws that are enacted by federal, state, and local legislators and enforced by the court system are known as
   - **a.** statutory laws
   - **b.** common laws
   - **c.** traditional laws
   - **d.** litigation

7. This occurs when a non-consenting patient is touched to give an unwanted treatment.
   - **a.** assault
   - **b.** battery
   - **c.** defamation
   - **d.** libel

8. Any attempt to restrain an individual or restrict his or her freedom is called
    a. negligence
    b. battery
    c. assault
    d. false imprisonment

9. A tort is any wrongful act that results in harm for which
    a. an apology must be made
    b. restitution must be made
    c. charges must be filed
    d. a prison sentence must be served

10. When a patient is incapacitated, providers are required to follow any instructions outlined in
    a. an advance care directive
    b. patient educational materials
    c. a will
    d. a consent form

Completion

11. Careless or senseless behavior by a health care practitioner that results in harm is called _____.

12. A provider who intentionally and unreasonably exposes a patient's body or reveals a patient's personal information without consent commits _____.

13. _____ sometimes referred to as private law, focuses on issues between private citizens, such as medical malpractice.

14. A patient's right to privacy is a basic civil right protected under _____.

15. Professional organizations establish _____ standards or codes to guide conduct in health care.

Short Answer

16. Who shouldn't be asked to sign a consent form?

_____

_____

17. What are two common forms of advance care directives used in health care?

_____

_____

18. What is a difference between laws and ethics?

_____

_____

19. Name at least three of the seven ethical principles and provide a description of each.

_____

_____

20. What are some of the benefits of joining a professional health care association?

_____

_____

INVESTIGATE IT

1. Do you know the history behind the introduction and passing of your state's Good Samaritan Act? Search the Internet and other available resources to learn more about the history of this act and what, if any, cases prompted its enactment. Use the search term *Good Samaritan Act* with your state's name to begin your Internet search.

2. There are a wide variety of health care-related professional associations. Do you know what professional associations are available for your intended health care profession? Search the Internet and other available resources to learn more about professional associations relating to your particular field of interest. Use the search term *professional association* and the name of your intended profession to begin your Internet search.

RECOMMENDED READING

Miller, Jennifer. *The DNA Age: Insurance Fears Lead Many to Shun DNA Tests*. Ethics Illustrated. Available at http://www.bioethicsinternational.org/blog/?p=471.

National Cancer Institute. *BRCA1 and BRCA2: Cancer Risk and Genetic Testing*. Available at http://www.cancer.gov/cancertopics/factsheet/Risk/BRCA.

U.S. Department of Health and Human Services, National Institutes of Health. *HIPAA Privacy Rule*. Available at http://privacyruleandresearch.nih.gov/.

U.S. Department of Health and Human Services. *Health Information Privacy*. Available at http://www.hhs.gov/ocr/privacy/hipaa/understanding/consumers/index.html.

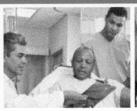
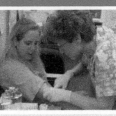
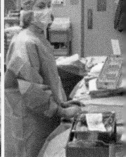

Human Growth and Development

CHAPTER OBJECTIVES

After careful study of this chapter, you should be able to:

❋ List factors influencing growth and development.

❋ Name major developments for each stage of life.

❋ Describe Kübler-Ross's stages of grief.

❋ Discuss the developmental theories of Erikson, Havighurst, and Freud.

❋ Describe each level of Maslow's hierarchy of basic human needs.

KEY TERMS

development
embryo (EM-bre-o)
fetus (FE-tus)
gestation (jes-TA-shun)

GROWTH AND DEVELOPMENT

Growth and development occur throughout the life span. *Growth* is an increase in body size or changes in body cell structure, function, and complexity. Development is an orderly pattern of changes in structure, thoughts, feelings, or behaviors resulting from maturation, life experiences, and learning. Growth and development result from the interrelated effects of heredity and environment.

Factors Influencing Growth and Development

Many factors influence both growth and development. An individual's growth and development might be facilitated or delayed by these factors:
- Heredity
- Prenatal factors, like the mother's age or health during pregnancy
- Caregiver factors, like mental illness
- Individual differences, such as vision and hearing impairments
- Health or illness
- Environment, including culture
- Nutrition

Because of a variety of factors and the complex ways in which they interact, each person's growth and development is unique within general patterns.

Stages of Growth and Development

Human development takes place in two overall periods, childhood and adulthood, each of which has several specific stages. Childhood includes these stages: embryo (the developing offspring during the first 8 weeks of life), fetus (the developing offspring from the beginning of the third month until birth), *neonate* (the child from birth to 28 days), infant, toddler, preschooler, school-aged child, and adolescent. The three remaining stages of growth and development are young adult, middle-aged adult, and older adult.

Embryo and Fetus

Pregnancy begins with fertilization of an ovum and ends with delivery of the fetus. During this approximately 38-week period of development, known as gestation, all fetal tissues develop from a single fertilized egg. Along the way, many changes occur. During the two stages of embryo and fetus, the following changes take place:
- All body organ systems grow and develop.
- By birth, the average infant weighs 7.5 pounds and is 20 inches long.

🔲 ZOOM IN

Genes, Environment, and Individual Differences

We're accustomed to being told that we look like someone in our family—that we have our grandmother's hair, for example, or our mother's eyes. Heredity determines many of a person's physical characteristics, and it influences many others, such as weight, body build, life span, and susceptibility to disease. But what about nonphysical traits? Can a person inherit a tendency toward calmness or an optimistic attitude, for instance?

A good way to study questions like these is to look at twins. *Identical twins* develop from a single egg cell fertilized by a single sperm cell that splits after fertilization to produce two distinct but genetically identical embryos. If heredity determined everything about us, identical twins would be the same in every way. In fact, identical twins have many similarities, but they're also different. They have different personalities and different likes and dislikes.

In an ongoing landmark project, researchers at the University of Minnesota have studied more than 10,000 twins. They've looked at identical twins, *fraternal twins* (twins that develop from different eggs fertilized by different sperm), and *virtual twins*—children the same age, reared in the same household, but not sharing genetic similarities, such as a natural and an adopted child.

Researchers have concluded that identical twins are much more alike than fraternal twins, even when they don't grow up together. Fraternal twins are much more alike than virtual twins. This similarity holds true for a wide range of characteristics, including personality traits like being introverted or extroverted and decision making.

Genetics may influence more of our personality and behavior than we might think, but environment plays an important part, too. For example, we inherit a potential for a given size, but our actual size is also influenced by nutrition, development, and general health. Scientists are still discovering how intimately related heredity and environment—nature and nurture—can be.

Neonate

At birth, the neonate must adapt to extrauterine life (life outside the uterus) through several significant physiologic adjustments. The most important occur in the respiratory and circulatory systems as the neonate begins breathing and becomes independent of the umbilical cord.

- The neonate displays certain reflexes, including sucking, swallowing, blinking, sneezing, and yawning.
- Body temperature responds quickly to environmental temperature.
- Senses are used to respond to the environment, see color and form, hear and turn toward sound, smell and taste, and feel touch and pain.
- Stool and urine are eliminated from the body.
- Both an active crying state and a quiet alert state are exhibited.

Infant

The infant stage lasts from 1 month to 1 year. Growth and development are extremely rapid at this stage.

- The brain grows to about half the adult size, and the heart doubles in weight.
- Height increases by 50 percent, and birth weight usually triples.
- At 4 to 6 months, teething begins.
- The infant learns to crawl, walk, and use building blocks and attempts to feed himself or herself.
- By 12 months of age, the infant can convey wishes through a few key words.
- Attachments and bonds to people are formed.
- The infant begins to discover his or her environment and to learn how to control it through play. Social play, like rolling a ball to someone, is motivated by a desire for pleasure and relationships with others. Cognitive play, like assembling a puzzle, is motivated by the desire to learn.

Toddler

From 1 to 3 years of age, a child is considered a toddler. Growth and development continue steadily but more slowly than in infancy.

- The brain grows rapidly.
- The arms and legs grow, and so do the muscles.
- The toddler learns to pick up small objects, walk forward and backward, run, kick, climb stairs, ride a tricycle, drink from a cup, use a spoon, turn pages, and draw stick people.
- By 2½ to 3 years of age, a toddler has bladder control during the day and sometimes during the night.

- By age 2, the toddler begins to use short sentences.
- The toddler has a sense of self and of gender identity.
- Increased independence from the mother begins.

Preschool Child

This stage is from 3 to 6. Growth and development are slower but still steady.

- By age 6, the head is close to adult size.
- The body is less chubby and becomes leaner and more coordinated.
- Baby teeth begin to fall out and are replaced by permanent teeth.
- The preschool child learns to skip, throw and catch a ball, copy figures, and print.
- Socialization with other children increases.
- Curiosity results in frequent questions and improved reasoning ability.

School-Aged Child

School-aged children, from 6 to 12 years, are typically sturdy and strong. Physical growth is relatively slow but continues steadily.

- The brain reaches 90 to 95 percent of adult size, and the nervous system is almost completely matured.
- Height increases by 2 to 3 inches, and weight by 5 to 7 pounds, per year.
- By age 12, a child has nearly all permanent teeth.
- The school-aged child thinks logically and uses inductive reasoning to solve new problems.
- Peer relationships become the major means of determining status, skill, and likeability.

Adolescent

Adolescence begins with puberty. It generally extends from 12 to 18 years of age, but this time period varies greatly with the individual. Adolescence is a period of rapid growth and development. Changes in the adolescent's body transform him or her in appearance from a child to an adult.

- The feet, hands, arms, and legs grow rapidly, accompanied by an increase in muscle mass.
- The genital organs mature, and secondary sex characteristics emerge, like breast development and menstruation in girls and facial hair growth and voice changes in boys.
- *Puberty* (the time when a person becomes able to reproduce) usually begins at 9 to 13 years in girls, with menstruation usually starting between 10 and 14. In boys, puberty usually begins at 11 to 14 years.

- The adolescent uses deductive, reflective, and hypothetical reasoning and abstract concepts.
- A characteristic of this stage is self-centeredness. Imaginary audiences and daydreaming are common.

Young Adult

Early adulthood extends from age 18 to about age 40. Full growth and development is complete by the mid-20s, and most body systems are functioning at maximum levels. Changes in weight and muscle mass result mostly from diet and exercise. As the young adult years progress, hair begins to thin and turn gray, and skin develops wrinkles. Young adults, compared to adolescents, are more creative in thought, more objective and realistic, and less self-centered. Major developments are choosing a vocation and establishing a family.

Middle-Aged Adult

Middle adulthood spans the ages of 40 to 65. The adult usually enters this phase of life functioning at near-peak efficiency. Middle adulthood is a period of gradual and individualized change. Some physical changes are a continuation of changes that began at the end of the young adult period. Women undergo menopause. Other changes, such as a gradual loss of hearing, described in the "Effects of Aging" sections of Chapters 25–29, generally start in middle age.

The middle adult years are often a time of increased personal freedom, economic stability, and social relationships. Other characteristic changes at this stage are increased responsibility and an awareness of one's own mortality.

Older Adult

Older adulthood usually begins at about age 65. Normal aging involves a decline in various functions, which is usually gradual unless it is impacted by illness. The "Effects of Aging" discussions in this and earlier chapters describe such changes. An older adult who has a strong sense of self-identity and who has successfully met challenges earlier in life will probably continue to do so. However, depending on the person's outlook on life and past ability to cope, events such as retirement, loss of health or income, and isolation can be devastating.

Death and Dying

Elisabeth Kübler-Ross studied people's emotional responses to death and dying in depth, and health care providers have used her findings extensively. Kübler-Ross identified these five stages of grief that people go through when they learn that they are going to die:

1. **Denial.** The person denies that he or she will die and may isolate himself or herself from reality. The person may think the physician made a mistake with the diagnosis.
2. **Anger.** The person expresses rage and hostility and adopts a "why me?" attitude.
3. **Bargaining.** The person tries to barter for more time: "If I can just make it to my son's graduation, I'll be satisfied."
4. **Depression.** The person goes through a period of grief before death, often characterized by crying and not speaking much.
5. **Acceptance.** When this stage is reached, the person feels tranquil. He or she has accepted death and is prepared to die.

The stages may overlap. In addition, any stage may last from as little as a few hours to as long as months. The process varies from person to person.

> **CHECK POINT**
>
> **1** What are the stages of childhood?
>
> **2** What are the major developments of the young adult years?

Theories of Development

Human development and behavior have been studied from many different perspectives. Psychologists and other experts have developed theories that explain human responses that might be expected at certain ages.

Erik Erikson

Psychologist Erik Erikson believed that development is a continuous process made up of distinct stages. Each stage is characterized by the achievement (or failure to achieve) certain developmental goals. The goals are affected by one's social environment and significant others. Erickson's eight stages are outlined in Table 12-1.

Robert J. Havighurst

Psychologist Robert J. Havighurst believed that living and growing are based on learning and that a person must learn continuously to adjust to changing societal conditions. He described learned behaviors as developmental tasks that occur at certain periods in life. Table 12-2 lists two examples of developmental tasks identified by Havighurst for each age group.

Table 12-1 Erikson's Eight Stages of Development

Stage	Developmental Task or Crisis	Indicators of Positive or Negative Resolution
Infancy	Trust vs. Mistrust	Learns to rely on caregivers to meet basic needs. Mistrust results from inconsistent, inadequate, or unsafe care.
Toddler	Autonomy vs. Shame and Doubt	Gains independence through encouragement from caregivers. If caregivers are overprotective or have expectations that are too high, shame and doubt might develop.
Preschool	Initiative vs. Guilt	Actively seeks out new experiences and explores the how and why of activities. If the child is restricted or reprimanded for seeking new experiences and learning, guilt might result, and he or she might hesitate to attempt more challenging skills.
School-Aged Child	Industry vs. Inferiority	Gains pleasure from finishing projects and being recognized for accomplishments. If the child is not accepted by peers or cannot meet parental expectations, feelings of inferiority and lack of self-worth might develop.
Adolescence	Identity vs. Role Confusion	Acquires a sense of self and decides what direction to take in life. Role confusion occurs when the adolescent is unable to establish identity and a sense of direction.
Young Adulthood	Intimacy vs. Isolation	Unites self-identity with identities of friends and makes commitments to others. Fear of such commitments results in isolation and loneliness.
Middle Adulthood	Generativity vs. Stagnation	Wants to contribute to the world. If this task is not met, stagnation might result. The person might become self-absorbed or regress to an earlier level of coping.
Later Adulthood	Ego Integrity vs. Despair	Thinking about life events provides a sense of fulfillment and purpose. If one believes that one's life has been a series of failures or missed directions, despair might prevail.

Table 12-2 Havighurst's Developmental Tasks

Age	Examples of Developmental Tasks
Infancy and Early Childhood	• Learning to walk and talk • Learning to relate emotionally to parents, siblings, and other people
Middle Childhood	• Learning to get along with children who are the same age • Developing basic skills in reading, writing, and mathematics
Adolescence	• Achieving a masculine or feminine gender role • Achieving emotional independence from parents or other adults
Young Adulthood	• Starting a family and rearing children • Getting started in an occupation
Middle Adulthood	• Accepting and adjusting to physical changes • Attaining and maintaining satisfactory occupational performance
Later Maturity	• Adjusting to decreasing physical strength and health • Adjusting to retirement and reduced income

Table 12-3 Freud's Stages of Development

Stage	Description
Oral (0–18 months)	The mouth (eating, biting, chewing, and sucking) is the main source of pleasure and exploration. The greatest need is security. Weaning causes a major conflict.
Anal (18 months–3 years)	Toilet training is an important issue, requiring delayed gratification.
Phallic (3–7 years)	The child has increased interest in gender differences. There is conflict and resolution of that conflict with the parent of the same sex, based on feelings of sexual possessiveness for the parent of the opposite sex. Curiosity about the genital organs and masturbation increase.
Latency (7–12 years)	In this stage, the child increasingly identifies with the parent of the same sex, which prepares him or her for adult roles and relationships.
Genital (12–20 years)	Sexual interest can be expressed in overt sexual relationships. Sexual pressures and conflicts typically cause turmoil as the adolescent makes adjustments in relationships.

Sigmund Freud

Freud's theory emphasizes the effect of instinctual human drives on behavior. Freud identified the underlying stimulus for human behavior as sexuality, which he called libido. *Libido* is defined as general pleasure-seeking instincts rather than purely genital gratification. Freud described a series of developmental stages, based on sexual motivation, through which all people must pass. Freud's theory is outlined in Table 12-3.

Maslow's Hierarchy of Basic Human Needs

Psychologist Abraham Maslow developed a hierarchy of basic human needs (Figure 12-1). Certain needs are more basic than others and must be met, at least minimally, before other needs can be considered. The five levels of needs are as follows:

Level 1: **Physiologic needs.** Examples of these needs are oxygen, water, food, elimination, sexuality, and physical activity. They must be met, at least minimally, to maintain life. Because physiologic needs are the most basic and the most essential to life, they have the highest priority.

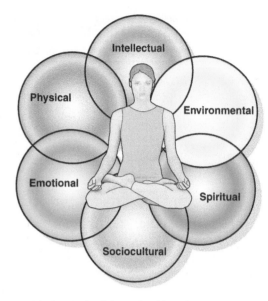

Figure 12-1 Maslow's hierarchy of basic human needs.

Level 2: **Safety and security needs.** Safety and security needs come next. These needs are both physical and emotional. Physical safety and security means being protected from potential or actual harm. Emotional safety and security involves trusting others and being free of fear, anxiety, and apprehension.

Level 3: **Love and belonging needs.** All humans have a basic need for love and belonging. These needs are the next priority. They include the understanding and acceptance of others in both giving and receiving love and the feeling of belonging to families, peers, friends, a neighborhood, and a community.

Level 4: **Self-esteem needs.** The next priority is self-esteem needs, which include the need to feel good about oneself, to feel pride and a sense of accomplishment, and to believe that others also respect and appreciate one's accomplishments.

Level 5: **Self-actualization needs.** The highest level of Maslow's hierarchy is self-actualization needs, which include the need for individuals to reach their full potential through development of their unique capabilities.

✓ **CHECK POINT**

3 What are the eight developmental tasks or crises in Erik Erikson's theory of development?

4 What are the five levels in Maslow's hierarchy of basic human needs?

Don't forget to visit thePoint· companion website for additional study resources!

CHAPTER HIGHLIGHTS

- Growth and development occur throughout life. They may be facilitated or delayed by heredity, prenatal factors, individual differences, caregiver factors, environment, and nutrition. Other factors that influence growth and development are health or illness and culture. Because of these interdependent factors, each person's growth and development are individual.
- Developmental theories attempt to explain human responses that might be expected at certain ages during life. Three important theories of human development were established by Erik Erikson, Robert Havighurst, and Sigmund Freud. Elisabeth Kübler-Ross identified five stages of grief, and Abraham Maslow developed a hierarchy of basic human needs.

REVIEW QUESTIONS

Matching

1. _____ This stage usually involves a gradual decline of function.
2. _____ At this stage, most body systems function at maximum levels.
3. _____ Menopause occurs at this stage.
4. _____ At this stage, the brain reaches 90 to 95 percent of adult size.
5. _____ At this stage, genital organs mature, and secondary sex characteristics develop.

   a. school-aged child **b.** adolescent **c.** young adult **d.** middle-aged adult **e.** older adult

Multiple Choice

6. Which of the following is a factor that might facilitate or delay growth and development?
   - **a.** heredity
   - **b.** environment
   - **c.** nutrition
   - **d.** all of the above

Completion

7. _____ is the time when the ability to reproduce begins.
8. _____ is an orderly pattern of changes in structure, thoughts, feelings, or behaviors resulting from maturation, experiences, and learning.

Short Answer

9. Compare and contrast Erikson's and Havighurst's theories of development at the level of young adulthood. Do you agree or disagree with their concepts? Explain your views.

   _____

   _____

10. Describe the five stages of grief, according to Elisabeth Kübler-Ross.

    _____

    _____

11. Describe the five levels in Maslow's hierarchy of basic human needs.

    _____

    _____

INVESTIGATE IT

1. Skin, eye, and hair color are examples of hereditary traits. What are some others? Use the Internet to find five to ten additional examples of hereditary traits. (Use the search phrase *hereditary traits*.) Make a list of these traits. Write a paragraph that explains what traits are and how they are inherited. Write another paragraph that identifies the traits you think you have inherited and from whom.

2. In 2003, scientists completed the mapping of the human genome. What are some implications for health care of genome research and discoveries? Read a news article on one of the following topics or a related topic:
   - The Human Genome Project
   - Epigenetics
   - Individual genetic profiles
   - Genetic testing
   - Use of genetic information by insurance companies or others
   - Privacy and confidentiality of genetic information
   - Selection of embryos based on desirable genetic characteristics

3. Identify significant developmental changes for five of your family members or friends who are at different ages across the life span. (For example, you might note that your preschool nephew is interacting increasingly with other children.)

4. Think of a health-care profession that interests you and that deals with patients of varying ages. What differences could you expect to encounter when working with adults and children as patients because of developmental differences?

RECOMMENDED READING

Berk, L. *Development Through the Life Span*, 4th ed. Boston: Allyn and Bacon, 2007.

Genetic Science Learning Center. Heredity and Traits. Last updated December 4, 2009. Available at: http://learn.genetics.utah.edu/content/begin/traits.

MSNBC. The Menstrual Cycle. Available at: http://msnbcmedia.msn.com/i/msnbc/Components/Interactives/Health/WomensHealth/zFlashAssets/menstrual_cycle_dw2%5B1%5D.swf.

MyHealthScore.Com. Female Reproductive System. Human Anatomy Online. Available at: http://www.innerbody.com/image/repfov.html.

MyHealthScore.Com. Male Reproductive System. Human Anatomy Online. Available at: http://www.innerbody.com/image/repmov.html.

NOVA. Life's Greatest Miracle. Available at: http://www.pbs.org/wgbh/nova/miracle/program.html.

WebMD. Conception Slideshow: From Egg to Embryo. Available at: http://www.webmd.com/baby/slideshow-conception.

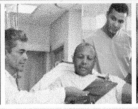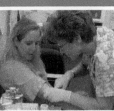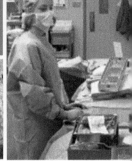

Diversity and Difference in Health Care

13

CHAPTER

CHAPTER OBJECTIVES

After careful study of this chapter, you should be able to:

✳ Name cultural and ethnic differences that you may encounter in the workplace and explain how they may relate to health care.

✳ Describe how people of different races and cultures vary physically and psychologically.

✳ Give examples of cultural differences involving reactions to pain, gender roles, time orientation, and food and nutrition preferences.

✳ Identify differences among individuals based on socioeconomic factors, age, and religion.

✳ Describe examples of diverse health care practices, including natural remedies and complementary and alternative treatments.

KEY TERMS

acculturation
cultural assimilation
cultural diversity
culture

dominant group
ethnicity
ethnocentrism

folk medicine
hereditary
immigrate

minority group
race
subculture

ealth care professionals interact with people from a variety of backgrounds and cultural origins. This is true of both the patients they care for and the people they work with. From genetic characteristics to cultural values and beliefs, diversity is evident throughout health care today.

In our society, cultural diversity is characterized by a wide range of distinctions, including:
● race
● national origin
● religion

● language
● physical size
● gender
● sexual orientation
● age

219

- disability
- socioeconomic status
- occupational status
- geographic location

Individual patients and providers both have their own beliefs and values, which give rise to personal principles. How a person perceives situations and other people is greatly influenced by their beliefs, including:
- cultural beliefs
- social beliefs
- religious beliefs
- personal convictions

As a rule, you should work to avoid ethnocentrism, the belief or assumption that a particular social or cultural group is superior in some way. Every person, whether an acquaintance, patient, or coworker, should be viewed as a unique, valuable individual. People shouldn't be judged based on cultural or societal differences. Such prejudging leads to—or results from—*stereotypes*, mistaken perceptions that are typically rooted in strong feelings and lack of knowledge. Instead, the differences among people should be appreciated and respected.

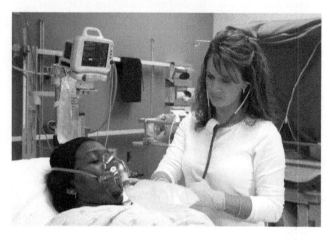

It is vital that you, as a health care professional, understand the different needs of a culturally diverse patient population.

Viewing and treating people as individuals is especially important for health care workers. Part of the health care provider's ethical code demands that everyone be treated with equal care and respect. This chapter focuses on diversity in patient care and the workplace.

CULTURAL AND ETHNIC DIFFERENCES

The U.S. is a multicultural, multiethnic, and multiracial country. Culture is a shared system of beliefs, values, and behavioral expectations that provide structure for daily living. Culture influences people's roles and interactions with others and is revealed in the attitudes, customs, and institutions unique to particular groups. Culture is influenced by, and rooted in, many aspects of human society, including:
- beliefs
- habits
- likes
- dislikes
- customs
- rituals

It is vital that you, as a health care professional, understand the different needs of a culturally diverse patient population. Following are some facts about culture:
- Culture is shared by, and helps provide an identity for, members of a cultural group. It guides group members into behaviors that are acceptable to the group.
- Culture influences the way people in a group view themselves, what expectations they have, and how they behave in response to certain situations.
- The practices of a particular culture often can be traced to the group's social and physical environment.
- Cultural practices and beliefs may evolve over time, but many traits remain constant.
- Each new generation learns the norms, or expected behaviors, of its culture through formal teaching and by watching the behavior of elders. Language is a primary means of transmitting culture.

Because a culture is made up of individuals, there are differences within each culture, as members reflect cultural attitudes or behaviors in varying ways. Therefore, you must be careful not to assume that every member of a particular culture or ethnic group is exactly the same.

While it is natural to note differences among individuals, you must never allow any preconceived notions about others to affect the quality of your work. By avoiding making judgments about others, you can learn to appreciate the things that make people different. This will help you treat everyone with the same care and respect. Health care professionals who are aware of, and understand, cultural differences provide better patient care.

Individuals may vary from their culture's norms. Within a given culture, smaller groups, or subcultures, also express cultural differences. A subculture is a group of people who are members of a larger cultural group, but whose attitudes and behaviors reflect different beliefs and values from those of the larger culture. A subculture might be based on occupational status or age. For example, nursing is a subculture of the larger health care system culture. In the U.S., teens and older adults are often regarded as subcultures of the general population. Subcultures can also be based on ethnicity or language.

Ethnicity involves a sense of identification with a group based on a common heritage. A person belongs to a specific ethnic group either through birth or through the adoption of that group's characteristics. People within an ethnic group generally share unique cultural and social characteristics, including:

- language and dialect
- religious practices
- literature
- folklore
- music
- political interests
- food preferences

The term *ethnicity* is often used interchangeably with the term *race*. However, these two terms do not mean the same thing. Race is normally based on specific physical characteristics, such as skin pigmentation, body stature, facial features, and hair texture. When people speak of racial groups in the U.S., they typically distinguish among whites, African Americans, American Indians and Alaska natives, Asian Americans, and native Hawaiians and other Pacific islanders (using Census Bureau categories). The U.S. government views Hispanics as an ethnic, rather than a racial, group.

Cultures include both dominant groups and minority groups. A dominant group is the group within a society that tends to control that society's values. Although the dominant group is usually the largest group in a society, it does not have to be. For example, from the time it was colonized until the early 1990s, South Africa's dominant group was made up of white people of European ancestry, despite the fact that this group accounted for only 13 percent of the country's population. The values of a dominant group strongly influence the value system of its society.

A minority group usually has some physical or cultural characteristics that identify the people within it as different from the dominant group, such as:

- race
- religion
- beliefs
- customs or practices

Some members of minority groups maintain their culture in the midst of the dominant culture. Others, however, lose the cultural characteristics that once made them different. This process is called cultural assimilation or acculturation. Assimilation occurs when an individual shifts his or her identity from the minority group

ZOOM IN

State Variations in Population Diversity

Cultural diversity varies greatly from state to state, and even from county to county within a state. While the range of patient diversity ultimately depends on the state or region in which a health care professional practices, all providers are likely to encounter a variety of different cultures and ethnicities in their health care careers.

According to U.S. Census Bureau statistics, white non-Hispanics make up approximately 79.6 percent of the population of the U.S. As indicated by the map below, Northern states have a higher than average percentage of white non-Hispanics, while Southern states have a lower than average percentage.

Percentages vary greatly from state to state. The smallest population of white, non-Hispanics is found in New Mexico (44.7 percent), California (46.7 percent), and Texas (52.4 percent). At the opposite end of the spectrum, the largest white, non-Hispanic populations are found in Maine (96.5 percent), Vermont (96.2 percent), and West Virginia (94.6 percent).

to the dominant group and adopts the values, attitudes, and behaviors of the dominant culture. When people immigrate, or settle in a new country, they may find that their values differ from those of the dominant culture. As immigrants go to work and to school and learn the dominant language, they often move closer to the dominant culture.

Living in a dominant culture that differs from one's own can produce feelings of psychological discomfort or disturbance called *culture shock*. The patterns of behavior that an individual learned were acceptable and effective in his or her native culture are often not suited to the new one. Culture shock often produces stress and may lead an individual to feel foolish, fearful, inadequate, embarrassed, humiliated, or inferior.

These feelings can lead to frustration, anxiety, and loss of self-esteem. These issues are intensified when the person is also trying to cope with a disease or illness. Health care professionals need to understand and appreciate the differences among cultural and ethnic groups. When put into practice, this understanding can help reduce a patient's stress and improve his or her care experience. Table 13-1 (following page) provides ten culturally sensitive questions health care professionals should consider when caring for patients from different cultural backgrounds.

Table 13-1 Questions about Health-Related Beliefs and Practices

1. To what cause(s) does the patient attribute illness and disease (e.g., divine wrath, imbalance in hot/cold or yin/yang, punishment for moral transgressions, hex, soul loss, pathogenic organism)?

2. What are the patient's cultural beliefs about the ideal body size and shape? What is the patient's self-image compared to the ideal?

3. What name does the patient give to his or her health-related condition?

4. What does the patient believe promotes health (eating certain foods; wearing amulets to bring good luck; sleep; rest; good nutrition; reducing stress; exercise; prayer; rituals to ancestors, saints, or intermediate deities)?

5. What is the patient's religious affiliation (e.g., Judaism, Islam, Pentacostalism, West African voodooism, Seventh-Day Adventism, Catholicism, Mormonism)? How actively involved in the practice of this religion is the patient?

6. Does the patient rely on cultural healers (e.g., curandero, shaman, spiritualist, priest, minister, monk)? Who determines when the patient is sick and when the patient is healthy? Who influences the choice/type of healer and treatment that should be sought?

7. In what types of cultural healing practices does the patient engage (use of herbal remedies, potions, or massage; wearing of talismans, copper bracelets, or charms to discourage evil spirits; healing rituals, incantations, or prayers)?

8. How do the patient and his or her family perceive health care providers? What type of care do they expect from health care professionals?

9. What comprises appropriate "sick role" behavior? Who determines what symptoms constitute disease/illness? Who decides when the patient is no longer sick? Who cares for the patient at home?

10. How does the patient's cultural group view mental disorders? Are there differences in acceptable behaviors for physical versus psychological illnesses?

From Andrews, M., & Boyle, J. (2002b). *Transcultural concepts in nursing care* (4th ed.). Philadelphia: Lippincott Williams & Wilkins.

Physical Characteristics

Human physical features have evolved over time as a response to environmental demands. Skin color is an example. Evidence suggests that humans first arose in Africa, and scientists believe that early humans had dark skin. Over time, however, some human populations have developed much lighter skin color. Scientists believe that this change was an adaptation to the environment. As populations moved to northern climates, they developed lighter skin to better synthesize vitamin D from sunlight. They needed this adaptation because northern climates have less sunlight throughout the year. Nose shape and size may also have evolved because of different climates in which human groups lived. These adaptations were natural changes that helped improve the lives and well-being of humans.

Studies have shown that certain racial or ethnic groups possess specific characteristics that make them more prone to developing particular diseases and conditions. Below are four examples of disorders that are, or may be, hereditary, or inherited genetically:

- *Tay-Sachs disease.* This condition is a rare genetic disorder that progressively destroys nerve cells in the brain and spinal cord. Infants born with this disease may develop normally for the first few months of their lives, but they later develop a growing inability to move and eventually die. The incidence of this disease has declined over the years due to genetic testing, but there is still no known treatment. Individuals of Eastern European Jewish descent are most likely to develop Tay-Sachs disease.

- *Keloids.* Keloids are an overgrowth of connective tissue that forms during healing from an injury to the skin. Rather than healing level with the surrounding skin tissue, the wound heals with a rough, lumpy, or elevated scar. People with dark skin are much more likely to develop keloids. The tendency towards keloids seems to run in families, suggesting a genetic cause. Scientists have not yet determined the genetic mechanism, however.

- *Lactase deficiency and lactose intolerance.* The milk of all mammals contains *lactose*, a sugar. The body needs the enzyme *lactase* to break down lactose during digestion. Without lactase, the lactose ferments in the intestines, resulting in gas, diarrhea, and bloating. Lactase deficiency and lactose intolerance are more common among certain groups, including Hispanic women and men and women of African, Chinese, and Thai descent. People with lactase deficiency can drink milk substitutes or dairy products that have been enriched with lactase.

• *Sickle cell anemia.* Sickle cell anemia is a hereditary disorder in which the body makes sickle-shaped, or c-shaped, red blood cells. These cells break down more rapidly than normal red blood cells. The sickle shape also prevents the red blood cells from moving easily through the smaller blood vessels in the body. This can cause blood vessels to be clogged by red blood cells, which can lead to many serious problems. Sickle cell anemia primarily affects people of African descent; Hispanics of Caribbean ancestry; and individuals with Middle Eastern, Indian, Latin American, Native American, or Mediterranean heritage.

Psychological Characteristics

In social interactions, people interpret the behaviors of others around them. This is true for both health care providers and patients. While you're assessing the attitude and behavior of a patient, the patient is probably evaluating your conduct as well.

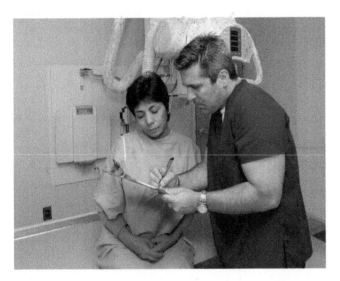

Health careers that involve patient care are rich with social interactions.

As a result, you need to remember that your view of the situation could differ from your patient's view. Even if a patient's concerns seem unreasonable or irrelevant, you must remember that these concerns are very real and important to the patient. In interactions with patients, then, you need to put aside your own opinions and try to look at the circumstances from the patient's point of view. Values and beliefs about health, illness, and treatments are shaped by cultural and ethnic influences.

You must not presume to know a person's true feelings or intentions based solely on gestures or body language. Your understanding of a patient's actions may be different from the patient's true intentions. Keep in mind that

ZOOM IN

Different Cultural Perspectives on Health

A male patient has been experiencing back pain on and off for several months. His care provider originally recommended physical therapy to treat his back problem, but so far, this has provided no significant relief. The provider next suggests that the patient consider skeletal traction. However, the patient wants to consult a folk healer.

While the care provider may not consider the folk healer to be a reasonable option, he or she must respect the patient's beliefs and be willing to discuss this possible course of treatment. As a result, the patient may be more willing to listen to the provider's reasons for favoring skeletal traction.

people may interpret behaviors differently. One person may feel that standing close to another person is a sign of respect. The other person, however, may view this as aggressive behavior. Some individuals consider a casual touch or direct eye contact to be courteous, while others find this same conduct disrespectful.

Reactions to Pain

Researchers have discovered that many of the expressions and behaviors of people in pain are culturally influenced. Some cultures allow, and even encourage, the open expression of pain, while other cultures frown on such open display.

Health care providers may assume that a patient who does not complain of pain is not experiencing any pain. As a result, a patient who deals with pain quietly and stoically may have his or her need for pain treatment ignored. If you are providing direct patient care, you should be sensitive to signs that patients are in pain, even if they do not complain of pain. On the other hand, you shouldn't consider patients who freely express their discomfort to be constant complainers whose requests for pain relief are excessive. Pain is a warning from the body that something is wrong. Pain is what a person says it is, and every complaint of pain should be assessed carefully.

Health care providers can follow these guidelines to treat patients with cultural sensitivity:

• Recognize that culture is an important part of an individual's approach to the world and that each person holds (and has the right to hold) his or her own beliefs about health.

- Respect the patient's right to respond to health care issues in whatever manner he or she wishes.
- Never stereotype a patient's perceptions or responses based on his or her culture.

Gender Roles

In many cultures, males are dominant and generally make decisions for all family members. In some Muslim families, for example, if approval for medical care is needed, the male head of the family gives that approval regardless of which family member needs care. In male-dominant cultures, women are usually passive. However, in other cultures, women are dominant and make the decisions.

Knowing which member of the family is dominant is an important consideration when planning patient care. If the dominant member is ill and can no longer make decisions, the whole family may be anxious and confused. If a non-dominant family member is ill, he or she may need help verbalizing needs, particularly if those needs differ from what the dominant member perceives as important.

Time Orientation

Americans are very time oriented. Many people—and almost all institutions—in the U.S. value promptness and punctuality. Whether arriving for an appointment, doing a job, or even meeting for recreation, being on time and getting the job done promptly are viewed as important.

In other cultures, punctuality and completing tasks within an allotted amount of time may not be valued as highly. For example, in some South Asian cultures, being late is considered a sign of respect.

Another cultural difference related to time involves perceptions of past, present, and future. While the dominant American culture is future oriented, other cultures are more concerned with the present or the past.

These cultural differences in time orientation can affect patient care. For example, a patient raised in a culture that focuses primarily on the present may find it difficult to understand the importance of planning for long-term care. With such patients, health care professionals may need to take some extra time to explain the seriousness of a medical situation and then follow up to ensure that the patient fully understands all instructions. (Chapter 16, "Health Care Communication," provides more information about communicating with patients.)

Cultural differences related to time can also surface in interactions between coworkers. A colleague who is habitually late for work or meetings may be viewed by others as lazy or irresponsible. However, that individual may be an extremely hard-working, responsible professional who simply comes from a culture that does not emphasize punctuality. Avoid making assumptions about others based solely on your own beliefs or cultural norms. This can lead to tensions in the workplace that produce unhealthy working conditions and can lead to poor patient care.

Food and Nutrition

Culture strongly influences food preferences, including both ingredients and how foods are prepared. Most cultures consider certain foods to be dietary staples. For example, rice is a staple of many Asian cuisines, while pasta is a staple in southern Italy. Be careful not to make assumptions, however. While many Hispanic cultures favor beans, not all Hispanic cuisine is the same. Mexican cooking, for example, features chili peppers and tortillas, while Caribbean Hispanics often pair beans with rice.

Health care providers who teach about diet should take these cultural differences into account. Dietary advice should also recognize cultural attitudes about the social significance and sharing of food. Table 13-2 provides some

Table 13-2 Cultural Influences that Affect Diet and Nutrition

1. Which foods are considered edible and which are not?
   - In France, corn is considered an animal feed, whereas corn is a commonly eaten vegetable in the United States.
   - Religious beliefs prohibit some Jewish, Muslim, and Seventh-Day Adventist patients from eating pork.
   - Patients who follow a vegetarian diet do not eat pork, beef, or chicken

2. What times and types of food are considered meals?
   - Anglo-Americans typically eat three meals a day, with foods such as bacon and eggs or cereal for breakfast, sandwiches and soup for lunch, and meat with potatoes and vegetables for dinner.
   - Vietnamese may eat soup for every meal.
   - Beans are a staple for meals among Mexican people.
   - People from Middle Eastern countries often eat cheese and olives for breakfast.
   - Native American and Latin American people usually eat two meals a day.
   - Rural southern African Americans may eat large amounts of food on weekends and less food at meals during the week.
   - Holy days or religious holidays influence food choices for almost all cultures.

culturally sensitive questions and facts to consider regarding diet and nutrition.

✓ **CHECK POINT**

1 Why is it important that health care providers not judge others based on their own cultural norms?

2 How should a health care professional react when a patient expresses what seem to be irrational concerns?

OTHER DIFFERENCES AMONG INDIVIDUALS

In addition to cultural influences on beliefs about health, illness, and treatments, other factors play significant roles in shaping every individual's view of health care. Economics, age, and religion all shape how patients and health care providers view one another. These same factors can also impact patient care.

Socioeconomic Factors

Family income affects individual health and access to health care. While most middle-class families have the resources for health care when needed, many poorer Americans do not. Studies have shown that people in upper-income groups tend to live longer and experience less disability than those in lower-income groups. Although a number of programs help families with low incomes meet their health care needs (see Chapter 19, "Health Care Economics"), many poorer Americans still go without regular health care.

Poverty particularly affects older Americans and families headed by single mothers. It often leads to inadequate care of infants and children, poor preventive care, poor diet, and homelessness. In addition, many poor families cannot afford the transportation they need to get to a health care provider. All of these factors affect health care.

Many poor families lack affordable or adequate housing, which can also affect the health of family members. When low-income housing is available, it may lack necessities like running water, heat, and electricity. To stretch their money and to pool resources, many poor people live in crowded conditions, with multiple families joining together in one household. Research has shown that people living in crowded conditions have a diminished sense of individuality. Crowded living conditions have also been associated with higher crime rates and can contribute to psychological problems, such as schizophrenia, alienation, and feelings of worthlessness. Such living conditions can also contribute to the spread of disease.

ZOOM IN

Poverty by Ethnicity

According to the U.S. Census Bureau 2007 estimates, around 18 percent of Americans live in poverty. When broken down by race or ethnic group, poverty rates show stark differences:

- White, non-Hispanics: 10.1 percent
- Asian Americans: 12.5 percent
- Hispanic Americans: 28.6 percent
- African Americans: 34.5 percent

Source: U.S. Bureau of the Census. *Current Population Survey, Annual Social and Economic Supplements.*

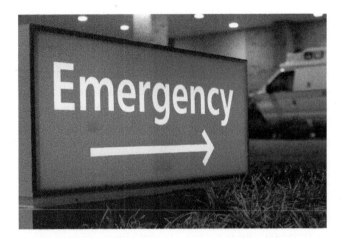

Many poorer American must go without regular health care, which may lead to ER visit that might otherwise have been preventable.

Age

An individual's age affects his or her health in different ways. Younger people have different health care needs from older adults. Adults are better able to communicate their symptoms and responses to medication than children, although some older adults may also have communication problems. Health care providers need to be sensitive to patients' changing physical and emotional needs as they grow older.

However, it is essential to not make assumptions about a patient based solely on his or her age. Physical fitness and levels of health vary at every age. Sixty-year-olds who exercise regularly and have no chronic conditions or disease may be healthier than younger adults who are obese and suffering from related conditions. Age is just one of many different factors that affect health.

◉ ZOOM IN

Religious Affiliation, Attendance at Religious Services, and Hospitalization

Researchers at the Duke University Medical Center examined a group of older patients to study the relationship between religious affiliation, attendance at religious services, and the use of acute hospital care. The study analyzed these variables for medical center patients aged 60 or older. Data on their use of acute hospital services during the prior year and the length of their stay at the medical center were also collected.

Findings showed that patients who attended religious services at least once a week were significantly less likely to have been admitted to the hospital in the previous year. They also had fewer overall hospital admissions and spent fewer total days in the hospital than those attending services less often.

Patients with no religious affiliation had significantly longer hospital stays—25 days, on average—than those with a religious affiliation, with stays averaging only 11 days. The correlation between religious affiliation and reduced hospitalization was even stronger when physical health and other variables were controlled. Among older adults in this study, at least, religious affiliation and practice was correlated with better health.

Religion

Patients' religious beliefs and values may affect how they wish to be treated by health care professionals. Health care providers must be sensitive to each patient's values and beliefs. For example, male Orthodox Jews may not be touched by women who are not members of their families. Because such patients would be uncomfortable interacting with a female care provider, it would be important to have a male health care professional attend to them.

✔ CHECK POINT

3 What potential impact could socioeconomic factors, age, and religion have on a person's health or interaction with health care professionals?

4 How might lack of affordable and adequate housing affect a person's health?

DIVERSITY IN HEALTH CARE PRACTICES

There are countless ways to describe or label health care practices and systems: modern, conventional, traditional, complementary, alternative, allopathic, homeopathic, and folk, to name a few. While modern medical care is the norm for health care in the U.S., many patients prefer other kinds of health care. These preferences may be the result of poverty, language, availability of different kinds of care, lack of insurance, and preference for familiar and personal care.

Some providers choose to combine their medical training with nontraditional healing techniques. For example, some physicians learn the Chinese practice of acupuncture.

Regardless of your own treatment philosophy, you must be open and accepting of other professionals who use different methods in certain situations. You must also be conscious of your own perceptions of health, illness, and health care practices.

Folk Medicine

Folk medicine is widely practiced in the U.S. and throughout the world. In general, folk medicine is a form of prevention and treatment that uses old-fashioned remedies and household medicines handed down from generation to generation within a particular culture.

In some cultures, the power to heal is thought to be a gift from God bestowed on certain people. People in these cultures believe that healers know what's wrong with them through divine revelation. A patient accustomed to traditional healers may consider health care providers incompetent if they ask a list of questions before treating an illness. They also might not understand the need to undergo some laboratory tests. Traditional healers speak the patient's language, are often more accessible, and are usually more understanding of the patient's cultural and personal needs.

Nontraditional healing includes several different therapies, such as:

- *Cutaneous stimulation.* This technique involves stimulating the skin through massage, vibration, heat, or cold to reduce the intensity of pain.
- *Therapeutic touch.* In this therapy, the healer uses touch to transfer energy to the patient in order to stimulate the patient's healing potential.
- *Acupuncture.* A method that originated in China, this therapy prevents, diagnoses, and treats pain and disease

by inserting special needles into the body at specified locations.

- *Acupressure*. In acupressure, the provider performs deep pressure massage at certain points in the body.

Natural Remedies

Throughout history, herbs have been a common method of treatment in many cultures. In fact, many medications used today are based on these traditional substances. If a patient normally drinks an herbal tea to alleviate symptoms, there's no reason why both the herbal tea and prescribed medications can't be used together, as long as the tea is safe to drink and its ingredients don't interfere with, or exaggerate the action of, the medication.

You should be prepared to work with patients who prefer natural remedies over more conventional medications. You must keep your own personal opinions or biases from coloring your interactions with patients. If a patient feels that you're ridiculing his or her treatment choices, the patient will be less likely to talk to you about other treatments or remedies in the future. This could have devastating effects on the patient's health.

Complementary or Alternative Medicine

As you may recall from Chapter 1, "Today's Health Care System," complementary or alternative medicine typically promotes healing through nutrition, exercise, or relaxation. Many complementary therapies are culturally based, and some of today's modern healing practices have

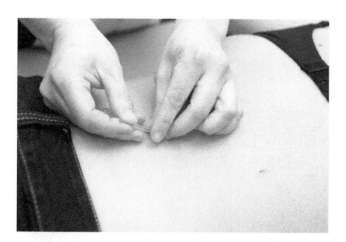

Acupuncture is a healing practice that originated in China but has now been incorporated into nontraditional western medicine.

ON LOCATION

Jehovah Witnesses and Transfusions

Many practicing Jehovah Witnesses consider it a sin to receive the blood of another person in a transfusion. As a health care worker, how would you feel if a patient refused a blood transfusion following an automobile accident? Based on your medical training, you may feel strongly that the blood could save the patient's life, but you also know that each patient has the right to make his or her own medical decisions. (For more on this right, see Chapter 11, "Law, Ethics, and Professionalism in Health Care".)

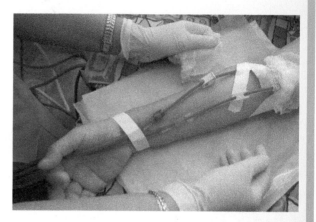

How would you react if a patient objected to a life-saving blood transfusion because of his religious beliefs?

historical roots in the complementary therapies of various cultural or ethnic groups. For example, Hawaiian medical practices have traditionally emphasized preventive medicine. An emphasis on preventive medicine is becoming more and more common in modern health care.

From African American faith healing to Asian Taoism, complementary and alternative medicine practices are as diverse as the cultures from which they originated. Table 13-3 (following page) lists some of the cultural factors that affect patient care, including both folk and traditional healing.

CHECK POINT

5 What are some of the reasons a person may prefer to use a health care provider outside the modern health care system?

6 Give four examples of traditional therapies classified as folk medicine.

Table 13-3 Cultural Factors that Influence Patient Care

Cultural Group	Family	Folk and Traditional Health Care	Values and Beliefs	Patient Care Considerations
White Non-Hispanic	• Nuclear family is highly valued • Older family members may live in a nursing home when they can no longer care for themselves.	• Self-diagnosis of illnesses • Use of over-the-counter drugs (especially vitamins and analgesics) • Dieting (especially fad diets) • Extensive use of exercise and exercise facilities	• Youth is valued over age • Cleanliness • Orderliness • Attractiveness • Individualism • Achievement • Punctuality	• Careful assessment of patient's use of over-the-counter medications • Nutritional assessments of dietary habits
African American	• Close and supportive extended-family relationships • Strong kinship ties with non-blood relatives from church or organizational and social groups • family unity, loyalty, and cooperation are important • Usually matriarchal	• Varies extensively and may include spiritualists, herb doctors, root doctors, conjurers, skilled elder family members, voodoo, faith healing	• Present oriented • Members of the African American clergy are highly respected in the black community • Frequently highly religious	• Many African American families may still use various folk healing practices and home remedies for treating particular illnesses. • Special care may be necessary for hair and skin. • Special consideration should be given to the sometimes extensive and frequently informal support networks of patients (i.e., religious and community group members who offer assistance in a time of need).
Asian (Beliefs and practices vary, but most Asian cultures share some characteristics.)	• Welfare of the family is valued above the person. • Extended families are common. • A person's lineage (ancestors) is respected. • Sharing among family members is expected.	• Theoretical basis is in Taoism, which seeks a balance in all things. • Good health is achieved through the proper balance of yin (feminine, negative, dark, cold) and yang (masculine, positive, light, warm). • An imbalance in energy is caused by an improper diet or strong emotions. • Diseases and foods are classified as hot or cold, and a proper balance between them will promote wellness (e.g., treat a cold disease with hot foods).	• Strong sense of self-respect and self-control • High respect for age • Respect for authority • Respect for hard work • Praise of self or others is considered poor manners • Strong emphasis on harmony and the avoidance of conflict	• Some members of the Asian culture may be upset by the drawing of blood for laboratory tests. They consider blood to be the body's life force, and some do not believe it can be regenerated. • Some members believe that it is best to die with the body intact, so they may refuse surgery except in dire circumstances. • Members of many Asian cultures seldom complain about what is bothering them. Therefore, the health professional must carefully assess the patient for pain or discomfort, such as facial grimacing or wincing and holding of the painful area.

Some Asians consider it polite to give a person the responses the person is expecting. Therefore, some Asian patients may provide misinformation in an effort to be respectful.

Some Asians refuse to have diagnostic studies done because they believe that a skilled and competent physician can diagnose an illness solely through a physical examination.

Some Asians may have a difficult time understanding the importance of taking a regimen of medications because many of their fold treatments involve the ingestion of only one dose of herbal mixtures.

Dietary counseling may be necessary if the patient is on a salt-restricted diet because many Asian foods have a high salt content related to the use of soy sauce.

It may be difficult to convince an asymptomatic patient that he or she is ill.

Special diet considerations are necessary if the patient believes in the hot/cold theory of treating illnesses.

Diet counseling may be necessary at times because many members have a normal diet that is high in starch.

Many Asian health care systems use herbs, diet, and the application of hot or cold therapy. Also many Asians believe that there are points on the body that are located on the meridians or energy pathways. If the energy flow is out of balance, treatment of the pathways may be necessary to restore the energy equilibrium.

Hispanic

Respect is given according to age (older) and sex (male).

Roman Catholic Church may be very influential.

God gives health and allows illness for a reason; therefore, may perceive illness as a punishment from God. An illness of this type can be cured through atonement and forgiveness.

Familial role is important.

Campadrazgo: special bond between a child's parents and his or her grandparents

Family is the primary unit of society.

Curanderas(os): folk healers who base treatments on humoral pathology—basic functions of the body are controlled by four body fluids or "humors":
(1) Blood—hot and wet
(2) Yellow bile—hot and dry
(3) Black bile—cold and dry
(4) Phlegm—cold and wet

The secret of good health is to balance hot and cold within the body; therefore, most foods, beverages, herbs, and medications are classified as hot (caliente) or cold (fresco, frio) (a cold disease will be cured with a hot treatment).

(continued)

Table 13-3 Cultural Factors that Influence Patient Care (continued)

Cultural Group	Family	Folk and Traditional Health Care	Values and Beliefs	Patient Care Considerations
Puerto Rican	• *Campadrazgo*—same as in Hispanic culture	• Similar to that of other Spanish-speaking cultures	• Place a high value on safeguarding against group pressure to violate a person's integrity (may be difficult for Puerto Ricans to accept teamwork) • Close-mouthed about personal and family affairs (psychotherapy may be difficult to achieve at times because of this belief) • Proper consideration should be given to cultural rituals such as shaking hands and standing up to greet and say goodbye to people. • Time is a relative phenomenon; little attention is given to the exact time of day. • *Ataques*—culturally acceptable reaction to situations of extreme stress, characterized by hyperkinetic seizure activity	• It may be difficult to teach Puerto Rican patients to follow time-oriented actions (e.g., taking medications, keeping appointments).
Native American (Each tribe's beliefs and practices vary to some degree.)	• Families are large and extended. • Grandparents are official and symbolic leaders and decision makers. • A child's namesake may become the same as another parent to the child.	• Medicine men (*shaman*) are heavily used. • Heavy use of herbs and psychological treatments, ceremonies, fasting, meditation, heat, and massages	• Present oriented. Taught to live in the present and not to be concerned about the future. This time consciousness emphasizes finishing current business before doing something else. • High respect for age • Great value is placed on working together and sharing resources. • Failure to achieve a personal goal frequently is believed to be the result of competition.	• The family is expected to be part of the care plan. • Note-taking often is taboo. It is considered an insult to the speaker because the listener is not paying full attention to the conversation. Good memory skills often are required by the caregiver. • Indirect eye contact is acceptable and sometimes preferred. • It often is considered rude or impolite to indicate that a conversation has not been heard.

- High respect is given to a person who gives to others. The accumulation of money and goods often is frowned on.
- Some Native Americans practice the Peyotist religion, in which the consumption of peyote, an intoxicating drug derived from mescal cacti, is part of the service. Peyote is legal if used for this purpose. It is classified as a hallucinogenic drug.

- A low tone of voice often is considered respectful.
- A Native American patient may expect the caregiver to deduce the problem through instinct and not through asking many questions and history taking. If this is the case, it may help to use declarative sentences rather than direct questioning.

Hawaiian

- Familial role is important.
- *Ohana*, or extended families, are jointly involved in child-rearing.
- Hierarchy of family structure, each gender and age have specific duties
- Closely knit families in small, isolated communities

- *Aloha*: a deep love, respect, and affection between people and the land
- Respect given to people and land
- Christian gods replaced the myriad of Hawaiian gods.
- Lifestyle more revered than compliance with health care issues.
- Present oriented, less initiative and drive rather than direction and achievement
- Death seen as part of life and not feared.

- *Kahuna La'au Lapa'nu* is the ancient Hawaiian medical practitioner.
- View patient's illness as part of the whole.
- Relationships among the physical, psychological, and spiritual
- Emphasis on preventive medicine
- Treatment uses more than 300 medicinal plants and minerals

- Many Hawaiians may still use folk healing practices and home remedies.
- Special consideration given to the extensive family network during hospitalization
- Acceptance from health care practitioners of current health practices and lifestyle

Appalachian

- Intense interpersonal relations
- Family is cohesive, and several generations often live close to each other.
- Older members are respected as providers.
- Tend to live in rural, isolated areas

- Independence and self-determination
- Isolation is accepted as a way of life.
- Person-oriented
- May be fatalistic about losses and death
- Belief in a divine existence rather than attending a particular church

- "Granny" woman, or folk healer, provides care and may be consulted even if receiving traditional care.
- Various herbs, such as foxglove and yellow root, are used for common illnesses, such as malaise, chest discomfort, heart problems, and upper respiratory infections.
- Older members may have had only limited contact with health care providers and be skeptical of modern health care.

- Treat each person with regard for personal dignity.
- Allow family members to remain with patient as support system.
- Acceptance from health care providers of current health practices and lifestyle
- Allow patients to make decisions about care.

Chapter Wrap-Up

Don't forget to visit the Point companion website for additional study resources!

CHAPTER HIGHLIGHTS

- Culture affects roles and interactions with others and is apparent in the values, attitudes, and behaviors of particular groups.
- Cultures include both dominant groups and minority groups. A minority group usually has some physical or cultural characteristics that identify the people within it as different from the dominant group.
- Ethnicity involves a sense of identification with a group, largely based on the group's common heritage.
- Race, ethnicity, and culture can influence an individual's physical characteristics. Membership in a particular race might make an individual more likely to develop a genetic condition that can affect his or her health.
- Health care professionals must understand that their view of a given situation could differ from their patient's view.
- Attitudes toward time, including punctuality and orientation toward the past, present, or future, vary culturally.
- Family income affects individual health and access to health care.
- Health care professionals need to be sensitive to patients' changing physical and emotional needs as they grow older.
- Patients' religious beliefs and values may affect how they wish to be treated by health care professionals.
- Methods for treating various illnesses have been passed down from generation to generation within many cultures, and members of those cultures may prefer to rely on such methods or to supplement their medical care with those techniques.

REVIEW QUESTIONS

Matching

1. _____ The presence of people from a variety of ethnic backgrounds and cultural origins in the same society

2. _____ A group of people who are members of a larger cultural group, but whose attitudes and behaviors reflect different beliefs and values from those of the larger culture

3. _____ The group within a society that tends to control that society's values

4. _____ Involves a sense of identification with a group based on a common heritage

5. _____ Belief or assumption that a particular social or cultural group is superior in some way

    a. ethnocentrism   **b.** cultural diversity   **c.** ethnicity   **d.** subculture   **e.** dominant group

Multiple Choice

6. Which of the following is NOT a reason that poor families often have poorer health than middle-class or upper-income families?
    a. lack of income
    c. lack of intelligence
    b. lack of transportation
    d. lack of adequate housing

7. Which of the following is an example of a physical or cultural characteristic that may identify members of a minority group?
   - a. race
   - b. religion
   - c. customs and practices
   - d. all of the above

8. Which of the following treatments involves inserting needles at specified locations in the body?
   - a. acupressure
   - b. acupuncture
   - c. cutaneous stimulation
   - d. therapeutic touch

9. A form of prevention and treatment that uses old-fashioned remedies handed down from generation to generation is known as
   - a. conventional medicine
   - b. modern medicine
   - c. folk medicine
   - d. mainstream medicine

10. The feelings of discomfort, stress, and sometimes inferiority that a person experiences when placed in a different culture is known as
    - a. ethnic cleansing
    - b. culture shock
    - c. stereotyping
    - d. cultural assimilation

Completion

11. In many cultures, males are _____ and make decisions about health care for the entire family.

12. A shared system of beliefs, values, and behavioral expectations that provide structure for daily living is known as _____.

13. Cultural _____ occurs when an individual shifts his or her identity from the minority group to the dominant group.

14. The hereditary disorder known as _____ affects the shape of red blood cells and interferes with circulation.

15. _____ is different from ethnicity and is normally based on specific physical characteristics, such as skin pigmentation, body stature, facial features, and hair texture.

Short Answer

16. What are stereotypes, and how might they interfere with good patient care?

_____

_____

17. How are racial groups typically classified in the U.S.?

_____

_____

18. In addition to cultural influences, what other factors play a significant role in shaping a person's view of health care?

_____

_____

19. Why might a patient accustomed to folk healers consider modern health care providers incompetent?

_____

_____

20. How might religion affect a person's health and health care?

_____

_____

INVESTIGATE IT

1. Ethnic diversity varies widely from city to city, region to region, and state to state. Using the Internet and other available resources, find out which cultures have been most influential in your home state's history. Are those same cultures evident today? For your Internet search, use the words *cultures* and *history*, followed by the name of your state.

2. Folk and traditional health care remedies are often passed down from generation to generation. Ask your parents or other family members about folk remedies that have been passed down in your family. Using the Internet and other available resources, research some folk remedies for conditions that you are interested in. Use the search terms *home remedies* or *natural remedies* to start your search.

RECOMMENDED READING

Koenig HG, Larson DB. Use of hospital services, religious attendance, and religious affiliation [abstract]. *South Med J*. 1998 Oct; 91(10):925–932. Available at http://www.ncbi.nlm.nih.gov/pubmed/9786287.

Taylor C. *Fundamentals of Nursing: The Art and Science of Nursing Care*. Baltimore: Lippincott, Williams, and Wilkins, 2008.

U.S. Census Bureau. Population and Household Economic Topics. Available at http://www.census.gov/population/www/pubs.html.

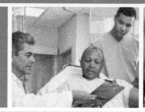
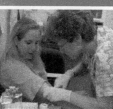
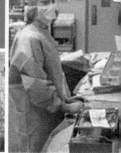

Teamwork and Leadership

CHAPTER OBJECTIVES

After careful study of this chapter, you should be able to:

* Explain the characteristics of effective teams.
* Give an example of how a health care team may be composed.
* Characterize the elements of team structure.
* List tips for effective teamwork.
* Explain how to manage conflict.
* Define leadership skills, styles, and responsibilities.

KEY TERMS

autocratic leadership
conflict
democratic leadership

directive leadership
group dynamics
health care team

laissez-faire leadership (le-sā-FAR)
leadership

multidisciplinary team
nondirective leadership
teamwork

When discussing teamwork, people often use sports examples. These examples are effective because the basic principles that make up a good sports team also apply to professional teams. Sports teams, military teams, academic competition teams, management teams, and health care teams all have one thing in common—they're made up of a group of individuals working cooperatively toward a common goal. In health care, teams can take various forms, including:
- administrative teams
- medical emergency teams
- hospital patient care teams
- physician's office teams
- dental office teams
- outpatient care teams

At the helm of any successful team is a good leader. Teamwork and leadership both play important roles in all health care careers.

DEFINITION OF A TEAM

The most basic definition of a team is two or more individuals organized to function cooperatively together. The way a team is organized depends on the purpose of the team.

Team Composition

Teams are composed of members who are focused on the same results. Whether the end result is a sports victory, a successful business project, or quality patient care, teams are organized to make the most of different members' strengths in order to achieve the team's goals.

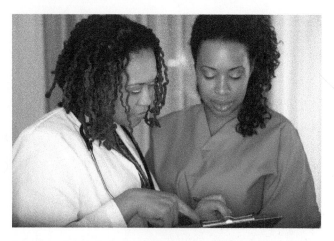

Teams are composed of members who are focused on the same results, even though their specific responsibilities may differ.

A health care team consists of health care professionals who often have a variety of health-related backgrounds, education, and experiences. The two main types of health care teams are those composed of individuals from the same profession and those that include individuals from more than one discipline.

One-Profession Team

A team consisting of professionals working within the same field is a one-profession team. A team leader or coordinator is responsible for organizing and overseeing a one-profession team. This person assigns tasks to individual members and serves as the central point of communication within the team.

A nursing team is a good example of a one-profession health care team. A nursing team may consist of a combination of nursing professionals:
- registered nurses (RNs)
- licensed practical nurses (LPNs)
- licensed vocational nurses (LVNs)
- certified nursing assistants (CNAs)

Each team member provides a different nursing-related service. These services are coordinated under the leadership of the RN, who outlines and implements patient care plans. This includes assigning team members tasks that utilize their individual abilities. Nursing team members all work toward the common goal of providing quality patient care.

Multidisciplinary Team

A multidisciplinary team is a cooperative group that includes professionals with different qualifications, skills, and areas of expertise. While each member has different capabilities, they generally complement each other. In health care, multidisciplinary teams provide comprehensive care. A cardiac rehabilitation team, for example, provides patients with physical, emotional, social, and occupational therapy after a heart attack. The common goal of this team is to restore the skills and abilities of the patient while providing care. This broad goal couldn't be achieved with members from only one health care area. Instead, a combination of specialists from a wide range of health care areas is needed. This team may consist of all or some of the members listed in Table 14-1.

Elements of Team Structure

The structure of a team, and how well the team members understand that structure, often determines whether or not a team is successful. Members are responsible for determining the team's purpose, specific goals, the roles of team members, and the functions of the team. It is very important for all team members to understand each element of a team's structure. If not, members risk wasting valuable time and resources working toward different objectives.

Team Purpose

A team's purpose needs to be defined. What is the reason for the team? What does it hope to accomplish? A team's purpose points all members in the right direction and determines how the team should develop and move forward. A health care team's general purpose is to provide or support patient care, although certain health care teams may have other specific purposes.

Team Goals

A properly functioning team requires all members to interact and coordinate their actions in order to achieve common goals or objectives. This means that decisions can't be made independently. Instead, decisions need to be made as a group, in the best interest of the team and its goals. To

Table 14-1 Potential Members of a Cardiac Rehabilitation Team and Their Responsibilities

Team Member	Responsibilities
Cardiologist	• Evaluate and treat patients with heart problems • Coordinate patient care services with other team members
Rehabilitation Nurse	• Specialize in rehabilitative care • Assist patients in achieving maximum independence • Provide patient and family education
Clinical Social Worker	• Professional counselor • Acts as liaison for the patient, family, and rehabilitation treatment team • Coordinates and provides support for discharge planning and referrals • Helps coordinate care with insurance companies
Physical Therapist and Physical Therapy Assistants	• Work to restore functions for patients with problems related to movement, muscle strength, exercise, and joint function
Occupational Therapist and Occupational Therapy Assistants	• Work to restore functions for patients with problems related to activities of daily living (ADLs) including work, school, family, and community and leisure activities
Registered Dietitian	• Evaluate and provide for the dietary needs of each patient based on the patient's particular medical and nutritional needs, eating abilities, and food preferences

accomplish the team's goals, all team members need to be willing to listen to the opinions of other team members.

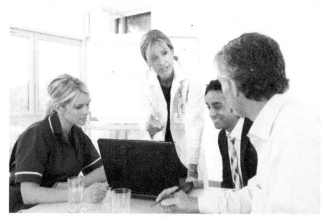

Health care teams interact to make decisions and coordinate care as a group.

Team Members' Roles

Teams typically include individuals possessing unique and distinct skill sets. The most productive teams have members with a balanced combination of talents and abilities, with each member contributing to the overall purpose. Members have roles within the team based on their strengths. Each member is expected to perform all relevant tasks to the best of his or her ability. Some roles within a team might be assigned, while others might simply be assumed by the person best able to carry them out at the time. Individuals may also have different roles

in different situations. General roles found within any team are:

• *Team leader.* Defines issues, sets the agenda, and coordinates work of team members.
• *Recorder or secretary.* Records the ideas of all team members; may act as a timekeeper during meetings.
• *Spokesperson.* Maintains contact with others on behalf of the group.
• *Resource.* Provides unique knowledge or expertise on a particular issue.
• *Implementers.* Carry out the specific activities, such as patient care, determined by the team.

Members bring a variety of personalities to a team, each playing an important role. For example, a *reflector* observes the group process while participating in team activities. This team member can report the results of these observations, providing insight into the way team members are working together. Another important role is that of the *optimist*. This team member has a positive attitude that encourages others to find solutions and overcome challenges. Another team member may play the role of *skeptic*, reviewing ideas for potential problems.

Every team member and every role is just as valuable as another. Depending on the purpose and goals of a team, roles may be added, adjusted, or removed. Some members may also assume more than one role on a team. Once members assume specific roles on a team, they're responsible for fulfilling the tasks relating to those roles. When members attempt to perform duties outside their roles, they risk steering the team away from meeting its goals. For example, if the secretary of a team attempts to coordinate patient care, this interferes with the team leader's role and may leave the recording duties unfulfilled.

Team Functions

Team functions are the activities that the team members must carry out to meet the team's goals. Because a team may have many different specific goals, certain team members will accomplish some of the goals, while other members will work on other goals. When health care professionals work as a team, they can focus their time and attention on performing the functions appropriate to their individual skills and experience. For example, while a registered nurse may actively implement certain medical interventions, a nurse assistant may provide the patient with hygiene care. Or when a dentist is about to perform a restoration procedure, a dental assistant may prepare the patient and organize the equipment needed for the procedure.

How well team members perform their assigned duties has a direct impact on other members, the team's goals, and the patient's care. Given the rapid advances in all areas of health care, team members must keep their knowledge and skills up to date. Through continuing education, they can learn about new methods and procedures, treatment options, and other health care advances.

Tips for Effective Teamwork

Being *on* a team does not necessarily mean that you are working *as* a team. Teamwork involves cooperating with other team members to accomplish the task at hand. Effective teamwork depends on open and honest communication, sufficient organizational resources, and mutual support among team members. Most importantly, effective teamwork requires understanding and recognizing the role and function of each member. By identifying each member's responsibilities, the health care team is able to deliver more efficient and thorough health care.

Meetings to Share Information

To work as a team, all team members need access to the same information. The best way to ensure this is through regular team meetings. The team leader or spokesperson should follow these guidelines when preparing team meetings:

- Set the meeting time and place in advance.
- Choose a day and time when all team members are available.
- If the team meets on a regular basis, schedule the meetings for the same day and time so that they become a regular part of every member's schedule.

- Distribute an agenda prior to the meeting. Agendas list the topics to be covered in the order they will be discussed. They also stimulate ideas and thoughts and help keep the team focused.

Group Communication

Communication is vital to the success of a health care team. Poor communication can lead to mistakes—and when health care is involved, mistakes can have very serious consequences. Team members must communicate in order to achieve the team's goals. (Chapter 16, "Health Care Communication" has detailed information on effective verbal and nonverbal communication.)

The more people involved in the communication process, the more complex it becomes. The most effective groups have members who communicate openly and honestly with one another. Good communication also helps team members build trust and mutual respect for one another. To promote good communication within a group, every team member should:

- listen with full attention to other members
- express ideas as clearly as possible
- encourage feedback on all ideas
- avoid letting negative emotions cloud communications

Tips for Contributing to a Team

How individual group members relate to one another is known as group dynamics. Although effective leadership helps a group reach its goals, the group's success ultimately depends on contributions by all of its members. A group with positive group dynamics will foster an atmosphere in which that can take place.

In effective groups, no member should dominate the group process. Everyone in the group should respect the views of other group members and feel comfortable voicing their own opinions. Table 14-2 lists some characteristics of effective and ineffective groups.

Conflict

Conflict, or a disagreement between team members, often occurs when a variety of personalities are brought together on a team. But disputes within a team aren't always a bad thing. They often reflect the passion that members feel for their vocation or their team's purpose. When health care professionals strive to provide the best possible care for their patients, disagreements are likely to result. Therefore, conflict management is an essential skill for all team members to find the solution that will most benefit the patient.

Table 14-2 Characteristics of Effective and Ineffective Groups

Element	Effective Group	Ineffective Group
Group identity	Group members value and "own" the goals of the group; goals are clearly defined.	The group's goals are not of great importance to the group's members.
Cohesiveness	Group members generally trust and like one another and are loyal to the group; they have a high degree of commitment and a high degree of cooperation.	Group members often feel alienated from the group and from one another. There is a low degree of commitment to the group and members tend to work better alone than with the group.
Communication	Honest and direct communication flows freely. Group members support, praise, and critique one another.	Communication is limited; members rarely share information about themselves. Some group members may restrict communication flow by dominating group discussions or preventing others from participating.
Decision making	Problems are identified; an appropriate method of decision making is used; the decision is implemented, and there is follow-up. Group commitment to the decision is high.	Problems are allowed to build without resolution, and little responsibility is shown for problem solving. Group commitment to a decision is low.
Responsibility	Group members feel a strong sense of responsibility for group outcomes.	Little responsibility for the group is felt by the group members.
Leadership	An effective style of leadership is used to achieve the desired goals.	Leadership is ineffective.
Power	Sources of power among group members are recognized and used appropriately. The needs or interests of members with little power are considered.	Power is used and abused to "fix" immediate problems. Little attention is given to the needs or interests of members with little power.

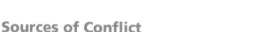

Sources of Conflict

Conflict may result from either substance—such as disagreements over what caused a patient's problem or how to address the problem—or personality differences. When team members have different ideas, opinions, and perspectives, disputes are bound to arise. Substance conflicts can be minimized, however, when members remain open-minded and respectful of one another.

Despite the term "health care team," many health care professionals spend most of their time working independently. This leads to limited opportunities for group conversation, which can create an atmosphere of distrust and suspicion. Coupled with differences in training, knowledge, and experience, a competitive work environment can develop. The end result may be an inability for team members to work together productively.

Managing Conflict

Health care professionals frequently encounter conflict between colleagues, patients, and themselves. Unresolved conflict can lower morale and threaten quality care. Problem-solving skills help manage conflict. Steps in problem solving include:

- *Assessing.* Gather information about the conflict.
- *Diagnosing.* Analyze the details about the conflict and the attitudes of the members involved to determine the cause of the conflict.
- *Creating a plan.* Determine the best method for resolving the conflict.
- *Implementing the plan.*
- *Evaluating the plan.* Review the effects of the attempted solution. Has the conflict been resolved?
- *Modifying the plan (if necessary).* Based on the evaluation, make any modifications or develop a new plan.

Depending on the situation, health care professionals may choose to work through these steps independently or as a group. Even if a conflict arises between only two members, the situation affects other team members as well. Therefore, it is often beneficial to discuss areas of conflict openly within a team setting. This builds understanding within the entire group and allows those directly involved in the conflict to hear different viewpoints, which may help lead to a resolution.

To prevent conflict in team meetings, the leader needs to keep the meeting focused on the agenda. All members of the team should be encouraged to participate. This

ON LOCATION

The Difficulties of Group Dynamics

The St. Elizabeth Diabetic Education Team is made up of seven health care professionals, including a registered nurse, a dietician, a physician, an optometrist, an occupational therapist, a pharmacist, and a patient educator. The team has been charged with researching and approving the purchase of a new style of blood glucose meter to be used throughout the hospital.

For the past month, the team has been meeting twice a week to test, discuss, and debate the pros and cons of various meters. The pharmacist has arrived at least 10 minutes late for nearly every meeting. The dietician spends most of the meetings taking phone calls. The patient educator, who is the team leader, knows that these behaviors are disruptive to the meetings, but because she avoids confrontation, she has ignored both problems. She also ignored the fact that the registered nurse told an off-color joke during the first meeting, which offended the optometrist. Those two team members haven't spoken to one another since.

After testing twelve different meters, the team narrowed the choices to three models at the last meeting. Realizing that the purchase deadline was near, the patient educator emailed team members to schedule a final team meeting for early the next morning. Unfortunately, two members would not be in the office that morning and could not attend the last-minute meeting.

The dietician spent most of the meeting talking on the phone, and the pharmacist arrived a full half hour late. For most part of the meeting, the team members debated the merits of each meter, while the patient educator simply sat back and listened. When the registered nurse announced that there was only one meter that she approved, the optometrist immediately said that he would never accept that particular meter. By the end of the meeting, the team was reduced to arguing over the different meters and was unable to reach a consensus decision.

- How can the team identify and resolve the conflicts and move on to a solution?
- What factors do you think might be creating problems within the group process?
- Why do you think the team is unable to reach a consensus?
- Do you think the group members' behaviors are creating difficulties within the group?
- Is there anything the team leader can do to help resolve the conflict?

---

ensures that everyone's opinion is heard. It also helps avoid situations in which one member feels animosity toward the group if it seems that his or her opinion isn't valued. All members of the group should feel free to communicate their thoughts and opinions without censorship or anger.

CHECK POINT

1 What four basic elements make up a team's structure?

2 What should every member do to promote good communication within a team?

LEADERSHIP

Leadership is the ability to influence others while working toward a vision or goal. Successful leaders can direct or motivate those around them to work toward the same objective. Health care providers become successful leaders when they:
- understand the complexity of coordinated care
- remain open to different points of view
- understand the interdependency of the health care team

The power to influence a group or team depends on a person's leadership style and skills. Health care professionals can use leadership skills to make many kinds of change in how health care is provided.

Leadership Skills

Whether leadership is direct or implied, leaders have power. The most effective group leaders use this power to encourage members to cooperate. Health care leaders need four basic leadership skills: communication skills, problem-solving skills, management skills, and self-evaluation skills.
- *Communication skills.* Leaders use communication skills to form strong interpersonal relationships with patients, peers, and colleagues. These skills also help establish and reach goals and improve the leader's own personal and professional growth.
- *Problem-solving skills.* Problem-solving skills allow leaders to analyze all sides of a problem before making a decision.
- *Management skills.* Management skills help leaders recognize and foster unique talents and skills in other team members and direct others toward goals. These skills

ZOOM IN

Building Teamwork and Leadership Skills

Student organizations provide a wealth of opportunities for students to begin building teamwork and leadership skills. Whether holding an office or simply participating in meetings and activities, participation in a student organization provides students with a chance to learn, while interacting with others who share a similar interest. Possibilities include:

- social organizations
- sports teams
- academic clubs
- religious groups
- political societies
- service organizations
- cultural associations

After entering your career, you can continue building your teamwork and leadership skills through participation in a professional organization. Nearly every health care field offers a local, state, national, or international association, many of which are discussed in Part IV, "Career Profiles: The Most In-Demand Professions." A few examples include

- American Association of Healthcare Administrative Management
- American Society of Radiologic Technologists
- National Association of State EMS Officials
- Society of Diagnostic Medical Sonography
- American Academy of Physician Assistants
- American Association of Medical Assistants
- American Medical Technologists
- American Optometric Association
- Association of Surgical Technologists
- National Association of Emergency Medical Technicians

also help leaders to stay organized, control finances, and use resources wisely.

- *Self-evaluation skills.* Self-evaluation skills help leaders to assess their own effectiveness and to accept criticism, as well as praise.

Leadership Styles

The complexity of the modern health care system allows for many different styles of leadership. Leadership is a behavior—something that an individual does to influence others. This influence can take many forms and requires much creativity, intellect, and savvy to manage the influence in positive directions. Different leadership styles are used in different situations and at different levels.

Autocratic Leadership

In the autocratic leadership style, also known as directive leadership, the leader assumes complete control over the decisions and activities of the group. A health care professional with this type of leadership style may be described as firm, self-assured, or even dominating. For example, Brian is a recovery nurse with nearly 15 years of experience. He discovers that a patient is bleeding excessively from a surgical incision and realizes that the patient needs immediate attention. Brian calls the unit coordinator and asks her to notify the surgeon of the problem. He then contacts an on-duty licensed practical nurse and a nursing assistant. He asks the nursing assistant to gather

the necessary supplies needed to care for the patient and then directs the licensed practical nurse to assist in stabilizing the patient. In this situation, Brian has assumed the autocratic style of leadership so that all of the necessary tasks can be accomplished immediately.

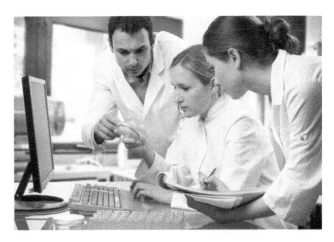

Leadership styles vary depending on personality, situation, and professional environment.

Democratic Leadership

The democratic leadership style promotes a sense of equality between the leader and other participants by sharing decisions and activities among all members of the team. The group and the leader work together to accomplish goals and outcomes that have been mutually agreed upon. Kathy, for example, is a head respiratory therapist who realizes that respiratory treatments aren't being given on time. Although she's not exactly sure why the treatments aren't being provided according to the schedule, she knows that the issue needs to be addressed. Kathy calls together the rest of the staff and leads a discussion to discover possible causes and solutions. In this situation, Kathy has assumed the democratic style of leadership to help motivate the staff to make sure that the treatment schedule is followed more closely.

Laissez-Faire Leadership

In the laissez-faire leadership style, also known as non-directive leadership, the leader hands power over to the group members. This approach encourages independent activity by group members, and its success depends on team members being able to direct their own activities. This leadership style is more effective when all team members are clinical experts with a thorough understanding of both clinical and administrative processes. For example, Lamar is the head of an occupational therapy department and wants to promote the use of a new treatment for brain injury rehabilitation. He posts an article related to this new technique on the hospital's intranet site. He's confident that the other therapists are professionals who want to improve their care and that they will choose to read and follow the findings within this new article.

Leadership and Management

While leaders are not always managers, managers are always leaders. Many health care professionals serve in management roles, often in addition to their professional roles. Managers generally have four functions:

- *Planning.* Managers are skilled at identifying problems and developing long-term goals, short-term objectives that build toward those goals, and strategies to achieve those objectives and goals. The plans they develop must fit within financial and workforce constraints.

- *Organizing.* Managers acquire, mobilize, and manage resources to carry out the planned strategies.
- *Directing.* Managers direct the work of others, instructing them about when and how to carry out tasks.
- *Controlling.* Managers monitor the work of those for whom they are responsible, by creating and implementing a method for evaluating the group's work. Managers need to stay focused on clinical quality and financial accountability.

Preparing for a Leadership Role

All health care professionals, to the extent that they work with others, can become leaders. Even students can begin to assume leadership roles, such as in their study groups or on team projects. To prepare for a leadership role, take some time to reflect on the following:

- *Identify your strengths.* Continually improve the things that you do best. Work on acquiring the skills and knowledge you need to maximize your strengths and remedy your bad habits. Honestly assess your "intellectual arrogance." Realize that being bright is not a substitute for knowledge.

- *Evaluate how you accomplish work.* We all try to work in ways that yield the best results for us. Do you work more productively in teams or alone? Are you more productive as a decision maker or as an advisor?

- *Clarify your values.* Working in an organization or a group whose value system is unacceptable or incompatible with your own can lead to frustration and poor performance. Identify your values and seek a work environment that fits those values.

- *Assume responsibility for relationships.* Cultivate relationships, and analyze the differences you may have with others. Know and understand the strengths, values, and work styles of your coworkers and managers.

✔ **CHECK POINT**

3 What four basic skills are needed by health care leaders?

4 What are three types of leadership styles?

Don't forget to visit thePoint companion website for additional study resources!

CHAPTER HIGHLIGHTS

- A health care team consists of members with a variety of health-related backgrounds, education, and experiences.
- The structure of a team, and how well the team members understand that structure, often determine whether a team is successful. The elements of team structure include the team's purpose, specific goals, the roles of team members, and the functions of the team.
- Effective teamwork requires open and honest communication, organizational resources, and mutual support among team members.
- Conflict management is an essential skill for health care professionals and involves finding the right solution for the situation.
- Leadership is the ability to influence others while working toward a vision or goal.
- The three main leadership styles are autocratic, democratic, and laissez-faire.
- Health care professionals who serve in managerial roles are responsible for planning, organizing, directing, and controlling.

REVIEW QUESTIONS

Matching

1. _____ Leadership style in which the leader assumes complete control over decisions and group activities

2. _____ Leadership style in which the leader and group work together to accomplish mutually agreed upon goals

3. _____ Two or more individuals organized to function cooperatively as a group

4. _____ Leadership style in which team members are allowed to act independently

5. _____ Depends on open and honest communication, sufficient organizational resources, and mutual support

   a. team   **b.** laissez-faire   **c.** autocratic   **d.** democratic   **e.** teamwork

Multiple Choice

6. A health care team consists of members with a variety of health-related
   - **a.** backgrounds
   - **b.** education
   - **c.** experiences
   - **d.** all of the above

7. This is to be expected when a variety of ideas and personalities are brought together on a team.
   - **a.** teamwork
   - **b.** conflict
   - **c.** democracy
   - **d.** all of the above

8. The ability to influence others while working toward a vision or goal is
   - **a.** planning
   - **b.** organization
   - **c.** leadership
   - **d.** all of the above

9. Which of the following is NOT an example of a team member role?
   - **a.** patient
   - **b.** spokesperson
   - **c.** resource
   - **d.** optimist

10. The most effective group leaders use power to encourage members to
    a. form similar opinions
    b. confront one another
    c. cooperate with one another
    d. define their own goals

Completion

11. A team's _____ points it in the right direction.

12. A team _____ defines issues, sets the agenda, and coordinates team members.

13. Team _____ are the activities that the team members must carry out to meet the team's goals.

14. A group of registered nurses working on a common problem is an example of a/an _____ team.

15. Teams made up of professionals with different qualifications, skills, and areas of expertise are _____ teams.

Short Answer

16. How could the fact that many health care professionals spend most of their time working independently of others create an atmosphere of distrust and suspicion?

_____

_____

17. Why is it useful to have regular meetings of a team occur on the same day and at the same time?

_____

_____

18. What role does the reflector play on a team?

_____

_____

19. What are the basic elements of team structure?

_____

_____

20. Why might a leader want to distribute an agenda to team members prior to a meeting?

_____

_____

INVESTIGATE IT

1. Self-evaluation is one means by which individuals can assess their leadership attitudes and skills. The following site provides four different questionnaires that can be used as self-evaluation tools: http://www.adv-leadership-grp.com/Self-Evaluations.html. Complete at least one self-evaluation questionnaire from this web site.

2. How good are you at managing and resolving conflict? Do you believe that in order for one person to "win," another person has to "lose"? Is conflict always a bad thing? Search the Internet and other available resources to find information about conflict management. Use the search terms *conflict management* or *conflict resolution* to begin your Internet search.

RECOMMENDED READING

Cook DJ, Griffith LE, Sackett DL. Importance of and Satisfaction with Work and Professional Interpersonal Issues: A Survey of Physicians Practicing General Internal Medicine in Ontario. *Can Med Assoc J* [serial online]. Sept. 15, 1995; 153(6):755–764. Available at http://www.pubmedcentral.nih.gov/picrender.fcgi?artid=1487276&blobtype=pdf.

Eade DM. Motivational Management: Developing Leadership Skills. Available at http://www.adv-leadership-grp.com/Motivational_Article.html.

Physical Medicine and Rehabilitation Team. [New York-Presbyterian Hospital web site]. Available at http://nyp.org/health/physical-medicine-rehabilitation-team.html.

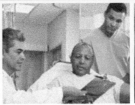
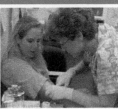
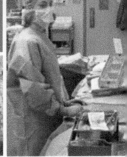
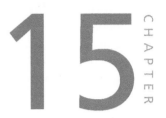

Critical Thinking and Problem Solving

CHAPTER OBJECTIVES

After careful study of this chapter, you should be able to:

* Define critical thinking.
* Discuss the importance of critical thinking in health care.
* Identify the characteristics of a critical thinker.
* Explain the basic problem-solving approach used in health care.
* Compare and contrast the basic problem-solving method with trial-and-error problem solving,

scientific problem solving, and intuitive problem solving.
* Explain the best way to study.
* Describe the features of a good study area.
* Outline the learning process and important strategies for learning.

KEY TERMS

acronym
acrostic
critical thinking

intuitive problem solving
perception phase
reception phase

scientific problem
  solving
selection phase

trial-and-error problem
  solving
working memory

Health care professionals work with patients whose health involves many different factors. They confront situations that require quick and clear-minded decision making. For these reasons, most health care professionals use critical-thinking and problem-solving skills every day.

Although critical thinking and problem solving are two separate skills, they're both useful tools for making good decisions and finding the best solution to a problem. Health care workers who can think critically and make good judgments based on the information at hand are better equipped to do their job well. This chapter discusses the use of critical thinking and problem solving in health care careers. It also describes study skills that will serve you now as a student and later in your career.

CRITICAL THINKING

As a health care professional, you should use critical thinking—continually and proactively *thinking* about the tasks at hand, applying your knowledge and skills in a thoughtful and "present" way—and not simply rely on rote actions and skills. Critical thinking, as defined by Dr. Richard Paul, Director of Research and Professional Development at the Center for Critical Thinking, is "a systematic way to form and shape one's thinking. It functions purposefully and exactingly. It is thought that is disciplined, comprehensive, based on intellectual standards, and, as a result, well-reasoned." Critical-thinking skills allow you to achieve results through focused thinking. Effective critical thinking in health care has four features:

- It is purposeful and results-oriented.
- It is based on principles of health care practice and the scientific method, which means that judgments are based on evidence rather than guesswork.
- It is guided by professional standards and ethics codes.
- It is self-correcting through constant reevaluation and reflects a desire to improve.

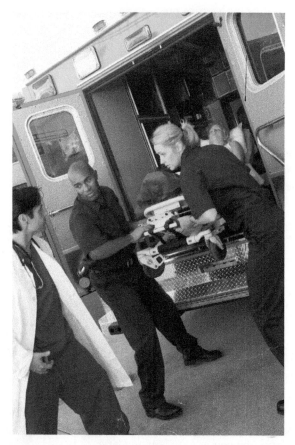

Critical thinking skills are crucial in emergencies and other high-pressure health care situations.

Analyzing and Evaluating Information

When you think critically, you analyze information objectively to form your own judgment about it. The information may come from your own observations, personal experience, and reasoning, or it may be data communicated to you by others. As a health care professional, you continually gather and analyze information and evaluate results on a daily basis. If you're able to think critically and make good judgments based on information you gather, you'll have a positive impact on patients' health.

Whether it involves a patient's medical history or an article to be read for class, the analysis process involves breaking information into parts that can be easily understood. For example, if you have been assigned to read articles on a topic and then give a class presentation, you must first ensure that you understand the information contained in each article. You can't talk about a subject if you don't fully understand it yourself. To do this, you must break the information into parts and ask a few basic questions:

- What is the main purpose of each article?
- What is the most important information in each article?
- What data support the main purpose of each article?
- What are the key concepts or most important ideas in each article? How do they relate to the article's main purpose?
- What message is the author trying to convey?

Health care professionals follow the same analytical process. When analyzing patient information, for example, you might ask these questions:

- What is the main purpose of this patient's visit?
- What is the most important information given by this patient?
- What data support the information presented by the patient?
- What are the key concepts or most important ideas learned from the information? How does each relate to the patient's purpose?
- What message is the patient trying to communicate?

To determine whether information you've gathered has value or relevance, you must evaluate it by assessing which conclusions are actually supported by facts and research.

Characteristics of a Critical Thinker

Critical thinkers have certain characteristics or qualities:
- fair-mindedness
- autonomy
- perseverance
- integrity
- creativity

- humility
- confidence

Fair-Mindedness versus Unfair-Mindedness

Critical thinking is not based on stereotypes or unreasoned opinions. Critical thinkers are open to all viewpoints and evaluate the viewpoints equally. This enables them to consider opposing points of view and understand new ideas fully before accepting or rejecting them. For example, a health care professional who thinks critically will listen to statements by the patient, members of the patient's family, and other health care professionals before reaching a conclusion.

Autonomy versus Conformity

In Chapter 10, "Personal Qualities and Professional Skills for Success," you learned about respecting patient autonomy—patients' rights to make decisions about their health care (even if you do not agree). Autonomy is also a component of critical thinking. To be a critical thinker, you must think for yourself and reach your own conclusions. Critical thinkers are committed to analyzing and evaluating beliefs and values; they do not simply accept established ways of doing things. Critical thinkers question when it's reasonable to question, believe when it's reasonable to believe, and conform when it's reasonable to conform. For a health care worker, thinking autonomously might mean, for example, being open to talking with a patient in a different manner in order to learn the patient's medical history. It may not be reasonable to always follow the same routine exactly the way you originally learned it.

Perseverance versus Laziness

Perseverance requires dedication and determination to find an effective solution to a problem. Important issues are often complex and confusing and require a great deal of thought and research in order to reach the best solution. It can be tempting to find the quickest, easiest answer when a situation becomes confusing or frustrating. However, the critical thinker will persevere to find the best solution. Suppose, for example, that an occupational therapist designs a set of exercises for a patient recovering from a stroke. If the therapist determines that the patient finds the exercises too difficult at this stage of recovery, he or she needs to persevere in developing a new set of steps.

Integrity versus Deceit

Integrity means that a person applies the same rigorous standards of proof to his or her own knowledge and beliefs as the person would apply to the knowledge and beliefs of others. Health care professionals who are critical thinkers question their own knowledge and beliefs as thoroughly as they challenge those of colleagues, patients, and others. For example, a dietetic technician believes that a certain type of low-fat diet is best for patients seeking to lose weight. However, reading an article about a new study comparing the varying effectiveness of different types of diets for different people may lead to reconsidering that belief.

Creativity versus Lack of Creativity

A critical thinker always questions the best way to accomplish any task. While critical thinkers value traditional solutions to problems, they also recognize that more creative solutions may be needed. For example, suppose a five-year-old boy has just had abdominal surgery. He needs to breathe deeply with an apparatus to help prevent pneumonia. He resists doing this, however, because it's painful and the apparatus upsets him. Rather than insisting that the boy use the apparatus, the respiratory therapist considers other, less intimidating methods that can help the boy breathe deeply. To solve the problem, the therapist obtains some bubble solutions and has the boy blow bubbles through a wand. Now the boy is breathing deeply while simultaneously having fun.

Humility versus Arrogance

People who are humble are aware of the limits of their own knowledge. Being willing to admit what you don't know is an important characteristic of a critical thinker. For example, Regina, a young woman right out of school, is hired as a radiologic technician at a local hospital. Recognizing that she is still learning, she doesn't simply forge ahead, assuming that she knows everything about her job. Instead, she asks her mentor for advice and guidance when she doesn't understand a directive or procedure.

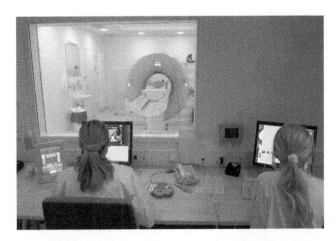

It is not a sign of weakness to ask a more experienced colleague or supervisor for help or guidance.

Confidence versus Distrust

Critical thinkers believe that well-reasoned thinking will lead to trustworthy conclusions, so they have confidence in the reasoning process. For example, Jeff, a dental hygienist who works with a dentist in private practice, sees a patient for prophylactic treatment while the dentist is out of the office and notes what may be an oral medical condition. Although not qualified to make a diagnosis, he takes the initiative to schedule the patient for another appointment with the dentist. With his 10 years of experience, he is confident in his ability to make this decision.

Improving Your Critical-Thinking Skills

How can you improve your critical-thinking skills? There's no one right answer to that question, but the first step is to be critical of your thinking—to think about how you think. Here are a few ideas to get you started thinking about your thinking:

- **Clarify your thinking.** What's the real meaning behind what people are saying in a conversation, a journal article, or a news story? What's the real meaning behind what you're saying? Summarize what you hear or read and ask for confirmation that you understood it correctly. Don't agree or disagree until you're sure that you understand what was said or what you've read. Conversely, when you are transmitting information, restate your point in different words or give examples to illustrate your point, and then ask those receiving the information to summarize or restate it.
- **Discipline your thinking.** Focus your thinking on what is relevant to the task at hand or the problem you're trying to solve. Be on the lookout for illogical leaps in thinking. Retain those thoughts that are logically connected to the main task or problem, but don't allow your mind to wander to unrelated thoughts.
- **Ask meaningful questions.** What types of questions do you typically ask? Are they superficial questions whose answers don't really increase your understanding, or are they penetrating questions that, when answered, lead to deeper understanding of an issue or clarification of a problem? Become a skilled questioner so that you can clarify situations, problems, and solutions more effectively. Don't simply accept how others portray situations or problems.
- **Be willing to change your mind.** It is human nature to believe that your thoughts and views are sound and accurate—and they may be. But other people often have better thoughts and views. Are you willing to consider the views of others? Be open to changing your mind when presented with good reasons to change it.

✓ **CHECK POINT**

1 What are the seven characteristics of critical thinkers?

PROBLEM SOLVING

Everyone solves problems (either effectively or less so) in both their personal and professional lives. While there are different approaches to solving problems, most health care professionals use the general problem-solving technique illustrated in Figure 15-1.

Basic Problem-Solving Approach in Action

The basic problem-solving approach involves five steps: (1) identify the problem; (2) gather information and identify

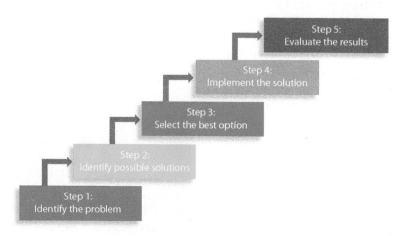

Figure 15-1 This basic problem-solving process is a logical, thorough method health care workers can use to analyze problems and identify the best solution.

possible solutions; (3) select the best option; (4) implement the solution; and (5) evaluate the results. To demonstrate the process, let's use an example to see it in action:

As a health care professional, you recommend that one of your patients attend a local support group that meets once a month. Your patient agrees, but he has no car, and the bus ride from his apartment to the meeting place is very long. The plan, then, seems unrealistic. This situation calls for problem solving.

- **Identify the Problem.** You begin by clearly defining the problem, so that you and the patient are focused on the same issue. In this example, the problem is the patient's lack of convenient transportation to the support group.
- **Gather Information and Identify Possible Solutions.** After identifying the problem, you need to gather all the pertinent data. Get all the facts that you can that relate to this situation. This step may take some time, but it will lay a solid foundation for your decision-making process. Collect data that can help you solve the problem. Ways to do this include:
  - Brainstorming in small groups
  - Collecting data from the patient through assessment
  - Conducting research
- Brainstorming encourages people to generate creative thoughts spontaneously, without stopping to analyze each idea. During brainstorming sessions, there should be no criticism of ideas. You are trying to open up possibilities and break down wrong assumptions about the limits of the problem. People may come up with ideas and thoughts that seem to be a bit shocking or crazy at first. Ideas should only be judged or analyzed at the end of the brainstorming session. At that point, you can change and improve them into possible solutions that are useful—and often quite original.
- Continuing with our example, you and the patient make a list of ways to solve the problem. These might include getting a ride from someone else attending the same meeting, getting a ride from a relative, taking the bus and bringing along a book to read during the trip, or finding a closer support group.
- **Select the Best Option.** From among the various ideas, choose the course of action that will provide the greatest chance for success. Consider the short- and long-term effects of each idea. In our example, you encourage the patient to decide which solution he thinks will work best. Because he enjoys reading, he decides that he can make good use of the time he spends riding the bus to and from meetings by reading.
- **Implement the Solution.** Some solutions provide immediate results, and some take a while to show results, so be sure to give the solution enough time to work. In our example, you encourage the patient to put this solution into action, reminding him to remain open-minded about it. You explain that he may need to try riding the bus a few times, especially if the trip seems too long or unpleasant at first. You point out that he may get used to it over time.
- **Evaluate the Results.** After allowing time for the solution to work, reassess the situation. Has the problem been solved? To conclude our example, after a period of time, you meet again with the patient to determine whether the goal has been reached. If the patient regularly attends the group, the problem is solved. If not, you encourage the patient to try another solution, and then schedule a follow-up appointment to reevaluate his situation.

Trial-and-Error Problem Solving

Trial-and-error problem solving involves testing any number of solutions until one is found that solves a particular problem. While this method may be a useful problem-solving technique for some aspects of everyday life—such as solving the problem of a boring diet by experimenting with different new foods—it is not an effective problem-solving technique for health care professionals, and it could be dangerous to patients. For example, it would be dangerous if you used trial and error to determine the food to supply a dehydrated and malnourished patient. Instead, you need to know, based on clinical research, exactly what food and fluid supplements are most likely to reverse the patient's deficiencies.

Scientific Problem Solving

Scientific problem solving is a systematic problem-solving process that involves the following seven steps:
1. problem identification
2. data collection
3. hypothesis formulation
4. plan of action
5. hypothesis testing
6. interpretation of results
7. evaluation

Scientific problem solving is a more complex version of the basic problem-solving method. Because of the rigorous demands of scientific proof, it is used in controlled laboratory settings to carry out experiments. For example, a clinical laboratory technologist working at a pharmaceutical company would use a process similar to this one. (Health care occupations in laboratory services are detailed in Chapter 6, "Laboratory and Pharmacy Services.")

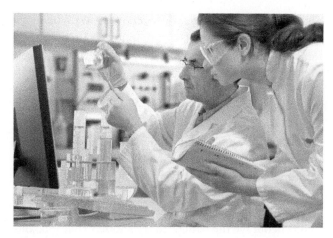

Because of the rigorous demands of scientific proof, scientific problem solving is used in controlled laboratory settings to carry out experiments.

Intuitive Problem Solving

While some health care theorists and educators argue that clinical judgments should be based on data alone, others acknowledge the role intuition plays in clinical decision making. Many health care professionals can describe situations in which an inner prompting led to a quick intervention that saved a patient's life.

When a person instinctively, without logical thinking, identifies a solution to a problem based on its similarity or dissimilarity to other problems, he or she is using intuitive problem solving. For example, a recovery room nurse who intervenes to help a postoperative patient whose condition is worsening, even before there are measurable signs of trouble, is using intuitive problem solving.

✓ **CHECK POINT**

2 What are the five steps of basic problem solving?

3 Where is the scientific problem-solving technique most often used?

STUDY SKILLS

Applying critical-thinking and problem-solving skills as you study will help you learn more successfully, both now and later in your chosen health care field. A career in health care involves life-long learning—and life-long studying—so it's important to learn effective study skills while you're still in school.

Many strategies can help both students and health care professionals make the most of their study time and resources. To some, studying is fairly straightforward. They simply gather their books and begin reading and taking notes. Others are less certain what it means to study. Studying involves four processes:

- refreshing one's memory
- taking in new information
- organizing and memorizing data
- making connections among information

Many individuals feel overwhelmed at the thought of studying an unfamiliar subject. Any little distraction can divert their attention and keep them from studying efficiently. To really learn and understand something, you first must learn the right way to study.

Study Area

You need a good place to study. Look for a location that is free of distractions. Ask yourself the following questions:

- Are there a lot of other people in the same area who could interrupt me?
- Are there things in the area that will distract me from studying?
- Is there a TV or radio in the area that might be turned on?
- Is there a phone that might ring too often?
- Is this area easy for me to get to regularly?
- Is the temperature comfortable? If it isn't, can I change it?
- Will cooking odors come into this area, making me feel hungry and distracted?
- Is this area big enough so that it won't get cluttered when I spread out all of my materials?
- Is there enough light so that I can read without straining my eyes?

The area should be large enough to arrange all study materials. For example, some students prefer to sit at a table when they study. This arrangement keeps them alert and focused, while helping them keep their materials organized. Other students, however, feel more comfortable sitting on a sofa, placing study materials on a coffee table or on the floor below. One place to avoid studying is in bed, where taking a nap may be too tempting.

To choose a good study area, you also need to think about the lighting, temperature, and surroundings.

Lighting

A good study area needs sufficient lighting that can be controlled. Light is very important. Too much will make your eyes hurt, while too little will force you to strain your eyes. The light should shine evenly over all your work and not directly into your eyes.

Temperature

Most people want to be comfortable when studying. Being too cold is distracting, and it is difficult to take notes with cold fingers. However, being too hot can cause heat stress, which impairs mental sharpness and can lead to drowsiness. For studying, the best temperature is between 65 and 70° F (18 to 21° C).

The best way to make sure that a study area is set to a comfortable temperature is to try it out yourself. A half-hour should be sufficient for you to judge whether the area's temperature is comfortable. Bear in mind that a nearby air conditioning or heating vent can make you too cold or too hot, or a nearby door may cause you to feel a draft.

Surroundings

A study area should be inviting. It should make you feel good and encourage you to want to spend time there. A pleasant space can make you more alert. The following tips will help you be more alert and avoid distractions while studying:

- Background music can promote relaxed alertness, which stimulates learning. It also may improve your recall. But avoid music that is too loud or that tempts you to sing along.
- Rather than music, some people like what is called white noise, such as a bubbling fountain or the hum of an electric fan. White noise blocks out other sounds without creating a distraction.
- To avoid the distraction of phone calls, leave your phone in another room, or turn it off and let an answering machine or voice mail take messages. Similarly, avoid reading or replying to text messages, sending emails, or engaging in other forms of social networking.
- Turn off the TV, or, better yet, study in a room without a TV.

Daily Preparation

Daily preparation helps you keep up with your coursework or job. To prepare for each day, make to-do lists and keep a daily planner. Then review all the resources related to the upcoming tasks, such as:

- reading texts
- reviewing notes
- studying patient files
- analyzing test results
- consulting fellow learners or colleagues
- examining additional resources

It is also wise to cover material in small amounts at a time. Information is more easily absorbed in chunks. Thus, reading short segments of a text or studying notes for brief periods of time is more effective than

long cramming sessions. Studying in one-hour sessions, with breaks between sessions, is a productive study schedule.

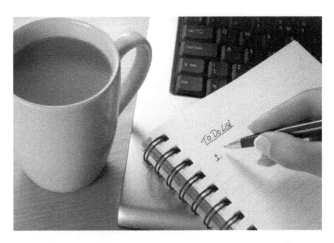

In school as well as in your career, you'll be more productive and focused if you start each day with a solid "to do" list.

ZOOM IN

More Study Tips

From books to web sites, many resources provide tips and tricks for improving study habits. In addition to the skills already covered in this chapter, here are more techniques for making the most of your study time:

- Think of studying as practice, not work—practice makes perfect.
- Remember that the quality of study time is much more important than the quantity.
- Study every day—make it a habit.
- Determine your best study time, and plan on studying at the same time every day.
- Study with a friend, colleague, or study group; compare notes and ask each other questions.
- Start with the most difficult tasks or assignments, and then move on to the easier ones; this focuses maximum brain power on the hardest tasks.
- Spend more time, not less, on the subjects you find most difficult.
- Try to recall the main points and as many details as possible after every study session.
- Try relating new information to something you already know.
- Ask a teacher, parent, colleague, or friend for help when you're unsure of something—asking questions is one of the most effective ways to learn.
- Plan a fun activity as a reward for when you're done studying.

The Learning Process

Learning involves much more than short-term memorization or "just knowing it for the test." To truly learn something, you must understand the subject fully, so that you can recall it and apply it when necessary.

The learning process begins when the brain receives information. This information can be received through a variety of ways, but reading is a very common one for students. Reading is more than simply running your eyes over a page. As you read, you should be asking yourself questions about the material. This helps ensure that you understand what you're reading. Many textbooks include review questions at the end of each chapter. Check your comprehension by trying to answer these questions, even if they haven't been assigned. If you're able to answer these questions correctly, you likely understand the material.

When reading material, you should:

- Pay special attention to bold and italicized print.
- Write main paragraph points in page margins or a notebook.
- Read everything, including tables, graphs and illustrations.

Whether through reading, listening, or using some other means, the process of learning information has three parts: reception, perception, and selection. In the reception phase, you take in information without yet knowing what it means. For instance, you may read about a symptom in your anatomy and physiology textbook, such as a "whooshing" sound coming from the bowel. However, you don't know what the sound means or what condition it represents. During the perception phase, you give meaning to the information. For example, your instructor may say that whooshing sounds might mean that the bowel is obstructed. You can now attach a meaning to the sound, and you begin to understand the symptom you've been reading about in your A&P textbook. Finally, during the selection phase, your brain recognizes information as important or unimportant. If you decide something is important, like the fact that whooshing sounds could mean an obstructed bowel, then that fact is processed for remembering. If you decide the fact is unimportant, you may forget it.

To ensure you remember information you've received, you should review it—ideally immediately after receiving it. It is a mistake to wait until just before an examination to begin reviewing.

To review something that you've studied, you rely on your working memory. The term working memory describes how the brain stores and retrieves information from short-term and long-term memory. Short-term memory is limited. It lasts as little as 15 seconds and can't store a great deal of information. In fact, research has shown that short-term memory can hold only five to nine chunks of information, depending on how well the information is grouped. For example, the numbers 1-9-2-9-0-0-7 are more easily remembered through grouping: 1929 and 007. These two groups are much easier to remember than all seven individual numbers. Grouping makes space for more data in short-term memory.

After information has been grouped, the brain either forgets it or moves it to long-term memory, where it's organized and stored for longer periods. How long depends on how completely the information is processed and how often you recall and use it. There are many ways to help move information from short- to long-term memory, but the best way is to recall or review the information immediately and often.

Sometimes, though, despite our efforts, information is forgotten. However, it may still be possible to retrieve that information. The next time you have trouble remembering something important, try these techniques to help you remember:

1. Say or write down everything you can remember about the information you're seeking.

2. Try to recall events or information in a different order.

3. Recreate the learning environment or relive the event. Include sounds, smells, and details about the weather, objects, or people who were there. Try to recapture what you said, thought, or felt at the time.

Different Strategies for Learning

Once information has been received and reviewed, the problem most people face is making sure the information stays in their long-term memory. This can be difficult, especially if the information isn't used regularly. Information is more easily forgotten when you're not very interested in the subject, when you lack a real purpose for learning, or when you have few or no connections between the memory and other pieces of information. However, you can use several fun strategies to help you store information in your long-term memory.

Make Associations

Making links between familiar items and new information helps you remember the new information. Once established, these links become automatic. Each time you recall a familiar item, you also remember the information associated with it.

Follow these steps to form associations as you study:

1. First, select the information to be remembered. For example, suppose you want to remember that osteoporosis causes a person's bones to become brittle.

2. Next, create an association to the information. You might associate the details about osteoporosis with the name of a person you know who has the condition. (Osteoporosis reminds me of Mary, who broke her hip. Osteoporosis → Mary → brittle bones.)

The most effective associations are personal, such as associating a song, a person, or a scent with the item being remembered. For some people, a certain smell takes them right back to a specific time in their past. When such people associate information with that smell, the memory of the information will be just as sharp.

Acronyms and Acrostics

Acronyms and acrostics are handy ways of recalling information, too. Acronyms are words created from the first letter of each word in a phrase or each item on a list. For example, ASAP is an acronym for the phrase "as soon as possible." The acronym *RICE* helps people remember the treatment of some musculoskeletal injuries:

- *R*est
- *I*ce
- *C*ompression
- *E*levation

Acrostics are phrases or sentences created from the first letter of each item on a list. In health care, a well-known acrostic helps identify the 12 cranial nerves: *On Old Olympus' Towering Tops, A Finn and a Swedish Girl Viewed Some Hops*. The initial letters stand for the nerves:

- *O*lfactory nerve
- *O*ptic nerve
- *O*culomotor nerve
- *T*rochlear nerve
- *T*rigeminal nerve
- *A*bduscens nerve
- *F*acial nerve
- *S*ensorimotor nerve
- *G*lossopharyngeal nerve
- *V*agus nerve
- *S*pinal accessory nerve
- *H*ypoglossal nerve

Acronyms and acrostics work especially well when it's hard to find a personal memory or other association for a piece of data. For example, it's probably difficult for someone to feel personal about the 12 cranial nerves. Acronyms and acrostics connect pieces of information to a new, but easily remembered, word or phrase, thus improving a person's ability to retain the information.

Flashcards

Flashcards are an effective study tool for learning new material or reviewing information. Write a term on one side of the card and the definition, formula, or other information about the term on the other side. When used with a partner, flashcards can be a fun review game. As a study partner holds up each card, attempt to recall the pertinent information. Mix up the cards to ensure that you understand each term separately, rather than as part of a certain sequence.

Music

Most people can still remember the lyrics of songs they heard years ago. Even if they haven't heard the song in years, hearing the first few notes may be enough to help them remember all of its lyrics. If they were asked to speak the lyrics, however, they might not be able to. The addition of a melody helps trigger memory. This principle can be applied to other information you need to learn. Making up a short jingle to go along with new material can make it much easier to recall the information later on.

Study Groups

Some people learn new information better by explaining it to someone else, like a classmate or coworker. By explaining it, they're actively processing the information, or thinking about it more clearly and deeply.

Studying in a small group can be helpful to all group members because everyone is "thinking out loud," sharing ideas, and learning from one another. Even if a study group is unable to answer everyone's questions, hearing others' thoughts on a subject is a good way to learn.

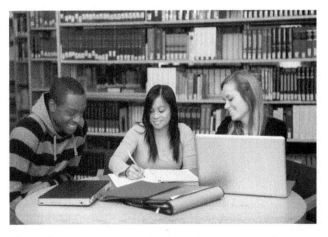

Studying in a small group can be helpful to all group members because interacting and sharing ideas can lead to participants learning from one another.

Getting the Group Together

A successful study group has members who reflect the four C's:

- Committed—truly interested in learning the material
- Contributing—willing to share their knowledge
- Compatible—able to overlook differences and focus on studying together
- Considerate—willing to arrive for studying on time

It is easier to stay on task when everyone in the group is interested in the same thing—studying. If the group becomes too large (more than four or five members), it should break into smaller groups. A smaller number makes it easier to review all the necessary material and answer each other's questions.

Making the Most of the Group Session

One of the greatest benefits of studying in a small group is the mutual support. Working in a group can also reinforce what you have learned and deepen your understanding of complex concepts. These tips will help you get the most out of study group sessions:

- **Determine objectives**. Group members need to know what they're going to achieve at each session. The group might want to pick a designated or rotating leader to set the objectives.
- **Prepare in advance**. Group members need to come to the study session prepared, by reading, reviewing notes, or doing whatever else needs to be done. This will help to make the most of everyone's time together.
- **Alternate instruction**. When group members take turns instructing the group, everyone in the group learns the material better.
- **Focus on the task**. The group needs to stay on the topic at hand. The group leader needs to steer the group back if it veers off that topic.

CHECK POINT

4 What are the important characteristics of a good study area?

5 List effective strategies for learning and retaining knowledge in long-term memory.

Don't forget to visit thePoint companion website for additional study resources!

CHAPTER HIGHLIGHTS

- Health care professionals should use critical thinking, a systematic way to form and shape one's thinking, and not simply rely on rote actions and skills.
- The characteristics of critical thinkers include fair-mindedness, autonomy, perseverance, integrity, creativity, humility, and confidence.
- The problem-solving technique used by most health care professionals involves five steps: (1) identifying the problem, (2) gathering information and identifying possible solutions, (3) selecting the best option, (4) implementing the solution, and (5) evaluating the results. Other problem-solving techniques include trial and error, scientific problem solving, and intuition.
- Studying involves four processes: (1) refreshing one's memory; (2) taking in new information; (3) organizing and memorizing data; and (4) making connections among information.
- A good place to study is free of distractions and has adequate space and lighting, a comfortable temperature, and pleasant surroundings.
- Learning involves much more than short-term memorization. When you truly learn something, you understand it fully, so that you can recall it and apply it when necessary.
- Strategies that can help you store information in long-term memory include making associations, using acronyms and acrostics, making flashcards, putting information to music, and studying in small groups.

REVIEW QUESTIONS

Matching

1. _____ Encourages people to generate creative thoughts spontaneously, without stopping to analyze each idea
2. _____ Being capable of thinking for oneself and reaching one's own conclusions
3. _____ Word created from the first letter of each word in a phrase or each item on a list
4. _____ Phrase or sentence created from the first letter of each item on a list
5. _____ Being open to all viewpoints and evaluating them equally

   a. fair-mindedness   **b.** acrostic   **c.** autonomy   **d.** brainstorming   **e.** acronym

Multiple Choice

6. Studying involves
   - **a.** refreshing one's memory
   - **b.** taking in new information
   - **c.** organizing and memorizing data
   - **d.** all of the above

7. When a person instinctively, without logical thinking, identifies a solution to a problem based on its similarity or dissimilarity to other problems, which type of problem solving is the person using?
   - **a.** trial-and-error
   - **b.** intuitive
   - **c.** scientific
   - **d.** brainstorming

8. Surveying material that has already been covered is called
   - **a.** reviewing
   - **b.** receiving
   - **c.** perception
   - **d.** selection

9. Where does the brain organize and store information for extended periods?
   a. long-term memory
   b. short-term memory
   c. working memory
   d. none of the above

10. Which type of memory can hold five to nine chunks of information, depending on how well the information is grouped?
    a. long-term memory
    b. short-term memory
    c. working memory
    d. none of the above

Completion

11. _____ thinking is a systematic way to form and shape one's thinking that functions purposefully and exactingly.

12. The basic problem-solving process includes identifying the problem; identifying possible _____; selecting the best option; implementing the solution; and evaluating the results.

13. _____ problem solving is a systematic problem-solving process used in controlled laboratory settings.

14. A good study area should be free of _____ and have adequate space and lighting, a comfortable temperature, and pleasant surroundings.

15. _____ memory describes how the brain stores and retrieves information from short-term and long-term memory.

Short Answer

16. Name at least five characteristics of critical thinkers.

   _____

   _____

17. What steps are involved in the scientific problem-solving process?

   _____

   _____

18. What are the four features of effective critical thinking in health care?

   _____

   _____

19. Briefly describe the three-part process of learning information.

   _____

   _____

20. What four elements should members of a successful study group possess?

   _____

   _____

Table 15-1 Characteristics of Critical Thinkers	
Rating	**Characteristic**
	Fair-mindedness—is open to all viewpoints and evaluates them equally
	Autonomy—thinks for oneself and reaches one's own conclusions
	Perseverance—persists to find an effective solution to a problem
	Integrity—applies the same rigorous standards of proof to one's own knowledge and beliefs as to those of others
	Creativity—questions the best way to accomplish a task and devises new or different approaches to solve a problem
	Humility—is aware of the limits of one's own knowledge and is willing to admit a lack of knowledge
	Confidence—believes that well-reasoned thinking will lead to trustworthy conclusions

INVESTIGATE IT

1. Characteristics of critical thinkers are summarized in Table 15-1 above. Think about situations where you either demonstrated or failed to demonstrate these characteristics. Using a scale of 1 to 7, with 1 meaning "almost never" and 7 meaning "always," rate how well you think you demonstrate each of the characteristics in the table. Then invite others who know you well to rate you, too. Did you and the others who rated you reach the same conclusions?

2. Puzzles, logic problems, and riddles are all fun ways to sharpen one's critical-thinking skills. Using the Internet and other available resources, find some interesting "brain teaser" exercises and use critical-thinking skills to solve them. A variety of puzzles can be found at the following web sites:

   - http://www.mathsisfun.com/chicken_crossing.html
   - http://www.brainbashers.com

RECOMMENDED READING

Elder L. Are you a critical thinker? Available at: http://www.csmonitor.com/2009/0312/p09s01-coop.html.

Olrech N. *Student Success for Health Professionals Made Incredibly Easy.* Baltimore: Lippincott Williams & Wilkins, 2008

Paul R. *Critical Thinking: How to Prepare Students for a Rapidly Changing World.* Santa Rosa, CA: Foundation for Critical Thinking, 1995.

Taylor C. *Fundamentals of Nursing: The Art and Science of Nursing Care.* Baltimore: Lippincott Williams & Wilkins, 2008.

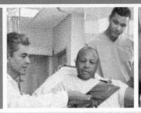
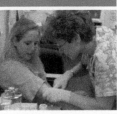
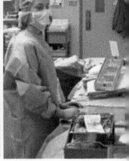

Health Care Communication

CHAPTER OBJECTIVES

After careful study of this chapter, you should be able to:

✳ Explain how the communication process is important in health care.

✳ Differentiate among the three most common modes of communication and how they are used in health care.

✳ Describe the different methods and types of patient communication.

✳ Communicate successfully with patients.

✳ Explain the importance of accuracy and security in health care recording and reporting.

✳ Identify the most common communication challenges in health care and know how to overcome them.

✳ Use good telephone manners in communication.

KEY TERMS

body language
channel of communication
chronological organization
clarification
communication

comparison organization
feedback
kinesics (ki-NĒ-siks)
message

non-language sounds
paraphrasing
problem-oriented organization

proxemics (präk-SĒ-miks)
reflecting
source

Communication, defined as an exchange of information, is important throughout the health care system. Whether your communication involves assessment, diagnosis, treatment, or documentation, you regularly share information about a patient's health or other information. Therefore, precision and confidentiality are imperative in all aspects of health care communications.

Excellent communication skills are crucial for all health care professionals. The clear and accurate transfer of information ensures that every person involved with a patient's care is using the same information. Breakdowns in communication in the form of incomplete patient histories, test inaccuracies, billing miscalculations, or treatment oversights can have devastating consequences. Prescription errors, misdiagnoses, or even death can result from communication failures.

COMMUNICATION PROCESS

The communication process involves the sending and receiving of information between two or more individuals It is the foundation of society and the most primary aspect of the patient-provider relationship. Without communication, it would be impossible to share experiences, gain knowledge, arrange treatments, or establish and maintain records. By nature, humans are social beings, and human needs are met through association with other humans. The ability to communicate is basic to human functioning and well-being.

In health care, the communication process often begins with a patient need that must be addressed. Three central elements are present within any communication process (Figure 16-1):

● sender—the person who transmits the message
● message—the information the sender conveys
● receiver—the person who gets the message

There is also a fourth, optional, element within the communication process:

● feedback—evaluation by the receiver and sender to verify that both understand the message that was sent

The communication process begins with a message. The sender, or source, of the message is the person or group that begins the communication process. The message comes from the source. It may be spoken words from a patient describing a symptom, information obtained during a consultation or telephone conversation, data entered in a patient's chart, written correspondence, or even a gesture.

Once a message is sent, the receiver interprets it. In most conversations, people shift back and forth

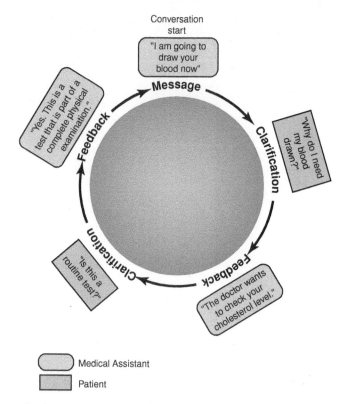

Figure 16-2   Example of flow of communication between a medical assistant and a patient.

between the roles of sender and receiver. Once you, as the receiver, understand the message, you decide how to respond. When you require clarification, or a better understanding of a message, your response is sent back to the sender. This is called feedback. For example, you might give a patient instructions about how to care for an incision at home—in which case you're the sender. The patient then asks a question that shows that he or she has not fully understood your instructions. This feedback from the patient gives you an opportunity to clarify your instructions. Figure 16-2 illustrates the flow of communication.

The channel of communication is the medium by which a message is sent. The most common channel is speaking. However, messages can also be sent and received through sight and touch. As a health care professional, you will use all three of these channels to communicate with patients and colleagues alike.

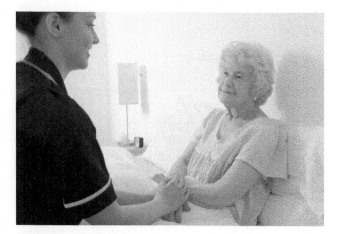

Figure 16-1   Communication in health care revolves around addressing patient needs.

✔ CHECK POINT

1 What three elements are present in all forms of communication?

2 What is the optional fourth element of communication?

ZOOM IN

Clear Communication

Anyone who has visited a physician is probably familiar with a standard physical exam. Although the steps in this exam are routine for many patients, you should not assume that all patients understand exactly what they're expected to do. Directions should be given clearly to patients throughout the exam.

For example, one procedure involves a nurse or doctor listening to a patient's lungs with a stethoscope, while instructing the patient to breathe deeply in and out. This procedure verifies that the lungs are clear, healthy, and functioning well. The practitioner also directs the patient to hold his or her breath for a moment.

Next, the patient is instructed to breathe out again. At this point in the exam, one might say to the patient, "I want you to expire now." Although this phrase is technically correct, the word *expire* has different meanings and may not be interpreted correctly by the patient. It would be much better to say, "You can breathe out now," or "I need you to exhale."

COMMUNICATION MODES

Information can be exchanged by different methods. The three most common modes of communication are:
- verbal communication
- nonverbal communication
- written communication

A sender's words (either verbal or written) and body language (nonverbal) often vary depending on the sender's socioeconomic background, culture, age, and education. For example, if you say, "I want you to expire now," some patients might think you mean "I want you to die," rather than "I want you to exhale"—the medical meaning of "expire" means something totally different from its other meaning, as understood by someone with a different background and education.

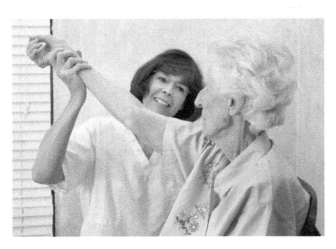
Verbal and nonverbal communication often happen at the same time.

Verbal Communication

In verbal communication, spoken words are used to exchange information. Because you choose the words you want to communicate, this is a deliberate form of communication. It is also the most common form of communication.

Good verbal communication skills are an important and necessary tool for all health care professionals. Whether scheduling appointments, providing patient education, arranging referrals, or sharing information with a colleague, you should follow a few simple verbal communication guidelines:
- Always use a polite tone. A pleasant manner of speaking helps put people at ease.
- Always use proper English. Using bad grammar or slang expressions implies that you are uneducated and unprofessional.
- Speak respectfully to colleagues and patients. Never "talk down" to someone.
- Avoid using an overly technical vocabulary. Many patients are unfamiliar with lengthy medical terms.

Tips for Successful Verbal Communication

Several factors are involved in successful communication between health care professionals and their patients and colleagues.

Language. The language a person uses often contributes to the first impression the person makes. Speaking clearly and concisely and using terms that patients can understand helps convey that you are competent, intelligent, and caring. For the most part, avoid medical terminology when speaking to patients. Instead, use normal, everyday language. For example, instead of saying, "The nurse will be catheterizing you tomorrow for a urinalysis," you might say, "Tomorrow the nurse will get a sample of your urine by putting a small tube into your bladder." As you speak, watch the other person to see whether your message is making the desired impression. If not, you should reword the message and try again.

Manner and Tone. The volume and tone of your voice can convey many things, including anger, caring, happiness, excitement, and much more. You can calm or agitate a patient with your tone of voice. If you drop a pile of paperwork into a patient's lap and say, "Fill this out; it's self explanatory," while using a hurried manner and tone, the patient hears, "I do not have time to deal with you right now, so do not ask any questions."

Competence. It is important for patients to trust your abilities as a health care professional, because they're putting their health and well-being into your care. You gain trust by being knowledgeable, honest, and dependable—in a word, competent. All information you give to patients should be up-to-date and accurate. You need to convey confidence and certainty in what you're saying, while still being able to acknowledge your limitations. When you say to a patient, "This is a new drug the doctor has ordered; let me tell you about it," you reassure the patient that you're not only knowledgeable, but very thorough in how you perform your job.

Verbal Encouragement. One easy way to make people feel good about a situation is through verbal encouragement. This is a great way to help patients feel like they're partners in health care communication. To encourage patients to speak openly, you should always appear receptive. Use verbal encouragement, such as saying "yes?" or "go on," to persuade patients to share all of their concerns before they begin patient treatment.

Humor. Mild and respectful humor can be an effective means of minimizing status differences between a patient and caregiver. You must be careful, however, and ensure that your comments are sensitive and respectful to all people. What one person may think is funny, another person may consider disrespectful or even hurtful.

Non-Language Sounds

Another form of communication, non-language sounds, may transmit messages unintentionally. Non-language sounds include sighs, sobs, laughs, grunts, and so on. These sounds can give spoken words very different meanings. For example, people who say, "Everything is fine," while sobbing, are sending a message that they may not feel fine at all.

Assertive Communication

When interacting with patients, family members, and colleagues, you should communicate in a way that demonstrates respect for all parties. Assertive behaviors,

ZOOM IN

Seeing Eye-To-Eye

Looking someone directly in the eyes has different meanings in different cultures. In the U.S., good eye contact usually implies that a person is honest and concerned. However, people from other cultures may feel differently about eye contact.

- In some cultures, including Asian and Native American cultures, direct eye contact is viewed as disrespectful. It may even seem sexually suggestive or aggressive.
- In other cultures, including Latino cultures, avoiding eye contact or casting the eyes downward is a sign of respect.

which are a hallmark of professional relationships, are different from aggressive behaviors, which are harsh and destructive.

The key to assertiveness is open, honest, and direct communication. "I" statements like "I feel . . ." and "I think . . ." play an important role in assertive statements. Table 16-1 gives examples of assertive and nonassertive speech.

The four basic components of an assertive response or approach are:
- having empathy
- describing feelings or the situation
- clarifying one's expectations
- anticipating consequences

For example, you might communicate in the following ways with your instructor:
- *Having empathy:* "I know you work hard each week to give us good clinical assignments."
- *Describing feelings:* "I want to share with you how the patient felt after I taught her to give her own insulin injection."
- *Clarifying expectations:* "I understand that each week I need to do teaching with my patients."
- *Anticipating consequences:* "Can we review the test together, as I did not do as well as I thought I would on it, and I'm afraid of not doing well in the course."

Characteristics of an assertive demeanor include having a confident, open body posture; making eye contact; using clear, concise "I" statements; and sharing thoughts, feelings, and emotions honestly.

An assertive work attitude is characterized by:
- a capacity to work with or without supervision
- the ability to remain calm under pressure
- a willingness to ask for help when necessary

Table 16-1 Examples of Assertive and Nonassertive Speech

	Assertive	Nonassertive
Health care worker to coworker	"I know we all lose track of time occasionally, but I'm finding it harder and harder to cover for you when you take extra time for lunch. I don't think it's fair for your patient and me to have to wait an extra 30 minutes every day for you to come back from lunch. Can we talk about this?"	"Huh? No, I didn't really mind. Luckily I wasn't too busy today." Thought: "What a sucker I am. Now I'll have to grab a quick bite so that I can get back on time."
Health care worker to another professional at a supervisory level	"I know we talked about this patient's condition before, but I've collected some new data. I believe a change in his treatment should be discussed."	"Um . . . yes I know you already changed the treatment. It's just that I thought it still wasn't working. Maybe I didn't give it enough time. Thanks for listening to me anyway. I'm sorry to bother you with this."
Student to Preceptor (Mentor/Trainer)	"Can you help me with this procedure? I reviewed the procedure steps, but I'd appreciate your talking me through this because I've never done it before."	"Uh . . . I'm sorry to be such a pain again. I have to do this procedure and don't know where to begin. I know you must be busy, but, uh, is there any way you might have time for me?"

- the ability to give and accept compliments
- honesty in admitting mistakes and taking personal responsibility for them

Active Listening

Active listening is necessary to ensure that messages are correctly received and interpreted. Failure to use active listening can result in poor patient care. By listening actively, you can help ensure that you understand completely what a patient or colleague is trying to communicate. As a result, you're more likely to gain valuable information.

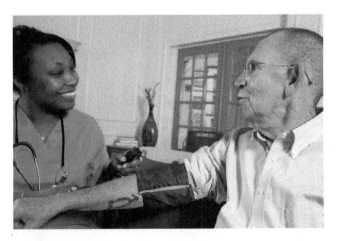

Being an active listener helps you establish positive relationships with patients and other health care workers.

Being an active listener helps you establish positive relationships with patients and other health care workers. Although you listen with your ears, you can't truly understand what another person is saying unless you also use your brain. You must concentrate to absorb what another person is saying. To listen actively, follow these guidelines:

- Give your full attention to the person who is speaking.
- Don't interrupt.
- Pay attention to the speaker's body language and nonverbal cues.

ZOOM IN

Digital Communication

In today's high-tech, fast-paced world, many of the messages people send and receive are handled digitally. Email, texting, and instant messaging are all common methods. Educational materials, seminars, and even continuing education courses can be accessed online without leaving the comfort of home or office.

Although technology brings efficiency and convenience to the process of exchanging information, health care professionals must not overlook the human element in communication. When delivering information, such as a patient's diagnosis, test results, or prognosis, the value of face-to-face contact between a health care professional and patient cannot be overstated. At the very least, important or sensitive information should be relayed through a telephone call. While digital communication is a highly effective tool for some aspects of health care, it must be used responsibly so that it does not diminish a patient's overall health care experience.

Nonverbal Communication

Nonverbal communication, also known as body language, relays a message without speaking or writing a single word. Because nonverbal behavior is less consciously controlled than verbal behavior, it often tells others more about what you're feeling than your spoken words. It is estimated that between 60 percent and 90 percent of your true emotions are conveyed through body language. For example, you may say to a patient, "I would be happy to sit here and talk with you"; but if you glance nervously at your watch every few seconds, you convey a different message to the patient. You should also pay attention to the patient's body language. For example, a patient's body language can provide feedback that shows whether they understand what you're saying or not. Table 16-2 lists a few examples of body language and what each of them can mean.

There are several different forms of nonverbal communication, including kinesics, proxemics, and touch. Eye contact is another important element of nonverbal communication.

Eye Contact

Maintaining good eye contact shows that you're interested in other people and what they're saying. When you look away during a conversation, you may give the impression that you think the speaker's message isn't important enough for your full attention. Likewise, good eye contact when you're speaking adds a sense of truthfulness to your message. If you look away from a patient or colleague while delivering a message, you will seem uncomfortable with what you're saying, and the receiver will become uncomfortable as well.

Table 16-2 Nonverbal Communication/Body Language Chart	
Body Movements or Expressions	**Meanings**
Leaning back in a chair, yawning, looking at a clock, shifting, or shuffling feet	● Boredom ● Fatigue ● Disinterest ● Impatience
Smiling, nodding agreement, keeping eye contact, and leaning forward	● Interest ● Enthusiasm ● Agreement ● Humor
Avoiding eye contact, frowning, scratching head, and pursing lips	● Confusion ● Disagreement ● Suppressing thoughts or feelings ● Anger ● Suspicion

Kinesics or Body Movement

One of the most powerful ways for a human to communicate nonverbally is through kinesics, or body movement. Body movements include facial expressions, gestures such as shrugging, and eye movement. Portrayed moods and emotions may either emphasize or contradict what's being said. Patients' faces often reveal their true inner feelings, such as anger, despair, or fear, which otherwise may be concealed in a conversation.

Proxemics or Personal Space

Personal space, or proxemics, is like an invisible bubble that surrounds you. If others move inside this bubble while talking to you, it may make you feel uncomfortable. Everyone's personal space is somewhat different. How close you normally stand to another person during a conversation most likely depends on your relationship with that person. Here are some interesting facts about personal space:

● Personal space is larger when talking to a stranger. For example, most people in the U.S. like to be about four to seven feet away from each other when holding a conversation with a stranger.

● The better you know the person you're talking with, the smaller the personal space can be between the two of you.

● Personal space is typically larger between two men than between two women.

● Personal space differs from culture to culture. For example, many Europeans are comfortable with a personal space that is about half of what Americans prefer. As a result, some Americans feel uncomfortable when talking with someone from Europe who is standing closer.

When you provide care or perform tests on a patient, you will probably need to enter that person's personal space. It is important that you approach the patient in a professional manner and explain clearly what you intend to do. Your explanation and professionalism will help the patient feel more comfortable and less anxious about what will take place.

Touch

Touch is experienced in many ways. Handshakes, pats, and kisses are just a few of the ways people communicate through touch. Research shows that touching can create either positive or negative feelings. Feelings are positive when a touch is perceived to be natural. On the other hand, when a touch is perceived to be manipulative or insincere, negative feelings will result. For some patients, a gentle touch provides emotional support. For others, however, it may produce a negative response.

When touching a patient, watch for nonverbal cues, such as expressions and body language, to determine how the patient feels about being touched.

Here are some guidelines to help you effectively transmit and receive nonverbal communications.

1. Maintain proper personal space, position, and posture. Your nonverbal communication is sending messages to the patient too.
   - Always look the patient in the face and be at eye level. Be aware of cultural differences when it comes to eye contact.
   - If the patient is sitting, you should sit too (if possible).
   - Use proper gestures.
   - Use touch, if the situation is appropriate.
2. Observe the patient's facial expressions and posture. People's nonverbal messages can differ from their verbal ones.
   - If the patient's nonverbal cues differ from what he or she is saying, ask appropriate questions to clarify the mixed message.
   - If a patient's verbal response still doesn't match what you're seeing, tell your supervisor of your concerns.

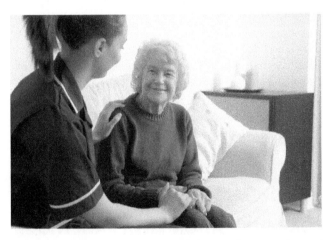

When touching a patient, watch for nonverbal cues, such as expressions and body language, to determine how the patient feels about being touched.

Written Communication

Another means of communication in health care is written communication. The ability to write clearly and accurately is important in the health care profession. As a health care professional, you may be responsible for one or more different types of written communications, such as:
- agendas for meetings
- letters
- messages
- patient charts
- consultation reports
- patient instructions
- laboratory reports

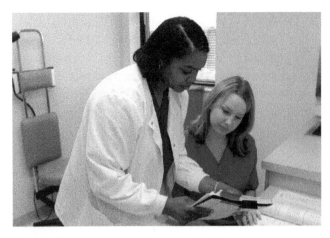

Patient charts and other written communications are key elements of health care communication.

Your written communication should be concise and use language that all parties will understand. Proper grammar may be even more important in written communication than in verbal communication. People may eventually forget about an incorrectly spoken word or term, but a written mistake will often be read many times. Grammatical errors reflect badly on the writer, as well as the writer's practice or office.

Also take enough time to ensure that every word is spelled correctly. Just one incorrect letter in a word can completely change the meaning of a medical term. Because written communications, like patient charts and lab reports, are accessed often, incorrectly spelled words can have devastating consequences for both health care professionals and patients.

Preparation is important for any form of written communication. Plan the content of a document before you begin to write. Written information should be organized logically. The three basic ways of organizing information in written communications include:
- **Chronological organization.** When information is written using chronological organization, items are presented in sequence, from the earliest date to the most recent date. For example, this organization might be used when writing about a physician's background in a brochure for new patients.
- **Problem-oriented organization.** When information is written using problem-oriented organization, a problem is identified and explained, and then instructions are given for correcting the problem. For example, a letter written to a patient reporting abnormal blood

test results would first state the problem, such as a low potassium level, then explain the possible causes of the problem, and finally suggest treatments and follow-up procedures.

- **Comparison organization.** When two or more pieces of information are compared, this is known as comparison organization. For instance, when a health care administrator writes a report to the board of directors that describes the pros and cons of two different electronic health record systems, this approach is being used.

The organization of written information is discussed in more depth in Chapter 17, "Medical Documentation."

Interoffice communications, such as memos and meeting notes, are typically less formal than other forms of communication, because they're not usually seen by patients or other professionals outside the practice. Nonetheless, they require the same preparation, composition, and editing as other written communications. Most computer software programs contain templates for the most common forms of written correspondence. These programs usually have a basic spell-check feature. Although this feature is helpful, a basic spell-check program cannot handle all medical terminology. Specialized medical dictionary software can be used when editing health care documents. These programs are discussed in Chapter 20, "Computers and Other Technology."

Medical Writing

Medical writing requires even more accuracy and clarity than business or personal correspondence. You must pay very close attention to detail when writing medical letters, reports, and other documents. These items may be placed in a patient's permanent medical record. Mistakes in written medical communications could cause injury or death, lawsuits, or professional harm to you or your employer. Some important guidelines for medical writing include the following:

Spelling. Always proofread your written communications. While the spell-check features in word-processing programs can be a great help, they are not a substitute for proofreading. For example, the spell-check feature in a word-processing program cannot find mistakes when words are spelled correctly but misused. For example, the term *mucus* refers to a sticky secretion, while the term *mucous*, spelled with the letter *o*, refers to the membrane that secretes mucus. If the word *mucus* is accidentally misspelled as *mucous*, the spell-check feature would consider the word correct, even though it is actually incorrect.

Capitalization. Pay special attention to how words and abbreviations are capitalized. Although a word may appear to be incorrectly typed or written, take the time to verify the information with the attending physician or other professional before changing it. For example, *m-BACOD* is a very different treatment from *M-BACOD*.

Abbreviations and Symbols. Using abbreviations and symbols saves time when making hand-written notes. However, when you are typing medical information, words should be spelled out. For example, *PM* (time) is commonly understood, but *NPO* ("nothing by mouth") is not. Most offices keep a list of approved abbreviations and symbols commonly used at the office. You should be familiar with the list at your office. (See Appendix D for a list of abbreviations and symbols commonly used in health care.)

Numbers. The numbers one through ten are usually spelled out in medical writing. There are exceptions, however:

- Units of measurement should always be written as numbers, no matter how small (for example, 5 mg).
- Numbers referring to an obstetrical patient's condition are not spelled out. (For example, the numbers in "the patient is gravid 3, para 2" should not be converted to words.)

CHECK POINT

3 What are the three most common modes of communication?

4 What are the four basic components of an assertive response or approach?

5 Why shouldn't you rely solely on a spell-checker to find spelling errors?

COMMUNICATION WITH PATIENTS

One of the most challenging aspects of working in any health care profession is communicating accurately and effectively with patients. Whether taking information from a new patient, discussing a course of treatment, or revealing test results, good communication between you and the patient is essential to the patient's care.

Patient Interviews

Many careers in health care require that you interview patients. You could be responsible for gathering initial information from a patient or for updating existing information. When conducting an interview, keep the following points in mind:

- Listen actively.
- Ask appropriate questions.
- Record information accurately.

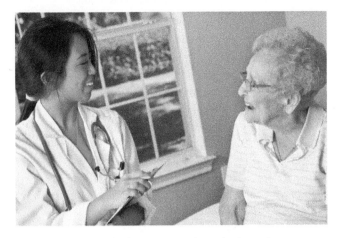

A typical task in many health care careers is conducting patient interviews.

During a patient interview, you must demonstrate professionalism and concern for the patient's privacy. Conduct the interview in a private area, and begin by introducing yourself. Being organized is the key to good interviewing. Know the questions that you're going to ask and the order of the questions before the interview begins. Be prepared to record patient answers, either on paper or electronically. (Chapter 17 provides in-depth information on medical documentation). Do not answer phone calls or attend to other distractions until you have completed the interview. Finally, when leaving the room, let the patient know who will be in next to see him or her and approximately how long it will take. For example, you might say, "Dr. Bradshaw will be in to see you next. It should be just a few minutes."

Basic Interview Techniques

The methods and procedures used during patient interviews vary by provider. However, you should be familiar with six basic interviewing techniques:

- reflecting
- paraphrasing
- clarification
- open-ended questioning
- summarizing
- silences

Reflecting. When you use open-ended statements to repeat back what you have heard from a patient, you are reflecting. With this technique, you do not complete a sentence but leave it up to the patient to do so. For example, you might say, "Mrs. Gomez, you were saying that when your back hurts you . . ." Reflecting encourages the

patient to make further comments and ensures that the patient's meaning is correctly understood. It also helps bring the patient back to the subject if the conversation begins to drift. Reflecting is a useful tool, but you should be careful not to overuse it, as some patients find it annoying to have their words constantly parroted back to them.

Paraphrasing. Restating or paraphrasing means using your own words or phrases to repeat what you have heard. Paraphrasing helps verify that you have understood correctly what has been said. It also allows patients the opportunity to clarify their thoughts or statements. A paraphrased statement typically begins with a phrase like "You're saying that . . ." or "It sounds as if . . . ," followed by the rephrased content.

Clarification. If you're confused about some of the information you've received from a patient, you need to ask the patient to give an example of the situation being described. For instance, you might ask, "Can you describe one of these dizzy spells?" The patient's example should help you better understand what the patient is saying. It also provides insight into how the patient perceives the situation.

Open-Ended Questioning. The best way for you to obtain information is by asking open-ended questions that require the patient to formulate an answer and provide details. Open-ended questions usually begin with the words *what*, *when*, or *how*. For example:

- "What medications did you take this morning?"
- "When did you stop taking your medication?"
- "How did you get that large bruise on your arm?"

Be careful about asking "why" questions, because they often sound judgmental or accusing. For example, asking "Why did you do that?" or "Why didn't you follow the directions?" may make patients feel that you are criticizing their behavior, and they may become defensive and uncooperative. Instead, you might ask, "What parts of the instructions were unclear?" or "How can we help you follow these instructions?"

Generally, avoid closed-ended questions that allow patients to give one-word answers like "Yes" or "No." For example, if you ask, "Are you taking your medication?" the patient may say "Yes" but may not be taking all of the medications that have been prescribed or may not be taking the proper dosage of each medication. However, by asking questions like "What medications do you take every day?" and "How many of those tablets do you take each day?" you will get answers from the patient that will give you a clearer understanding of whether the patient is taking the correct dosage.

However, keep in mind that sometimes closed-ended questions are necessary. For example, you might ask, "Are you still having pain?" after administering medication. Still, in many cases you might need to follow up with open-ended questions.

Summarizing. Use the summarizing technique to review the information that you have obtained and to give the patient another chance to clarify statements or correct misinformation. This method also helps you organize complex information or events in sequential order. For example, if a patient has been feeling dizzy and stumbling a lot, you might summarize by saying, "You told me that you have been feeling dizzy for the past three days and that you often stumble as you're walking. Is that correct?" The patient then has a chance to verify the information or correct something you may have misunderstood.

Silences. Periods of silence sometimes occur during an interview. Some people are uncomfortable with prolonged silences and feel a need to break the silence with words. However, silences can be beneficial. They are a natural part of conversation and can give patients time to formulate their thoughts, reconstruct events, evaluate their feelings, or assess what has already been said. During moments of silence, you can gather your own thoughts and formulate any additional questions you may have.

New Patient Interviews

New patient interviews cover several topics, and patient information is recorded in a patient medical record. (You will learn more about new patient interviews in Chapter 17.) Topics covered during a new patient interview include the patient's medical and family history, a brief review of body systems, the patient's social history, and medications the patient is taking. Important information that you need to obtain from a patient during a new patient interview is listed in Table 16-3.

Established Patient Interviews

An interview of an established patient, or a patient that you or your practice has seen before, is quite different. When interviewing an established patient, you will:

- Review the patient's chart for information about health problems.
- Make a list of questions to ask the patient in order to update health information, including current medical problems and any changes in health.
- Confirm that the patient is still on the medications and treatments listed in the chart.
- Ask about any known allergies.
- Record patient information.

Table 16-3 Key Subjects in a New Patient Interview

Key Subjects	What You Need to Know
Medical History	Any hospitalizations and dates Any surgeries and dates Any chronic problems
Female Patients	Any pregnancies and complications Any miscarriages, stillbirths, or abortions
Family History	Age and health of parents (if deceased, cause and age at death) Age and health of brothers and sisters Any genetic problems in family
Body System Review	General questions about all body systems: cardiovascular, pulmonary, integumentary, musculoskeletal, sensory, neurological, gastrointestinal, immune, endocrine, urological, and reproductive
Social History	Alcohol use Tobacco use Any drug use Hobbies Education Employment
Medications	Any prescription medicines (when taken and how much) Any over-the-counter medicines (when taken and how much) Any vitamins and herbal supplements

Patient Education

Patient education is more than just telling a patient which medications to take or suggesting which lifestyle behaviors to change. Effective communication is the key component in educating patients and includes:

- helping the patient accept illness
- involving the patient in the knowledge-gaining process
- providing positive reinforcement

Both active listening and interviewing skills are central to the patient education process. You also need to be aware of current medical issues, discoveries, and trends, as well as useful community services that are available in your area (Table 16-4).

The patient education process includes these five steps:

1. **Assess.** Collect information about the patient's current health care needs and abilities.

2. **Plan.** Establish goals and objectives. These are more valuable and meaningful when patient input is included.

ON LOCATION

Handling Patients' Questions

Assume you are working in a physicians' office where you're one of the first contacts with patients. The next patient is a woman in her early 30s who recently gave birth. She has only lived in town for a few months, and this is her first visit to your office. Immediately after you introduce yourself, the patient begins telling you the reasons for her visit and asks a barrage of questions:

"I've been having pains in my neck, chest, abdomen, and legs off and on for the past six months. The pains seem to be worse at night. I've been so busy with our recent move and our two-month old baby that I really haven't had time to see a doctor about this before now. I'm very concerned it could be something serious. Do you think the pains are all related? Or could my chest pains be caused by a heart problem? My father suffered from heart disease. I wonder if the headaches are related to stress. But if they're stress related, would I also have pains in my chest, abdomen, and legs? Diabetes runs in my family. Could my symptoms be related to that?"

Because she is a new patient, you need to collect her complete medical history before the doctor performs an exam. Once the medical history is taken, how would you respond to the questions she's asked so far?

Remember that it is inappropriate for you to respond to most of her questions. You should explain that she will have an opportunity to ask the doctor her questions.

3. **Implement.** Begin the training process, ensuring that the lines of communication between you and the patient remain open.

4. **Evaluate.** Determine how well the patient is adapting to the course of action and whether or not the patient is applying the new information to daily life.

5. **Document.** All conversations, events, and results related to the patient education process should be accurately recorded.

If possible, find a quiet room where you can talk with the patient. Allow sufficient time so that the patient does not feel rushed or interrupted. Patients should feel that

Table 16-4 Guidelines for Identifying and Using Community Resources

Being aware of community resources is important to your role as a patient educator. Follow these guidelines to develop and use a list of community resources.

1. Determine what types of resources are most useful for the patients your employer sees. This often depends on your employer's medical specialty, but patients also may have needs that are not directly related to their medical problem. Services that might help with such needs are:
   - support groups and services for people with serious and potentially fatal diseases such as cancer or MS
   - support groups and services for people suffering from various types of abuse
   - services such as meals-on-wheels that help people who are ill or older
   - services for hearing- or sight-impaired people or those with mental disabilities.

2. Create a contact list of sources from which to create a list of community services. Such a contact list might include:
   - social services departments at local hospitals
   - the local public health department
   - nursing home associations
   - local charities and church organizations
   - community service numbers in the local phone book
   - the Internet

3. Contact these resources to create a list of community services complete with addresses, email addresses, and phone numbers. Keep this list on your computer so that it can be routinely updated. You can create a binder of this information or print it as needed.

4. Provide patients with a printed list of specific services from your general list, according to their needs. Answer any questions they may have.

5. Offer to make the first contact for the patient. Recognize, however, that patients may prefer to do this themselves.

6. Document in the patient's chart that the information was provided.

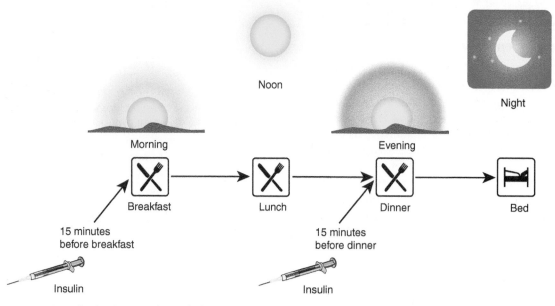

Example of a pictogram that might be given to patients to help them understand medication administration.

they can ask follow-up questions until they are comfortable with the information that they are learning.

Provide information in a clear, concise, and sequential manner. In addition to verbal instructions, give written instructions to help the patient remember the information after leaving the office. Keep informational handouts up to date and available for easy distribution. Information can also be posted on a practice's web site.

Once the educational materials have been reviewed, ensure that there is enough time for the patient to process the new information. Always encourage questions. Even if the patient has no questions, you should ask open-ended questions of your own. This helps ensure that the patient understands all of the information he or she has just received. Finally, make sure that the patient understands that it is okay to call the office with any additional questions that may arise later.

CHECK POINT

6 When conducting an interview, what three points should the provider keep in mind?

7 What is the key component in educating patients, and what does it include?

RECORDING AND REPORTING

Assessment of a patient's needs and condition requires accurate documentation. Most patients receive care from more than one health care professional, so it is extremely important that patient information is passed on to others accurately. To ensure both consistent care and patient safety, patient information needs to be recorded completely and precisely, with no room for misinterpretation by other health care professionals. And because patient information is confidential, it is vital that you record this information only in secure and appropriate locations.

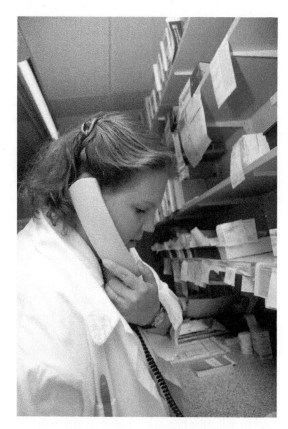

It's important to record accurately information received over the telephone.

ZOOM IN

**Tips for Keeping Patient
Communications Confidential**

All patient communication is confidential. In fact, a patient's right to privacy and confidentiality is a basic civil right protected under the Health Insurance Portability and Accountability Act (HIPAA). HIPAA regulations are discussed in more detail in Chapter 11, "Law, Ethics, and Professionalism in Health Care."

Patient information is sometimes discussed unintentionally, however. To avoid breaching confidentiality unintentionally, follow these guidelines:

- Never discuss patient problems in public places, such as elevators or parking lots. A patient's friends or family members might overhear a conversation and misinterpret what is said.
- Close the glass window between the waiting room and the reception desk and keep it closed unless you are talking directly with a patient at the window.
- Keep your voice low and calm so that you will not be overheard by others.
- When calling coworkers over an office intercom, never use patients' names or reveal patient information. Avoid saying anything revealing, such as "Bob Smith is on the phone and wants to know if his strep throat culture came back." Instead, you should say simply, "There's a patient on line 1."
- Before going home, destroy any slips of paper in your pockets that may contain patient information, such as reminders or other notes.

Any actions you take concerning a patient should also be recorded. This information is often recorded in a narrative manner. When a patient calls or emails the office, the conversation should be immediately documented in the patient's chart. Documentation is discussed in detail in Chapter 17.

 CHECK POINT

8 Why does patient information need to be recorded completely and precisely?

COMMUNICATION CHALLENGES

There are many different barriers to good communication. No matter how hard you try, patients may not always receive your message the way you intended, and you may not always understand what patients are telling you.

Patients may misunderstand your message for any number of reasons. As mentioned earlier, many patients do not understand complex medical terms. Avoid using medical terminology when speaking with patients.

Distractions also can lead to misunderstanding. Both health care workers and patients can be easily distracted. When you become too busy and distracted, you are less likely to ensure that patients understand all of the information you've transmitted. Many factors, such as pain or hunger, cause patients to be distracted. When patients are distracted, they are less likely to focus on what you're saying.

Environmental noise often causes distractions. Health care facilities are full of sounds. Noise can come from many sources, including other patients, stations where health care workers interact, and cleaning services. When possible, speak with patients in quiet, private areas.

Language barriers also present communication challenges. When a patient does not speak or understand English well enough for effective communication, an interpreter may be necessary. Use caution when a family member is a patient's interpreter, however. Patients over 18 years of age must give written permission allowing the family member access to their medical history. Otherwise, the family member is prohibited by HIPAA from participating in any provider-patient conversations.

Hearing-impaired patients present a special communication challenge. Impairments range from partial to complete hearing loss and may prevent patients from being able to communicate with health care professionals. When communicating with a hearing-impaired patient, gently touch the patient to gain his or her attention if needed. Always talk directly in front of the patient so that he or she can read your lips. Short sentences, spoken clearly, and written words and picture boards can also be helpful.

People with brain injuries, Alzheimer's disease, strokes, or other diseases often have difficulty with normal thought processes. They also may have trouble speaking and may become disoriented. People with these and other cognitive difficulties should be accompanied by someone with an appointed power of attorney, so that you can speak with that person on their behalf.

Illnesses, financial matters, and time spent waiting are just a few of the issues that can make patients angry or upset. Never be defensive with a patient. Instead, let patients know how long they may have to wait for you or for the next health care professional that they will be seeing. Upfront information about the cost of the visit and payment options, when appropriate, can help combat the financial distress a patient may be experiencing.

Sometimes you will find yourself treating patients who are experiencing grief. Patients may be grieving the loss of a loved one, or they may be grieving their own personal health issues. You should allow grieving patients an opportunity to talk about their feelings. Terminally ill patients may want to discuss their fear of dying and their concern for surviving loved ones. Dying patients may choose to talk to you, because they may want to spare their families' feelings. You need to allow patients time to discuss their emotions and listen actively to what they have to say.

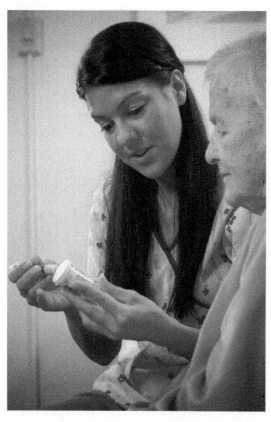

Remember that some patients may have difficulty understanding information or instructions.

CHECK POINT

9 What are some barriers to communication?

10 What factors can cause a patient to be distracted and less able to focus on what you're trying to communicate?

TELEPHONE MANNERS

The telephone is an important means of communication for many health care professionals. You must be able to communicate a positive image through the telephone.

ZOOM IN

Triaging Incoming Calls

Assume you work as a medical assistant in a busy medical practice. The telephone has four incoming lines, which allow several patients to call at once. Suppose the following calls were on the lines at the same time:

- **Line 1:** The caller wants to make an appointment for her son, who has a 101.3° fever but no other serious symptoms.
- **Line 2:** The caller wants to see the physician this afternoon. He's having chest pains.
- **Line 3:** The caller is upset because she's been disconnected three times. She has a question about her bill.
- **Line 4:** The caller needs a prescription refill.

You must triage these calls—that is, you must sort them into order of importance. Which call should be handled first? Which second? Which last?

- Talk to the caller on line 2 first. Any possible life-threatening situation must have top priority. Follow your office policy for emergencies in handling this call. In some offices, you would transfer the call to a nurse, who would assess the situation. In others, you would advise the patient to call 911.
- Take caller 3 next. The longer she waits, the more upset she'll be. That will make her more difficult to please.
- Then make the appointment for caller 1, following your office policies on patient care issues.
- The caller on line 4 is last because he has the least urgent need.

One tip for triaging calls is to keep a notebook by the phone. You can use it to make notes about who is calling and why. This will help you remember the details and decide which call is most urgent.

This is sometimes more difficult than in face-to-face communication. You need excellent verbal skills to project a caring and professional attitude while talking on the telephone. Even though a patient can't see the person on the other end of the phone, if you're smiling, you're more likely to project a cheerful and professional image when you're talking on the phone.

The tone of your voice and the quality of your speech shapes the impression you send over the telephone. Follow these guidelines when answering the phone:

- Answer the phone promptly—by the second ring if possible.

- Identify yourself and your office to the caller. This lets the caller know that he or she has reached the correct number.
- Always speak politely, even if the call has interrupted work. Never allow your voice to show impatience or irritation.
- Never answer a phone call and immediately put the caller on hold. Instead, first ask the caller if he or she would mind holding. Both courtesy and the patient's well-being require waiting for an answer to ensure that there isn't an emergency before putting a caller on hold.

CHECK POINT

11 Why can communication by telephone be more challenging than face-to-face communication?

12 Why is it important for you to identify yourself and your office when answering the telephone?

Chapter Wrap-Up

Don't forget to visit the Point companion website for additional study resources!

CHAPTER HIGHLIGHTS

- Communication is important throughout the health care system, and good communication between a provider and patient is essential to good patient care.
- The communication process involves the sending and receiving of information between two or more individuals. It consists of three central elements—the sender, the message, and the receiver—and often includes a fourth element, feedback.
- The three basic communication modes are verbal, nonverbal, and written.
- Verbal communication involves the use of spoken words.
- Assertive communication and active listening are important aspects of verbal communication.
- Nonverbal communication, also known as body language, relays a message without speaking or writing a single word. Three forms of nonverbal communication include kinesics (body movement), proxemics (personal space), and touch.
- Medical writing requires accuracy and clarity. Mistakes in written medical communications could cause injury or death, lawsuits, or professional harm to you or your employer.
- When conducting a patient interview, be an active listener, ask appropriate questions, and record answers accurately.
- The interview process for a new patient is quite different from that for an established patient.
- Effective communication is the key component in patient education.
- To ensure both consistent care and patient safety, patient information must be recorded completely and accurately.
- There are many barriers to good communication, including the use of medical terms, distractions, environmental noise, language barriers, hearing impairments, brain injuries and other cognitive difficulties, anger, and grief.
- The telephone is an important means of communication for many health care professionals, so they must be able to communicate a positive image through the telephone.

REVIEW QUESTIONS

Matching

1. _____ Body movement
2. _____ Both active listening and interviewing skills are central to this process.
3. _____ The person or group that begins the communication process
4. _____ Include sighs, sobs, laughs, grunts, and so on.
5. _____ Personal space

   a. non-language sounds   **b.** source   **c.** proxemics   **d.** kinesics   **e.** patient education

Multiple Choice

6. Health care workers regularly communicate with patients and other professionals regarding
   - **a.** assessment
   - **b.** diagnosis
   - **c.** treatment
   - **d.** all of the above

7. Which of the following elements is NOT present within *every* communication process?
   - **a.** message
   - **b.** feedback
   - **c.** receiver
   - **d.** sender

8. Using your own words or phrases to repeat what you have heard is called
   - a. reflecting
   - b. paraphrasing
   - c. comparison organization
   - d. problem-oriented organization

9. In health care, a message can be
   - a. a patient describing a symptom
   - b. information obtained during a telephone conversation
   - c. a gesture
   - d. all of the above

10. Using open-ended statements to repeat back what you have heard is called
    - a. reflecting
    - b. paraphrasing
    - c. comparison organization
    - d. problem-oriented organization

Completion

11. The three most common modes of communication are verbal, _____ and written communication.

12. _____ listening ensures that health care professionals understand completely what a patient or colleague is trying to communicate.

13. Maintaining good _____ shows that you're interested in what other people are saying and adds a sense of truthfulness to your message.

14. Nonverbal communication, also known as _____, relays a message without speaking or writing a single word.

15. Health care providers need excellent _____ skills to project a caring and professional attitude while talking on the telephone.

Short Answer

16. What are some of the possible consequences of communication failures?

   _____

   _____

17. Why does nonverbal behavior often reveal more than verbal behavior?

   _____

   _____

18. Why is proper grammar important in written communication?

   _____

   _____

19. What are some of the common communication barriers between a provider and patient?

   _____

   _____

20. How does the interview of an established patient differ from that of a new patient?

   _____

   _____

INVESTIGATE IT

1. Complete the following communication/interpersonal skill survey. How well do you really communicate with others? Do you communicate well at work? At home? Read each question below and then put a circle around the letter that best describes you. *Be honest with yourself.*

   A = Always/Usually   B = Sometimes   C = Seldom/Rarely

   1. I am not afraid to ask questions when I do not understand something.
      A   B   C

   2. I repeat what someone has said in my own words to check my understanding.
      A   B   C

   3. I notice people's body language.
      A   B   C

   4. I give clear, brief directions.
      A   B   C

   5. I listen carefully and speak clearly.
      A   B   C

   6. I ask questions in a way that is easy to understand.
      A   B   C

   7. I clearly state my opinions and give good reasons to back them up.
      A   B   C

   8. I respect other people's right to their opinions.
      A   B   C

   9. I listen carefully to others when they disagree with me.
      A   B   C

   10. I accept and think about constructive criticism.
       A   B   C

   Use what you have learned about your communication and interpersonal skills to help you improve in your weakest areas. Making changes in these areas will help you become a more effective health care professional.

RECOMMENDED READING

Bub B. The Lament, Hidden Key to Effective Listening. *Health Care Communication Review* [serial online]. Summer/Fall 2005;5(2):PS1-2. Available at http://www.healthcarecommunication.org/pro/hcrps/v5n2ps.pdf.

Kale-Smith G. *Medical Assisting Made Incredibly Easy: Administrative Competencies*. Baltimore: Lippincott, Williams, and Wilkins, 2008.

Kronenberger J. *Comprehensive Medical Assisting*. Baltimore: Lippincott, Williams, and Wilkins, 2008.

Smith M., Segal J. Supporting a Grieving Person: Helping Others Through Grief, Loss, and Bereavement. Available at http://www.helpguide.org/mental/helping_grieving.htm.

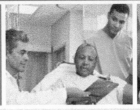
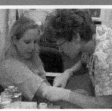
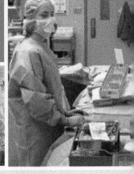

Medical Documentation

17

CHAPTER

CHAPTER OBJECTIVES

After careful study of this chapter, you should be able to:

* State the purposes of medical documentation.
* Explain the advantages of computerized medical record systems.
* Distinguish the different types of information found in patient records.

* Identify the characteristics of good medical documentation.
* Define the various types of progress notes.
* Explain why military time is used in health care documentation and interpret military time designations.

KEY TERMS

charting by exception
  format
familial

military time
narrative format

problem-oriented medical
  record (POMR)
SOAP format

source-oriented medical
  record (SOMR)

orking with medical documents is one of the most important tasks for any health care professional. Good medical documentation is essential to the smooth operation of any medical facility. Whether they are entering, editing, filing, searching, or retrieving patient records, health care providers are accountable for the safe and secure handling of medical documents. Health care professionals must adhere to the privacy rules of the Health Insurance Portability and Accountability Act (HIPAA) when working with patient information. (See Chapter 11, "Law, Ethics, and Professionalism in Health Care," for more detailed information on HIPAA.) This is true whether the record is in written or electronic form.

The average patient record contains many documents: insurance forms, patient health records, physician orders, notes, test reports, and more. This documentation forms a patient's permanent health record. In addition to communicating information between health care professionals, patient records are also legal documents. These uses, and the other purposes of medical documentation, are discussed in this chapter.

Medical documentation can be handwritten, but most facilities use an electronic medical record system to manage and retain patient information. This chapter discusses how computerized documentation has transformed patient recordkeeping. The chapter also explains the types of information in medical records and the characteristics of good medical documentation. Finally, it examines the different types of notes found in patient records and explains the use of military time.

PURPOSES OF DOCUMENTATION

Well-organized medical documentation serves many purposes. Two key purposes are communicating with other health care professionals and describing a patient's current medical condition and history. Other, less obvious, purposes include the roles these records play in processing reimbursement requests, maintaining a legal record, educating, and supporting research.

Communication

The primary purpose of medical documentation is to help health care professionals communicate with one another. Most patients receive care from more than one source, and these providers are rarely in the same room at the same time. For this reason, it is essential that all providers have access to the same, up-to-date patient information.

For example, a patient visits a physician once a year for a routine physical exam. This exam provides a convenient occasion to review prescription medications that the patient regularly takes. If the patient mentions the need for a new blood pressure prescription to the nurse, a sequence of steps would follow, in which medical documentation would play an important part:

- The nurse searches the patient's medical records to identify which blood pressure medication was last prescribed and notes that the patient needs a new prescription written before a particular date.
- While reviewing the patient's medical records, the doctor sees the nurse's note. The doctor then reviews the patient's current weight and other vital signs to verify that the dosage is still correct. Because the patient's last cholesterol test showed an elevated cholesterol level, the doctor decides to order a new test before renewing the prescription for the blood pressure medication.
- The laboratory technician running the blood test views the prescription drug history in the patient's medical record. This information allows the technician to interpret substances that may appear in the

blood test results. After examining the test results, the technician sees that the patient's cholesterol level has increased. He or she notes this result in the patient's medical record.

- The physician sees the technician's note and determines that the patient needs medication to treat high cholesterol, as well as high blood pressure. Because a new drug is available to treat both issues, the doctor sends a prescription for that new medication to the patient's pharmacist.
- The pharmacist checks the patient's medical history for any known allergies or for other prescriptions that can cause a drug interaction. Finding none, the pharmacist fills the new prescription.

With so many different health care professionals relying on the information contained in a patient's medical record, it is imperative that each and every detail in these records be entered correctly and clearly. The patient's health and well-being depend on the accuracy of his or her medical records.

Assessment

As health care team members gather assessment data about a patient, the information is placed directly in the patient's medical record. Assessment data includes such information as:

- vital signs (respiration rate, blood pressure, pulse, and temperature)
- circumstances surrounding the visit
- symptoms experienced
- medical history

Once recorded, the information becomes part of the patient's permanent medical record. This documentation gives health care professionals the ability to compare patient data from one visit to another. Current and past assessment information offers vital clues that providers can use to determine the right diagnoses and treatment plans.

Quality Assurance

Another important role of medical documentation is to provide evidence of the quality of care a patient received and the competence of the professionals who provided that care. For example, in a health care audit, a committee may choose to review patient records. In that case, several medical records are randomly selected and reviewed for evidence that the health care professionals met certain standards of care. (If deficiencies are found, in-service training can be used to remedy a problem and to improve the quality of care.) Accrediting agencies might also review medical documents to determine whether a particular institution is meeting its standards.

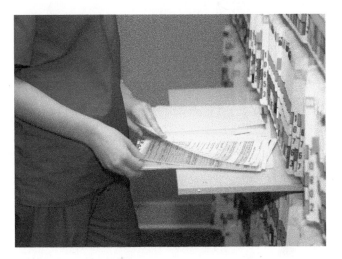

Patient medical records are a cornerstone of medical documentation.

Reimbursement

Patient records are also used to verify the care a patient received when a provider seeks reimbursement from an insurance policy or government plan. The documentation contained in a patient's medical record is used to determine the reason for a patient's visit, the type of care given, any diagnosis made, any tests that were ordered, and any treatments that were provided. The plan administrator's decision about how much the plan will pay for the services is based on this information.

Most medical record systems assign a code to each service that a patient receives. These codes are then submitted directly to the insurance company or government plan for review. Medicare, Medicaid, workers' compensation insurance, and private insurance companies review the billing codes, along with the patient's actual records, if necessary, to ensure that all requirements of the plan have been met before issuing a payment.

Legal Record

Health care professionals are required to adhere to certain legal, moral, and ethical standards when managing medical documentation. Any disregard for these standards may result in a breach of contract by the provider. A breach of contract may expose the patient to embarrassment or harm and leaves the health care professional vulnerable to fines or lawsuits.

Patient records are legal documents and are admissible as evidence in court proceedings. Because records document a patient's health status and history and the type of care received, they are useful if a health care professional is charged with improper care or malpractice. Patient medical records can also be used when a patient makes accident or injury claims. (See Chapter 11 for more information about the legal aspects of health care.)

Education

A great deal can be learned from reading a patient's medical record. As a result, providers often use patient medical records as educational tools to help train new people in the field. Patient records may also be used during the clinical portion of many health education programs.

Research

Health care-related research is sometimes carried out through the study of patient records. Researchers often learn how best to recognize or treat health problems by examining similar cases.

Data gathered from groups of patient records is helpful in determining:
- significant similarities in disease presentation
- contributing factors
- effectiveness of therapies

CHECK POINT

1 What is the primary purpose of medical documentation?

2 Name one other purpose of medical documentation and briefly explain how medical documentation serves this purpose.

COMPUTERIZED DOCUMENTATION

Advances in computer technology, medical recordkeeping software, and file-transfer security are convincing more and more health care institutions to convert from a paper-based patient chart system to an electronic format. One of the chief improvements provided by computerized systems is ease of access. Handwritten charts are available to only one person at a time and only to those who have physical access to the location where they are stored. Computerized documentation, on the other hand, allows multiple users in different locations to access portions of the same record simultaneously. Electronic documentation is also available through laptops, tablet computers, smart phones, and other hand-held devices, which allows health care workers to view, search, edit, and share patient information remotely.

From medical histories to test results, computerized documentation systems manage a diverse collection of information. Records are stored in various formats, depending upon the software and computer system the health care facility uses.

Computerized documentation offers several advantages over traditional paper charts:

- Information is easy to store and retrieve.
- Nearly unlimited file space is available.
- Electronic records are easy to backup for added security.
- Information is easily added or attached to patient records.
- Charting is easier to read.
- Data can be entered into a computer more quickly than it can be written.

Health care facilities also use computers to order supplies and services for patients, to store billing and financial data, and to maintain health care information. While studies show that some health care professionals are not making the change to electronic health records as readily as they could, the number of providers going paperless is expected to grow as a new generation of health care professionals enters the workplace. At some point in the near future, almost all health care professionals will work with a computerized and paperless record system. (See Chapter 20, "Computers and Other Technology," for more detailed information on computerized health records.)

The increasing use of computerized patient information systems has brought about the need for policies and procedures that ensure the privacy and confidentiality of patient information. These policies should specify which types of patient information can be retrieved, by whom, and for what purpose. As with paper documents, patient consent is necessary for the use and release of any electronic information that can be linked to the patient.

Several health care associations, including the American Health Information Management Association (AHIMA), offer guidelines and strategies for safe computer recordkeeping. (See Chapter 20 for more information on computer security.) Recommendations include the following:

- Never give a personal password or computer signature to anyone, including other health care professionals.
- Do not leave a computer terminal unattended after logging on.
- Follow the correct protocol for correcting errors. To correct an error after it has been stored, add a note reading "mistaken entry" to the item, then add the correct information, the date, and your initials. If the record was added to the wrong patient file, add a note reading "mistaken entry—wrong chart" and initial.
- Allow only authorized personnel to create, change, or delete records.

- Ensure that stored records are backed up regularly; follow the facility's procedure.
- Do not leave patient information displayed on a monitor within view of others.
- Keep a running log of any electronic copies made of computerized files.
- Never use email to send protected health information, unless it has been encrypted.
- Follow the health care agency's confidentiality procedures for documenting sensitive material, such as diagnosis of acquired immunodeficiency syndrome (AIDS) or human immunodeficiency virus (HIV) infection.

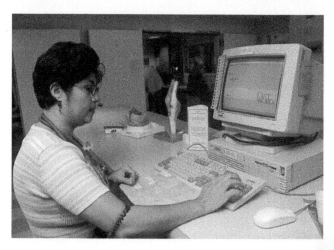

Computerized documentation offers several advantages over traditional paper charts.

CHECK POINT

3 What are some advantages that computerized documentation offers over handwritten charts?

4 What matters should be specified in privacy policies for computerized patient information?

TYPES OF INFORMATION IN PATIENT RECORDS

A patient's medical record is a compilation of health-related information. It is the only permanent legal document detailing a patient's medical history, test results, and interactions with health care professionals. But it is not just one lengthy document or even one type of document. It is a collection of many types of documents, each designed to collect and store certain kinds of information. The basic document types are discussed in this section.

Admission Sheet

An admission sheet is commonly used to gather information from the patient before the visit with the provider.

Some health care agencies mail these forms to new patients before their scheduled visit. This ensures that patients know what information is needed. Admission information includes the patient's:

- demographic data, such as name, address, and phone number; Social Security number; birthdate; marital status; gender; race; and employer's name, address, and phone number
- insurance information, including the primary health insurance carrier; policy number; insurance company's address and phone number; co-payment or deductible information (if applicable); and secondary insurance information (if applicable)

Established patients are required to update their admission information on a regular basis, typically once a year. A great deal of patient information can change in a year, including address, phone number, and insurance coverage. Having patients fill out new forms regularly ensures that the provider has the most up-to-date information on file.

If a patient has health insurance, most health care facilities also require a copy of the patient's insurance card. If the facility has a paper-based records system, a photocopy of the card's information, front and back, is added to the patient's file. If an electronic system is used, the card is scanned into the computer and added to the patient's file.

Graphic Sheet (Flow Sheet)

Whether a patient is being treated for a routine illness, a yearly check-up, or an illness that requires longer term care, vital signs are commonly taken and recorded at the beginning of each visit or at regular intervals (such as in the case of a hospitalized patient). Vital sign measurements include respiration rate, blood pressure, pulse, and temperature. Providers also typically weigh the patient and listen to the patient's breathing and heartbeat with a stethoscope. This information is entered into the patient's record, either as notes or on a graphic sheet (flow sheet)—a grid-like form used to record and monitor specific patient variables over time.

The graphic sheet contains a history of the patient's vital signs, along with the date they were taken. Since fluctuations in these measurements may affect a person's health, this information is reviewed for significant changes. By using a graphic sheet, providers can quickly spot changes over time. In a paper-based system, the provider plots the information (respiration rate, pulse, temperature, weight, and so forth) on the graphic sheet; in a computerized system, the software automatically creates a graph or table from the information the provider enters.

Physician's Orders

The physician's orders section of the patient record documents any orders for patient care. This section may include orders for medications, treatments, tests, and follow-up care.

This information is very precise and detailed. It includes all information relating to the order, such as medication dosages, treatment specifics, type of testing to be conducted, and dates for follow-up care. If entered electronically, providers can send this information automatically to other health care professionals, such as pharmacists, specialists, and laboratory technicians. This helps eliminate human error caused by lost paperwork or misread orders.

Progress Notes

Progress notes record each contact a provider has with the patient, whether in person or by phone, mail, or email. In this section, the provider summarizes any findings that resulted from the contact, including the effects of treatments, changes in condition, and other provider observations.

This information provides a snapshot of the patient's treatment, progress, and any issues. The provider records the date and time of each entry, along with his or her name. This is especially important in a hospital setting, where several different health care professionals typically access the patient's medical record throughout any given day.

Progress notes do not follow a standard format, and handwritten notes in a paper medical record may be difficult for others to read. For these reasons, electronic record systems are especially useful for progress notes. Such systems leave little room for misunderstandings or other human errors. Progress notes are discussed in more detail later in the chapter.

Medical History and Examination Sheet

Medical history and examination sheets vary from institution to institution, but these forms generally contain these elements:

- patient history
- family history
- social history
- results of physical examination
- current medical condition

The patient history section addresses the patient's current and prior health status and helps the provider plan appropriate care for any present illness. Information in this section typically includes the following:

- allergies
- immunizations
- childhood diseases
- current and past medications
- previous illnesses
- surgeries
- hospitalizations

Family history plays an important role in a patient's health because some diseases and disorders have hereditary tendencies—that is, a greater likelihood of developing these diseases or disorders is transmitted from parent to offspring. Other diseases tend to occur often in a particular family. These are known as familial diseases. The family history includes the cause of death of family members.

The social history information covers a patient's lifestyle, such as marital status, occupation, education, and hobbies. It also may include information about the patient's diet, use of alcohol or tobacco, and sexual history. This information helps providers understand how the patient's lifestyle may affect an illness, as well as how an illness and any treatment may affect the patient's lifestyle. The social history also may provide a guide for patient education, because some behaviors, such as tobacco use or a diet high in fat, may contribute to health problems.

Reports

The reports section of a patient's record contains any reports or findings from tests or laboratory work, such as blood tests, electrocardiographs (EKGs), x-rays, CT scans, or magnetic resonance images (MRIs). This section includes tests conducted both in the provider's office and at other facilities. Copies of any consultation reports from other providers are included as well.

Correspondence and Miscellaneous Documentation

A patient's medical record should also contain copies of all correspondence relating to the patient's care. This includes any correspondence between providers and the patient, letters or memos a provider sends to others concerning the patient, and any correspondence regarding the patient received from other providers.

Signed consent forms, including a signed copy of the HIPAA privacy notice, are also included in a patient's medical record. If the patient has provided instructions regarding end-of-life decisions, copies of these documents are retained in the record as well. These might include organ donation forms, a living will, and a durable power of attorney for health care.

✓ **CHECK** POINT

5 Name at least two types of information contained in a patient's medical record and briefly describe each type.

6 Name five elements that are generally included on a medical history and examination sheet.

CHARACTERISTICS OF GOOD MEDICAL DOCUMENTATION

With both paper-based records and electronic systems, the characteristics of good medical documentation are the same. Documents should be accurate, complete, concise, legible, and well organized. When working with a patient's record, always remember these principles. Also remember that the purpose of medical documentation is to create a record of the patient's health care. Therefore, *all* patient-related documentation must remain a part of the patient's medical record permanently.

Accuracy

Patient medical records are a key ingredient of proper care for patients. Unfortunately, there are often crucial omissions in medical documentation, along with repetitions and inaccurate entries. Although some errors are minor, other errors can seriously and negatively affect patient care.

In addition to putting a patient at risk, errors undermine a provider's credibility. With medical documents, health care professionals should make sure that:

- All entries include only facts.
- Correct spelling, medical terms, abbreviations, and acronyms are used.
- Errors are marked through with a single line and identified with the word "error" in a paper-based system. The professional making this change should add his or her initials plus the date and time of the change above the error. As stated earlier, to correct an error in a computerized system, add a note reading "mistaken entry" to the item, then add the correct information, the date, and your initials. If the record was added to the wrong patient file, add a note reading "mistaken entry— wrong chart" and initial. Keep in mind that erasing (in a paper-based system) or deleting (in a computerized system) is not acceptable in medical documentation.

Information must be documented in the proper location. The first rule of accuracy is to make sure that the information is recorded in the correct patient's record. In paper-based systems, this means checking to make sure that the name at the top of the chart matches the patient. With an electronic system, providers should always double-check to ensure that they are working with the correct patient's file.

Completeness

Medical documentation must include all relevant data, so that it paints a complete picture of all the care provided to a patient. The file must include phone messages, emails, and other correspondence. Conversations between providers and the patient should be documented, including any questions or concerns the patient has. Any notes relating to the patient's care, including dates and times of the care, are also necessary. When reports or tests are included, supporting documentation, such as x-rays and other images, must also be included.

Conciseness

Although medical records are complete, entries should be brief. Only relevant information is required, and that information should be expressed using partial sentences and phrases. Because a medical record belongs to only one person, it is not necessary to use the patient's name in entries. The term *patient* is adequate as a reference.

Abbreviations and acronyms are acceptable, but if they are not used correctly, they can contribute to misunderstandings and errors. Therefore, only universal abbreviations and acronyms should be used. Some institutions keep a running list of approved abbreviations and acronyms. If you are unsure about whether other providers will understand the meaning of a particular abbreviation or acronym, don't use it. A good rule of thumb is this: When in doubt, spell it out.

Legibility

Many notes and data in a patient's medical record will eventually be read by different health care professionals. If the writing is difficult to read, there is a good chance that the information will not be correctly understood by others. This increases the possibility of mistakes and miscalculations. With paper records, take time to ensure that your writing is neat and legible.

In some electronic systems, users write information with a stylus, rather than a keyboard. If the user's handwriting is messy, the software may not recognize the data

ON LOCATION

Use of Abbreviations

After working as a certified nursing assistant (CNA) at the same assisted living facility for nearly 12 years, Debbie recently completed the courses necessary to become a registered nurse (RN). She then accepted an RN position in the office of a primary care physician. This office charts patient medical records electronically, and Debbie is unfamiliar with the system.

As a learning activity, she is assigned the task of updating a few patient files on her first day. She quickly realizes that the personnel in her new office use many abbreviations with which she is unfamiliar. For example, one patient's medical record reads, "Pt complains of H.A. relieved by NTG. No N-V-D-V. Previous adm for PTCA 1988, PMH-P.E. 1992, EHL 1999, and LPI 2005. Takes Dig., heart."

- Debbie is unsure of whether *H.A.* stands for heart attack or headache. Her previous health care facility used *H.A.* for headache, but she knows that *NTG*, which follows the *H.A.* abbreviation, is a common abbreviation for nitroglycerin, which is used to treat people with heart-related issues.
- She has no idea what *N-V-D-V* stands for.
- She's uncertain whether *P.E.* means pulmonary emboli or physical exam.

What should Debbie do?

entries and may ask the user to enter it again. This helps ensure accurate information.

Organization

Good medical documentation is well organized and easy to navigate. Patient records are usually organized in one of two ways:

- The problem-oriented medical record (POMR) organizes information by the patient's problem. The patient's medical problem is listed on the first page of the record and assigned a number, and all documentation about that problem is assigned the same number. When the problem no longer exists, that information is recorded in the progress notes and an *X* is marked next to the problem on the list. A POMR is divided into sections: (1) problem list, as described above, contains every problem the patient has that requires medical treatment; (2) database, which contains items such as the patient's medical history, review of systems, and lab reports; (3) treatment plan, which includes tests and treatments that each problem

Table 17-1 Guidelines for Documentation

Content

Enter information in a complete, accurate, concise, current and factual manner.

Record patient findings (observations of behavior) rather than your interpretation of these findings.

Avoid words such as "good," "average," "normal," or "sufficient," which may mean different things to different readers.

Avoid generalizations such as "seems comfortable today." A better entry would be "on a scale of 1 to 10, patient rates back pain 2 to 3 today as compared with 7 to 9 yesterday; vital signs returned to baseline."

Note problems as they occur in an orderly, sequential manner; record the treatment provided and the patient's response; update problems or delete as appropriate.

Chart precautions or preventive measures used.

Document all medical visits and consultations of which other health care providers should be aware, either because of their impact on the patient or because of the care the patient now requires.

Document in a legally prudent manner. Know and adhere to professional standards and agency/institutional policy for documentation.

Document your concerns regarding questionable medical orders or treatment (or failure to treat). Factually record the date and time the health care professional issuing the orders was notified of the concern and the professional's exact response. If this occurs by phone, have a coworker listen to the conversation and cosign the note. If your supervisor was contacted, document this. Documentation should give legal protection to you, other caregivers, the health care agency or institution, and the patient.

Avoid the use of stereotypes or derogatory terms when charting.

Timing

Record information in a timely manner. Follow your employer's policy regarding the frequency of documentation and modify this if changes in the patient's status warrant more frequent documentation.

Indicate in each entry the date and both the time the entry was written and the time of pertinent observations and interventions. This is crucial when a case is being reconstructed for legal purposes.

Most health care institutions use military time, one 24-hour time cycle, to avoid confusion between a.m. and p.m. times. (Military time is discussed later in this chapter.)

Document medical interventions as closely as possible to the time of their execution. The more seriously ill the patient, the greater the need to keep documentation current. Record all significant data before leaving for a break or at the end of the workday.

Never document a medical intervention before carrying it out.

Format

Check to make sure you have the correct patient record before recording information.

Record information on the proper form as designated by the health care institution's policy.

Print or write legibly in dark ink to ensure permanence. Use correct grammar and spelling. Use standard terminology, only commonly accepted terms and abbreviations and symbols. Alternately, follow computer documentation guidelines.

Date and time each entry.

Record medical interventions chronologically on consecutive lines. Never skip lines. Draw a single line through blank spaces.

Accountability

Sign your first initial, last name, and title to each entry. Do not sign notes describing interventions not performed by you that you have no way of verifying.

Do not use dittos, erasures, or correcting fluids. A single line should be drawn through an incorrect entry and the words "mistaken entry" or "error in charting" should be printed above or beside the entry and signed. The entry should then be rewritten correctly.

Identify each page of the record with the patient's name and identification number.

Recognize that the patient record is permanent. Follow the health care institution's policy pertaining to the color of ink and the type of pen or ink to be used. Ensure that the patient record is complete before sending it to medical records.

Confidentiality

Patients have a moral and legal right to expect that the information contained in their patient record will be kept private. Become familiar with the health care institution's policy and pertinent legislation about who has access to patient records, other than the immediate caregiving team, and the process used to obtain access.

Most health care institutions allow students access to patient records for educational reasons. Students using patient records are bound professionally and ethically to keep in strict confidence all the information they learn by reading patient records. Actual patient names and other identifiers should not be used in written or oral student reports.

ZOOM IN

Lawsuit Protection and Charting

A thoroughly documented patient record can be a health care provider's greatest defense against claims of negligence and malpractice. When faced with a lawsuit, full and correct documentation can be used to defend against any claims of wrongdoing. While memories fade over time, medical records are permanent. If a lawsuit goes to a jury years after the fact, the patient's medical record needs to provide a clear picture of the care that was given. Therefore, follow these guidelines with medical records:

- Include all important details.
- Use language that's descriptive and respectful.

- Be objective and discreet when entering information into a patient medical record. You do not know who will eventually read the chart. A belligerent patient may appear drunk but should not be described as such, unless you are certain of that condition. It is possible that the patient may be suffering from a reaction to a medication.
- If possible, enter notes directly into an electronic medical record. If notes must be handwritten, make certain they're legible.
- If an error is made, do not alter the record. Instead, cross out the error using a single line and label the original notation as an error. Initial the change and include the date and time. A more detailed explanation may be required for significant errors.

---

has required; and (4) progress notes, which are numbered and grouped together.

- The **source-oriented medical record (SOMR)** groups information by type instead of by problem. For example, all radiology reports are filed in one group, all lab reports are filed in another group, and so on.

Regardless of the organization method used, there is one rule that is always followed: The most recent information always appears first in its section—that is, the most recent documentation is filed on top of existing documentation. This creates a reverse order of information—the farther back you go in each section, the older the information is.

All entries should have a date and time stamp and should be signed or initialed by the health care professional. Also, information should never be charted ahead of time; data should only be entered after an event occurs. Table 17-1 provides medical documentation guidelines regarding content, timing, accountability, and confidentiality.

CHECK POINT

7 What are the five characteristics of good medical documentation?

8 In medical documentation, what is the first rule of accuracy?

TYPES OF PROGRESS NOTES

The progress notes section in a patient's medical record documents each contact made between any health care professional and the patient. This section of the patient's record summarizes all relevant activities and is used by health care professionals from many different disciplines. There are three types of progress notes:

- narrative notes
- SOAP notes
- charting by exception

Some facilities use lined paper with two columns for progress notes. The date and time of the contact are written in the narrow left column, and the notes about the contact are written in the right column. Other offices use plain or lined paper without columns. In an electronic health record, vital signs and information provided by the patient may be recorded in progress notes.

Regardless of the format, the date, time, signature, and credentials of the individual entering the data are always included. Electronic health records have a function by which users sign electronically.

Narrative Notes

Some providers document visits in a narrative format. The narrative format is the oldest and least structured medical documentation style. It is simply a paragraph indicating the contact with the patient, what was done for the patient, and what outcomes resulted. Narrative notes are time-consuming to write and can be difficult to read.

SOAP Notes

Problem-oriented charting is one of the most common methods of documenting patient visits. The **SOAP** format has four parts, which make the acronym *SOAP*:

- *s*ubjective data
- *o*bjective data
- *a*ssessment
- *p*lan

Mamie Parrish

10/17/03	Pt. Called c/o fever, sore throat. Asked to speak to Dr. Johnson. Instructed patient to come in for exam; explained that Dr. Johnson cannot treat her over the phone. Given appt for tomorrow at 10:00 a.m.
10/18/03	Pt. called and stated that she felt "90% better". Appt. canceled.
	Jennifer Wise, CMA

12/05/03	Office Visit
SUBJECTIVE:	Pt presents c/o of bad pain in RLQ x 2 days.
OBJECTIVE:	Vital signs: T-101.3, P-94, R-16, BP-112/76. Urine pregnancy test was done, negative. Urine dip was negative for blood and WBC, pH 7.0, Urine was clear. Blood was sent to the laboratory for CBC with diff.
ASSESSMENT:	Pain in RLQ. Possible appendicitis vs. ovarian cyst.
PLAN:	Tylenol 650 mg suppository given now. Will await lab results and notify patient with further instructions at that time.
	James Owens, MD

| 12/16/03 | Lab work normal. Called pt. Per Dr. Johnson and instructed to notify us if her fever is not gone tomorrow. Patient states, "I guess I feel some better." Pt. will call office p.r.n. |
| | *Melissa Hurley, RMA* |

Figure 17-1 Sample Notes in the SOAP Format

Figure 17-1 shows a sample page from a patient record that follows the SOAP format.

Subjective Data

The subjective part of the record includes any statements from the patient describing his or her condition. Notes in this section include any symptoms the patient mentions, using the patient's exact words. For example, "I started feeling a sharp pain in my lower abdomen area a couple of days ago. I've been vomiting all night and have had diarrhea for the past two days. The last thing I was able to eat was crackers at dinnertime last night."

Objective Data

The objective part of the record includes information from the health care professional's observations of the patient. This includes any data the health care worker can measure, see, feel, or smell. It also includes test results and vital signs, if applicable. For example, an entry might say, "The patient appears weak, pale, and slightly dehydrated and has lost three pounds since her last visit."

Assessment

The assessment portion of the record contains the patient's diagnosis, based on the analysis of the subjective and objective data. If a final diagnosis can't be made yet, the provider lists possible disorders to be ruled out, for example, "Possible viral infection."

Plan

The plan is a description of what should be done about the problem. This includes any diagnostic tests, treatments that will be given, and any follow-up required, such as: "Stool culture, CBC with diff, BRAT diet, and Imodium for the next 48 hours. Call office if symptoms worsen; return to office if patient not well by the end of the week."

Charting by Exception

The charting by exception format is an abbreviated documentation method that makes use of well-defined standards of practice and documents only significant or abnormal findings. This is a strictly problem-oriented method of charting. As more facilities move to electronic medical records, charting by exception is becoming more common. This approach offers several benefits, including:

- decreased charting time, which frees more time for direct patient care
- greater emphasis on significant data
- easy retrieval of significant data
- timely bedside charting
- standardized assessment
- greater interdisciplinary communication
- better tracking of important patient responses
- lower costs

✓ CHECK POINT

9 What are the three basic styles of progress notes?

10 In "SOAP format," what is SOAP an acronym for?

MILITARY TIME

Times are entered into a patient's medical record for a variety of reasons. Time entries specify when an action was taken or when it should begin. It is extremely important to indicate time correctly. Most health care institutions use military time, a 24-hour time cycle that counts the hours of the day from 0000 (12:00 a.m.) to 2359 (11:59 p.m.). This prevents any confusion between a.m. and p.m. times (Table 17-2). A digital watch with a military time display will help you make the mental shift to the military time used in health care.

Table 17-2 24- to 12-Hour Time Conversion

Military or 24-Hour Time	12-hour Time
0000	12 a.m. (midnight)
0100	1 a.m.
0200	2 a.m.
0300	3 a.m.
0400	4 a.m.
0500	5 a.m.
0600	6 a.m.
0700	7 a.m.
0800	8 a.m.
0900	9 a.m.
1000	10 a.m.
1100	11 a.m.
1200	12 p.m. (noon)
1300	1 p.m.
1400	2 p.m.
1500	3 p.m.
1600	4 p.m.
1700	5 p.m.
1800	6 p.m.
1900	7 p.m.
2000	8 p.m.
2100	9 p.m.
2200	10 p.m.
2300	11 p.m.

✓ CHECK POINT

11 What time format do most health care institutions use? Why?

12 What is 11:00 a.m. in military time? 3:30 p.m.?

Chapter Wrap-Up

Don't forget to visit thePoint companion website for additional study resources!

CHAPTER HIGHLIGHTS

- Medical documentation serves many purposes, including communication, assessment, quality assurance, reimbursement, legal record, education, and research.
- Many health care institutions are converting from paper-based records to electronic formats.
- Medical records can include an admission sheet, graphic sheet, physician's orders, progress notes, medical history and examination sheet, reports, correspondence, and other documents.
- Good medical documentation is accurate, complete, concise, legible, and organized.
- The progress notes section in a patient's record documents each contact made between a health care professional and the patient and can be written in narrative, SOAP, or charting by exception format.
- Most health care institutions use military time in medical records.

REVIEW QUESTIONS

Matching

1. _____ Source of privacy rules health care professionals must follow
2. _____ Primary purpose of medical documentation
3. _____ Abbreviated documentation method that makes use of well-defined standards of practice
4. _____ Source of guidelines on security measures for electronic health records
5. _____ Traditional method for recording progress notes, which recounts interactions with patients in paragraph form

    a. communication **b.** AHIMA **c.** narrative format **d.** HIPAA **e.** charting by exception

Multiple Choice

6. Documentation in a patient's medical record forms the patient's
   - **a.** HIPAA file
   - **b.** assessment chart
   - **c.** permanent health record
   - **d.** progress notes

7. Which of the following is NOT true of computerized records?
   - **a.** Information is easy to store and retrieve.
   - **b.** The records never contain errors.
   - **c.** Nearly unlimited file space is available.
   - **d.** Information is easily added or attached to patient records.

8. Why are patients asked to fill out new admissions forms each year?
   - **a.** to ensure having up-to-date information
   - **b.** to provide baseline data for research
   - **c.** to see if their answers are consistent
   - **d.** to meet government mandates

9. Which of these is NOT part of a patient's social history?
   - **a.** marital status and number of children
   - **b.** use of alcohol or tobacco
   - **c.** age and gender
   - **d.** occupation and education

10. Which of these is the *best* advice about the use of abbreviations and acronyms?
    a. They should be used in print but not electronic records.
    b. They are the best method for achieving conciseness.
    c. They should be avoided in patient records for legal reasons.
    d. They should only be used if they will be understood and are from an accepted abbreviations list.

Completion

11. A patient's _____ include respiration rate, blood pressure, pulse, and temperature.

12. Patient records are used to verify the care that a patient received when _____ is being sought from an insurance policy or government plan.

13. Patient records are _____ documents and are admissible as evidence in court proceedings.

14. Regardless of the method used to organize a patient record, the most recent information always appears _____ in its section, thus creating a _____ order of information—the farther back you go in each section, the older the information is.

15. In military time, 4:45 p.m is written as _____.

Short Answer

16. What documents may be found in a patient's medical record?

    _____

    _____

17. How do researchers benefit from medical records?

    _____

    _____

18. In terms of access, how do handwritten charts compare to computerized records?

    _____

    _____

19. What is the proper procedure for handling an error in a paper medical record?

    _____

    _____

20. Name the four parts of the SOAP format and briefly describe each part.

    _____

    _____

INVESTIGATE IT

1. If careless wording is used, statements found in a patient's medical record may be misinterpreted by others. An account of a serious situation can become humorous or offensive if not carefully described. Go to the following web site: http://www.medleague.com/Articles/humor/charting_bloopers.htm. Choose a category and then read through some of the humorous statements that have been found in medical records. Consider how each statement could be rewritten to ensure that it is interpreted correctly and seriously, rather than humorously.

2. A well-documented patient medical record is a valuable tool for health care professionals facing charges of negligence or malpractice. Conduct research using the Internet or other sources to learn about medical documentation mistakes that can work against a provider in a legal proceeding. The following web site provides a good starting point: http://www.maureenkroll.com/Charting-Rules-to-Keep-You-Legally-Safe.htm.

RECOMMENDED READING

Buchman M. *Medical Assisting Made Incredibly Easy: Clinical Competencies*. Baltimore: Lippincott Williams & Wilkins, 2008.

Cascardo DC. Steps medical practices can take to minimize their malpractice risks. Available at: http://www.pmandr.com/medical_practice_management/malpractice_%7c_legal/steps_medical_practices_can_take_to_minimize_their_malpractice_risks.html.

Kale-Smith G. *Medical Assisting Made Incredibly Easy: Administrative Competencies*. Baltimore: Lippincott Williams & Wilkins, 2008.

Kronenberger J. *Comprehensive Medical Assisting*. Baltimore: Lippincott Williams & Wilkins, 2008.

Taylor C. *Fundamentals of Nursing: The Art and Science of Nursing Care*. Baltimore: Lippincott Williams & Wilkins, 2008.

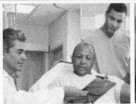
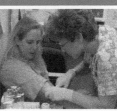
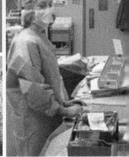

Safety and Infection Control

CHAPTER OBJECTIVES

After careful study of this chapter, you should be able to:

✷ Describe the role of the Occupational Safety and Health Administration and the Centers for Disease Control and Prevention in workplace safety and infection control.

✷ Explain the basic principles of health care safety.

✷ Identify the most common safety precautions and preventive actions used in health care.

✷ Outline how infectious diseases are transmitted.

✷ Explain how to prevent the spread of infectious disease.

KEY TERMS

aerobic (ār-Ō-bik)
airborne disease
anaerobic (AN-ār-Ō-bik)
antiseptics
bactericidal (bak-TĒR-i-SĪ-dăl)
bacteriostatic (bak-TĒR-ē-ō-STAT-ik)

blood-borne disease
  carrier
Centers for Disease Control
  and Prevention (CDC)
disinfection
exposure report
germicidal
hepatitis
host

human immunodeficiency
  virus (HIV)
incident report
medical asepsis (MED-i-kăl
  ā-SEP-sis)
nosocomial infection (NŌ-sō-KŌ-mē-ăl in-FEK-shŭn)

Occupational Safety and
  Health Administration
  (OSHA)
pathogens
sanitization
sterilization
vector
virus

All health care professionals are responsible for promoting safe and healthy care environments. Without proper safety and infection control, patients, health care workers, and visitors are all at risk of injury or infection. Health care workers also need the skills and abilities to respond safely and effectively in a crisis situation.

ROLE OF REGULATORY AGENCIES

Regulatory agencies, such as the Occupational Safety and Health Administration (OSHA) and the Centers for Disease Control and Prevention (CDC), provide safety rules and regulations for many workplaces. Most workplace injuries and disease transmissions in health care facilities can be prevented by strict adherence to guidelines issued by OSHA and the CDC.

Occupational Safety and Health Administration (OSHA)

The Occupational Safety and Health Administration (OSHA) is the main federal agency responsible for ensuring the safety of workers through the enforcement of safety and health legislation. By law, a health care facility must establish practices to keep employees healthy and safe. These written practices must be included in a policy or procedure manual or a separate infection control manual. These manuals should be kept where employees and OSHA inspectors can find them easily.

Centers for Disease Control and Prevention (CDC)

The Centers for Disease Control and Prevention (CDC) is a U.S. government agency dedicated to the prevention and control of disease, injury, and disability. Part of the Department of Health and Human Services, the CDC has developed guidelines to provide the widest possible protection against the spread of infection. CDC officials recommend that health care workers handle all blood and other body fluids, tissues, mucous membranes, and broken skin as if they contained infectious agents. These guidelines are described more fully in the section "Preventing the Spread of Disease" later in this chapter.

> ✓ **CHECK POINT**
>
> **1** What role does OSHA play in workplace safety?

PRINCIPLES OF SAFETY

Safety and security are basic human needs that help form the foundation of health care. While safety concerns vary depending on the type of health care facility and the needs of patients, health care professionals in any setting can help reduce patient risk.

Developmental Considerations

Health care needs and safety risks change as a person ages. From infancy to old age, each developmental stage carries its own particular risks. To ensure that an environment is safe and secure, health care workers need an awareness of potential hazards for each development stage. Here are just a few examples of factors to consider:

- The growth and development of an unborn child can be harmed by exposure to drugs, alcohol, or smoke.
- For children, potential hazards multiply as their motor skills develop and their environment expands.
- Adolescents face dangers when they abuse drugs or alcohol or engage in high-risk sexual activity.
- Older adults are particularly at risk of serious injury from falls, because their bones are more fragile. Abuse of older adults is also a growing problem that affects approximately five percent of older Americans.

Health care providers often work with patients and family members to eliminate or reduce risks to health and safety in the home and health care facilities.

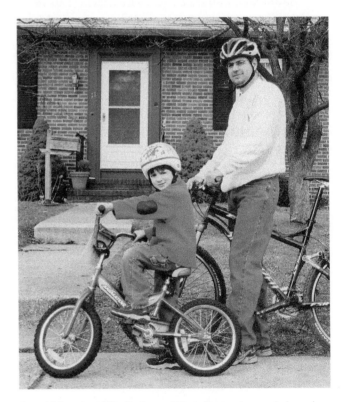

As a child's motor skills develop and his environment expands, hazards multiply.

Factors Affecting Safety

Both physiological and environmental factors can affect people's safety. Physiological factors are how people's bodies function. Environmental factors are conditions in the world around them.

Physiological Factors

The human body includes several systems that control every function—walking, talking, breathing, seeing, hearing, remembering, and so on. Two of these systems, the musculoskeletal and neurological systems, work together to help people detect and react to safety issues. Another factor affecting safety is fatigue.

Musculoskeletal System. Bones, joints, and muscles all make up the musculoskeletal system—the parts that provide movement, support, and protection for the human body. Any disruption or injury to these parts, such as arthritis, a broken bone, or a damaged muscle, can affect a person's mobility. This, in turn, may directly affect the person's ability to respond to hazardous situations and thereby increase the risk of injury.

Aging causes significant changes in the musculoskeletal systems of older adults. Their bones and muscles both grow weaker, and they also experience stiffness in their joints. All of these factors increase the risk of injury.

Neurological System. The neurological system, or nervous system, consists of the brain, spinal cord, and nerves that run throughout the body. These organs and tissues regulate nearly all body functions and enable humans to process information. A properly functioning nervous system allows people to think clearly, recall past events, imagine solutions, and solve problems. These functions can promote safety. Impairment to the nervous system, whether due to biochemical or psychological causes, illness, normal aging changes, or the influence of drugs or alcohol, can interfere with judgment and motor control and lead to harmful consequences.

Fatigue. Someone suffering from extreme weariness or exhaustion is experiencing *fatigue*. Fatigue can result from physical or mental activity and affects a person's ability to respond effectively. It often leads to poor perception of danger, faulty judgment, and inadequate problem solving.

Environmental Factors

Environmental factors vary from place to place. In the home, workplace, or community, environmental factors can affect health and safety.

Home. Adequate ventilation that provides plenty of clean air is essential for any home. A properly maintained heating system is also important. Leaks in natural gas or propane-fueled heating systems can lead to carbon monoxide poisoning or an explosion. Home carbon-monoxide detectors can alert homeowners to this danger.

Well-maintained electrical systems and appliances reduce the risk of accidental fires. Smoke detectors can alert people when fires do occur. All potentially toxic substances should be properly labeled and stored out of the reach of children.

Workplace. People who work in hazardous conditions, such as dust, chemicals, noise, heights, and dangerous machines, have a higher risk of injury in the workplace. Jobs requiring heavy lifting and repetitive motion may also lead to injuries. Federal and state regulatory agencies set workplace safety standards that employers must follow. Workers and managers have a responsibility to comply with these standards by following basic safety precautions, such as wearing protective masks, ear plugs, safety goggles, and harnesses. All of these practices help reduce the risk of workplace injury. (Safety standards related to health care facilities are discussed in more detail later in this chapter.)

Decreasing Equipment-Related Accidents

Use equipment only for the use for which it was intended.

Do not operate equipment with which you are unfamiliar.

Handle equipment with care to prevent damaging it.

Use three-prong electric plugs whenever possible.

Do not twist or bend electric cords. The wires inside the cord may break.

Be alert to signs that indicate equipment is faulty, such as breaks in electric cords, sparks, smoke, electric shocks, loose or missing parts, and unusual noises or odors. Report signs of trouble immediately.

Make certain that electric cords are not in a position to be pulled or trapped when equipment or furniture is moved, which can damage cords and create electrical or fire hazards.

Be alert for wet surfaces on areas where electric cords or connections are present.

Implement a process for reporting and addressing problems with equipment.

Community. Communities that are safe and secure provide a healthier environment. Negative environmental factors, such as air pollution, crime, hazardous waste sites, and dilapidated housing, increase the health risks of people in a community. The level of sanitation also affects a community's safety. Lack of sanitation may spread disease and infection. Proper sanitation includes a clean water supply, an adequate sewage system, and absence of insects and rodents.

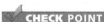
CHECK POINT

2 Why might safety precautions in a pediatrician's office be different from those in an assisted-living facility?

SAFETY PRECAUTIONS AND ACTIONS

Health care workers should be familiar with safety precautions and preventive actions for a variety of situations. These precautions ensure the safety of health care workers as well as patients.

Patient Safety

Patients are far less likely to experience accidental injuries when they're familiar with their surroundings. Patients new to a health care facility should be oriented to its layout, safety features, and equipment. An explanation and demonstration of the adjustable bed and side rails, call system, telephone, television, and bathroom will help a patient adjust to a new environment. When patients are transported from one place to another, safety straps and side rails should be used to ensure that patients remain secure.

A patient's *identification bracelet* also helps ensure safety. This bracelet contains information that must be verified by all health care personnel interacting with the patient—whether administering medications, delivering meals, or providing treatment. By following this precaution, each provider ensures that he or she is dealing with the correct patient.

Preventing patient falls must be a priority in any health care setting. Falls can be caused by many factors, including the effects of medication, debris on the floor, and inappropriately placed equipment. Health care professionals must be alert to potential hazards, even in areas not often frequented by patients. Health care workers should check all areas periodically to make sure that there are no magazines or trash on the ground, tables too close to each other, or large potted plants too close to seats. All of these are hazards that might cause falls.

Health care professionals are also responsible for making sure that the equipment they use is free from defects. They should also use the equipment properly, following all instructions in the procedure manual. If they have any questions about equipment use, they should ask their supervisors.

Health Care Worker Safety

Health care workers must also be aware of the risks to their own safety. Health care workers who work directly with patients are involved with positions and movements that can lead to injury. Safety precautions, such as good posture and proper body mechanics and ergonomics, can reduce a health care worker's risk of injury. Lifting devices can help prevent back injuries.

Other common risks to health care worker safety, including exposure to pathogens, chemicals, and radiation, are discussed in later sections in this chapter.

Fires

Careless smoking, faulty electrical equipment, and combustion of anesthetic agents are the most common causes of fires in health care facilities. Regular servicing of electrical equipment and strict smoking policies can help reduce the risk of fires. All health care professionals are responsible for patients' safety and need to be familiar with the facility's fire safety plan, emergency exits, the location and operation of fire extinguishers, and any special instructions for reporting a fire.

Many health care facilities base their fire response procedures on the acronym *RACE*:

Rescue anyone in immediate danger.

Activate the fire code system and notify the appropriate person.

Confine the fire by closing doors and windows.

Evacuate patients and other people to a safe area, or extinguish the fire if safe to do so.

There are three classes of fire:
- A—Ordinary combustibles: wood, cloth, paper, plastic
- B—Flammable liquids
- C—Live electrical

Fire extinguishers marked with an "A" extinguish with ordinary water, by cooling and smothering the fire. Type "A" extinguishers should *not* be used on flammable liquids or live electrical fires. "BC" extinguishers can be either dry chemical or carbon dioxide extinguishers. They are used for extinguishing flammable liquids or electrical fires and should *not* be used for ordinary combustibles. Type "ABC" fire extinguishers, the most common kind used in health care facilities, contain a material similar to baking soda that can be used on any type of fire. To operate a fire extinguisher, always read the directions first and then remember the acronym *PASS*:

Pull the locking pin.

Aim the nozzle at the base of the fire.

Squeeze the handle.

Sweep from side to side.

Electrical Hazards

Injury and even death can result from overloaded electrical circuits, faulty appliances, frayed wires, and careless use of electrical equipment. Electrical devices and cords should not be handled with wet hands or while wearing wet shoes. Health care professionals can protect themselves and patients from dangerous electrical shocks by keeping their hands dry when using machinery and by mopping up spilled fluids. They should also ensure that all plugs are grounded (three-pronged) and should report any equipment damage. Electrical equipment should be serviced regularly.

Oxygen

Supplemental oxygen is considered a medication and must be ordered by a health care professional. While vital for life, oxygen also supports combustion. To prevent fires and injuries, the following precautions should be taken:

- Avoid open flames in the room of a patient receiving oxygen.
- Place "No Smoking" signs in conspicuous places in the patient's room or home. Inform the patient and visitors that oxygen accelerates combustion and could produce a fire from even a small spark.
- Check to see that all electrical equipment used in the room is grounded, in good working order, and emits no sparks.
- Avoid synthetic fabrics that build up static electricity.
- Avoid using oils in the area. Oil (such as petroleum jelly) can ignite spontaneously in the presence of oxygen.

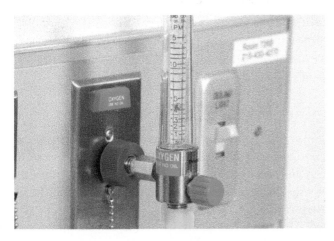

While oxygen is vital for life, it is also combustible. Safety procedures must be followed in the presence of supplemental oxygen.

Chemical Hazards

Chemicals pose another risk to safety in the workplace. Common hazardous chemicals found in health care settings include:

- Alcohol, used as a disinfectant (flammable)
- Ethylene oxide, used for sterilizing purposes (an eye irritant and also potentially explosive and flammable)
- Housekeeping products used for cleaning and disinfecting (potential eye, skin, and respiratory tract irritants)
- Various gases used as anesthetics or fuels for gas-powered equipment (potentially combustible and asphyxiating)

Health care personnel who work with these chemicals must understand the potential hazards and follow warning labels. They need to know how to use and dispose of the chemicals safely and what to do if an accident occurs. They should be especially cautious about mixing two chemicals together.

Radiation

Although the risk of radiation injury in most communities is low, health care professionals should be familiar with the common sources and effects of radiation exposure. The international symbol shown in Figure 18-1 marks areas where radioactive substances are used. Radioactive implants or ingestion of radioactive materials can make a person a source of radiation.

Health care professionals who work in areas where radiation or radioactive substances are used generally wear a radiation detection badge to assist the facility's radiation safety officer in monitoring exposure levels. The officer collects these badges periodically to determine exposure levels. In this way, the facility can ensure that staff members are staying within safe limits of exposure.

The three cardinal rules of radiation protection are:

- Minimize time of exposure to the source.
- Maximize distance from the source.
- Use appropriate shielding.

Regular inspection and servicing of equipment and licensing of x-ray and pharmacy technicians help minimize

CAUTION

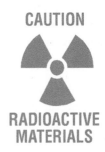

RADIOACTIVE MATERIALS

Figure 18-1 International Radiation Symbol.

the risk of radiation exposure to patients and other health care professionals. Providers should use lead shields or lead aprons when in close contact with a patient exposed to radiation. They should also wear gloves to prevent skin contact with any substances that might contain radiation, such as urine, stool, saliva, or blood.

Workplace Violence

The National Institute for Occupational Safety and Health (NIOSH) defines *workplace violence* as "violent acts (including physical assaults and threats of assaults) directed toward persons at work or on duty." Like workers in most settings, health care workers face a significant risk of job-related violence. Assaults, in particular, are a serious hazard in the health care industry. Work-related assaults in health care settings occur in relation to several factors, including:

- the prevalence of handguns and other weapons among patients, family members, and friends.
- the increasing use of hospitals by police and the criminal justice system for criminal holds and the care of acutely disturbed, violent individuals.
- the increasing number of mentally ill patients being released from hospitals without follow-up care. (These patients have the right to refuse medicine and can no longer be hospitalized involuntarily unless they pose an immediate threat to themselves or others.)
- the presence of drugs and money in hospitals, clinics, and pharmacies, making them likely robbery targets.
- the unrestricted movement of the public in clinics and hospitals.
- long waits in emergency or clinic areas that lead to frustration over the inability to obtain needed services promptly.
- the increasing presence of gang members, drug or alcohol abusers, trauma patients, and distraught family members.
- isolated work with clients during examinations or treatment.

To prevent or reduce violent workplace incidents, OSHA encourages health care employers to have a written violence prevention program and incorporate it into the organization's overall safety and health guidelines.

Emergency Action Plan

To prevent confusion or misunderstandings during a fire, explosion, or other emergency, all employees of a health care facility should be provided with a written set of emergency procedures. According to OSHA requirements, an *emergency action plan* should contain the following:

- a preferred method for reporting fires and other emergencies
- an evacuation policy and related procedures
- emergency escape procedures and route assignments, such as floor plans, workplace maps, and safe or refuge areas
- names, titles, departments, and telephone numbers of individuals to contact, both within and outside the facility, for additional information or explanation of duties and responsibilities under the plan
- procedures for employees who remain in the facility to continue or shut down critical operations, operate fire extinguishers, or perform other essential services
- designated rescue and medical duties for each employee

While not required by OSHA, facilities also often include the following in their action plan:

- the site of an alternative communications center to be used in the event of a fire or explosion
- a secure onsite or offsite location to store originals or duplicate copies of patient records, accounting records, legal documents, emergency contact lists, and other essential records

---

✓ CHECK POINT

3 Regarding fires, what does RACE mean?

4 Why do some health care professionals routinely wear radiation detection badges?

INFECTIOUS DISEASE

Disease prevention is a major focus for all health care professionals. Diseases carried by one person can infect another when pathogens, or disease-causing microorganisms such as bacteria or viruses, are passed from person to person. Pathogens are found naturally in almost all environments. Some are beneficial, while others are not. Some are harmless to most people, and others are harmful to many people. Still other pathogens are harmless except in certain circumstances.

Infectious Microorganisms

Some of the most prevalent agents that cause infections are bacteria, viruses, and fungi. *Bacteria*, the most significant and most commonly observed pathogens in health care institutions, are categorized by their shape, their reaction to a Gram stain test, and by their need for oxygen. Most bacteria require oxygen to live and grow and are referred to as aerobic. Those that can live without oxygen are called anaerobic bacteria.

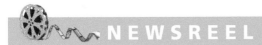

Antibiotic-Resistant Organisms

A significant and disturbing trend is the development of pathogens that are resistant to antibiotics. This resistance has resulted from the use of broad-spectrum antibiotics, which allowed the bacteria that survived to develop defenses against the antibiotics. As a result, resistant organisms, such as methicillin-resistant *S. aureus* (MRSA), have emerged. This organism, which is resistant to the antibiotic methicillin, became a common cause of postoperative infections.

Physicians seemed to have solved the problem when they began using a different antibiotic—vancomycin. In 2002, however, the first case of vancomycin-resistant *S. aureus* (VRSA) was reported.

These antibiotic-resistant organisms are a formidable challenge for health care professionals. Researchers continue to investigate new antibiotics that may become alternatives for treating drug-resistant bacteria.

A **virus** is the smallest of all microorganisms, visible only with an electronic microscope. Many infections are caused by viruses, including the common cold and the deadly acquired immunodeficiency syndrome (AIDS). Antibiotics have no effect on viruses, but some medications are effective with some viral infections. When given during the incubation period of certain viruses, these medications can shorten the length of the illness.

Fungi, or plantlike organisms (molds and yeasts), are present in the air, soil, and water and can also cause infection. Some examples of infections caused by fungi include athlete's foot, ringworm, and yeast infections. These infections are treated with antifungal medications. Many fungal infections are resistant to treatment, however.

An organism's potential to produce disease in a person depends on a variety of factors:
- the number of organisms in the exposure
- the *virulence* of the organism, or its ability to cause disease
- the relative strength of the individual's immune system
- the length and intimacy of the contact between the person and the microorganism

The Chain of Infection

The *chain of infection* is often thought of as a series of links through which a pathogen spreads from one person to another. Pathogens move along the chain's five links sequentially (Figure 18-2). Breaking the chain of infection at any link helps stop infectious disease from spreading. The five links are:
- reservoir
- exit from reservoir
- vehicle of transmission
- portal of entry
- susceptible host

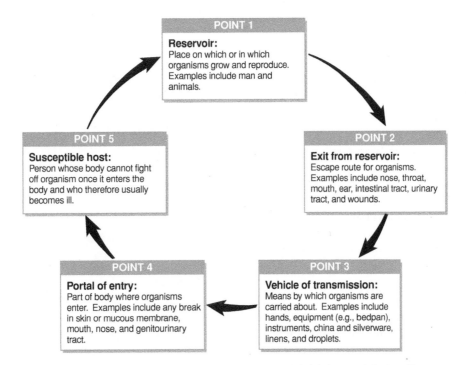

POINT 1

Reservoir:
Place on which or in which organisms grow and reproduce. Examples include man and animals.

POINT 2

Exit from reservoir:
Escape route for organisms. Examples include nose, throat, mouth, ear, intestinal tract, urinary tract, and wounds.

POINT 3

Vehicle of transmission:
Means by which organisms are carried about. Examples include hands, equipment (e.g., bedpan), instruments, china and silverware, linens, and droplets.

POINT 4

Portal of entry:
Part of body where organisms enter. Examples include any break in skin or mucous membrane, mouth, nose, and genitourinary tract.

POINT 5

Susceptible host:
Person whose body cannot fight off organism once it enters the body and who therefore usually becomes ill.

Figure 18-2   Chain of infection. Breaking the chain at any link helps stop infectious disease from spreading.

Reservoir

The *reservoir* is the person who is infected with the pathogen, or the carrier of the disease. Whether or not the carrier shows signs of infection, the pathogen uses the carrier's body as a source of nutrients and an incubator where it can grow and reproduce.

Exit from the Reservoir

A carrier can pass the disease along to others only if the pathogen has a means of exit from the reservoir. Pathogens can exit through mucous membranes of the nose and mouth, the openings of the gastrointestinal system (mouth or rectum), or an open wound.

Vehicle of Transmission

The third link in the chain of infection is the vehicle of transmission—the way by which the pathogen leaves the reservoir and spreads through the environment. Vehicles include direct contact between an unclean hand and another person or object. Mucous or air droplets from the oral or nasal cavities are excellent vehicles for many pathogens. Sneezing or coughing without covering the nose and mouth transmit pathogens into the environment and endanger potential hosts.

Portal of Entry

The route by which a pathogen enters a potential host is the fourth link in the chain of infection. When contaminated air droplets are inhaled, the respiratory system is the portal of entry. When the pathogen enters the body through contaminated food or drink, the portal of entry is the gastrointestinal system. Any break in the skin or mucous membranes can also be a portal of entry for pathogens.

Susceptible Host

The final link in the chain of infection is the susceptible host. The host is the person to whom the pathogen is eventually transported after leaving the reservoir host. If the conditions in the susceptible host promote reproduction of the pathogen, the susceptible host becomes a reservoir host and the cycle may repeat.

Modes of Transmission

The vehicle that spreads the pathogen is often called the *mode of transmission*. To understand how to break this link in the infectious cycle and prevent the spread of disease, you must understand the different modes of transmission of pathogens.

Direct Transmission

Contact between the infected reservoir host and a susceptible host constitutes *direct transmission*. This type of transmission may occur when a person touches contaminated blood or body fluids, shakes hands with someone who has contaminated hands, inhales infected air droplets, or has intimate contact, such as kissing or sexual intercourse, with someone who carries a pathogen.

Indirect Transmission

Indirect transmission can occur through contact with a vehicle known as a vector. Vectors include contaminated food or water; disease-carrying insects; and inanimate objects like soil, drinking glasses, and improperly disinfected medical instruments. While visible blood and body fluids are obvious sources of infection, many infectious organisms remain viable for long periods on surfaces that are not visibly contaminated.

Sources of Transmission

Most reservoir hosts are humans, animals, and insects. Human hosts include (1) people stricken by an infectious disease; (2) those who are carriers of a disease but not ill from it; and (3) those who are incubating the disease but not yet exhibiting symptoms. This last group can transmit the disease even though they're asymptomatic (have no symptoms). Animal sources, which are less common, include infected dogs, cats, birds, cattle, rodents, and animals that live in the wild. Diseases that may be transmitted to humans from infected animals include anthrax and rabies.

In addition to flies and roaches, which carry many diseases, many other insects are disease vectors. They may feed on the blood of an infected reservoir host, and then when they bite a human, they pass the pathogen to that person Ticks and mosquitoes may transmit diseases, including Lyme disease (ticks) and malaria (mosquitoes). Table 18-1 lists some common diseases and their methods of transmission.

Infectious Disease in Health Care Settings

While disease-producing microorganisms are found naturally in any number of environments, these pathogens generally occur in even higher numbers in health care settings. The reason is obvious: many people suffering from diseases caused by these microorganisms come to health care facilities for treatment and bring the microorganisms with them. Health care-associated

Table 18-1 Common Communicable Diseases

Disease	Method of Transmission
AIDS	Direct contact with infectious body fluids, or contact with contaminated sharps
Chicken pox (varicella)	Direct contact or droplets
Cholera	Ingestion of contaminated food or water
Diphtheria	Airborne droplets, infected carriers
Hepatitis B	Direct contact with infectious body fluid
Influenza	Airborne droplets, infected carriers or direct contact with contaminated articles such as used tissues
Measles (rubeola)	Airborne droplets, infected carriers
Meningitis	Airborne droplets
Mononucleosis	Airborne droplets or contact with infected saliva
Mumps	Airborne droplets, infected carriers, or direct contact with materials contaminated with infected saliva
Pneumonia	Airborne droplets or direct contact with infected mucus
Rabies	Direct contact with saliva of infected animal such as an animal bite
Rubella (German measles)	Airborne droplets, infected carriers
Tetanus	Direct contact with spores or contaminated animal feces
Tuberculosis	Airborne droplets, infected carriers

infections, known as **nosocomial infections**, are among the greatest risks posed to patients in health care settings (Figure 18-3).

The two main ways that diseases are transmitted are by air and by contact with blood or other body fluids.

An **airborne disease** spreads from person to person through droplets in the air. The pathogen is released into the air when an infected person sneezes or coughs and is transmitted to another person who inhales those droplets or touches a surface where the droplets have settled.

Tuberculosis (TB) is one common, and sometimes deadly, airborne disease that attacks the lungs and other parts of the body. TB is most often spread when a contagious person coughs, sneezes, or talks and is most likely to attack a person with a weakened immune system. There are many other common airborne diseases:

- chickenpox
- common cold
- diphtheria
- influenza
- measles
- meningitis
- pneumonia
- whooping cough (pertussis)

A **blood-borne disease** is spread from person to person when an infected person's blood or certain other body fluids come into contact with the mucous membranes or bloodstream of an uninfected person. Health care professionals can be exposed to blood-borne diseases through needlesticks or other skin punctures, mucous membranes, and breaks in the skin.

Three blood-borne pathogens pose great risk to health care professionals: HIV, hepatitis B, and hepatitis C. **Human immunodeficiency virus (HIV)** is a virus that slowly wears down a person's immune system and, in most cases, causes the person to develop acquired immune deficiency syndrome (AIDS). Patients with AIDS, if untreated, have such severely weakened immune systems that they eventually fall prey to infections and die.

Hepatitis causes inflammation of the liver. While this disease can sometimes be caused by alcohol or drug abuse, it's primarily caused by a virus. There are several

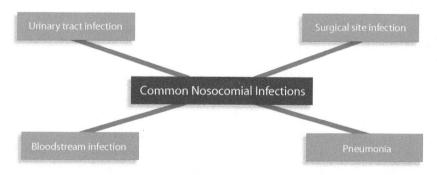

Figure 18-3 Health Care-Associated Infections.

different forms of the hepatitis virus, the most common being hepatitis B and hepatitis C. Although both viruses can spread through similar methods, hepatitis B is frequently spread through sexual contact, and hepatitis C is generally spread through the sharing of needles.

To avoid the spread of HIV, hepatitis, and other blood-borne diseases, needles should never be shared. A latex barrier, such as gloves or a condom, should be used to prevent contact with an infected person's body fluids.

OSHA requires that newly hired medical office employees who may be exposed to blood have special training to prevent infection by these diseases. That training must also be repeated every year to include any new policies recommended by OSHA, the CDC, the Department of Health and Human Services, or the U.S. Public Health Service. Training should include these key points:

- descriptions of blood-borne diseases, how they're transmitted, and related symptoms
- kinds of protective equipment available and the location of this equipment in the medical facility
- information about the risks of contracting hepatitis B and about the HBV vaccine

EXTRA EXTRA INTERESTING FACTS ABOUT THE INFECTIOUS PROCESS

Did you know that

- people in modern society are more vulnerable to the spread of infectious disease as a result of population crowding and easy travel?
- some types of infections, such as HIV, affect the entire body, while others, such as severe acute respiratory syndrome (SARS), affect only one organ or system of the body?
- localized infections, such as the common cold, occur more frequently in the upper respiratory tract (nose, nasal cavity, and throat)? Upper respiratory tract infections are among the most common infections in the world.
- the hepatitis B vaccine is the most widely used vaccine in the world? More than one billion doses have been given around the world. The vaccine, which is usually administered to infants, is a series of three shots given over a six-month period and provides a lifetime of protection. You cannot get hepatitis B from the vaccine because there is no human blood or live virus in the vaccine. The hepatitis B vaccine is considered the first anti-cancer vaccine because it protects against a hepatitis B infection, which is the primary cause of liver cancer.

- the facility's exposure control plan and post-exposure procedures, along with follow-up care if an exposure occurs

✓ CHECK POINT

5 Briefly explain the chain of infection.

6 What is a reservoir, and what are the three most common reservoir hosts?

PREVENTING THE SPREAD OF DISEASE

Most health care professionals take precautions when dealing with patients known to be carriers of infectious microorganisms, but many of these same precautions should be taken when treating any patient. It is estimated that health care workers treat five unknown carriers for every patient known to be infectious. Therefore, knowledge and use of effective infection control is essential with *all* patients.

Standard Precautions

Standard precautions are a set of procedures recognized by the CDC to reduce the transmission of microorganisms in any health care setting. Health care workers need to use standard precautions when touching blood, body fluids, damaged skin, or mucous membranes. The CDC recommends these procedures:

- Wash hands with soap and water after touching blood, body fluids, secretions, or other contaminated objects—whether gloves were worn or not.
- Use an alcohol-based hand rub to decontaminate hands even if they're not visibly dirty or contaminated.
- Wear clean, nonsterile examination gloves if coming into contact with blood, body fluids, secretions, mucous membranes, damaged skin, or contaminated objects.
- If potentially infected substances have been touched, change gloves between procedures, even if procedures involve the same patient.
- Wear equipment to protect eyes, nose, and mouth and a disposable apron or gown to protect clothing when performing procedures that may splatter blood or other body fluids.
- Do not sterilize and reuse single-use items, but dispose of them properly.
- Take precautions to avoid injury when a procedure involves needles or sharp instruments—before, during, and after the procedure.

- Do not recap used needles or bend or break them.
- Dispose of syringes, needles, and other sharps in a puncture-resistant sharps container as close as possible to where the procedure was performed.
- Use barrier devices when performing rescue breathing.
- Do not eat, drink, or put anything into your mouth while working in a clinical area.

Medical Asepsis

Measures taken to control and reduce the number of pathogens present in an area or on an object are called medical asepsis. Commonly called *clean technique*, these measures do not guarantee that an object or area is free from *all* microorganisms. However, medical asepsis helps prevent the transmission of microorganisms from one person or area to another within a health care facility.

Whether at home or in a health care facility, proper and thorough hand washing remains the best way to avoid the transfer of microorganisms and break the chain of infection. Hands should be washed:

- before and after every patient contact
- after coming into contact with any blood or body fluids
- after coming into contact with contaminated material
- after handling specimens
- after coughing, sneezing, or blowing your nose
- after using the restroom
- before and after going to lunch, taking breaks, and leaving for the day

Cleaning common areas within a health care facility can also help stop the spread of disease. These areas include examination and treatment rooms, waiting or reception areas, and clinical work areas. Dust and dirt are vehicles for transmission of microorganisms and should be cleaned regularly from all surfaces, including the floor. Health care professionals should teach patients and their caregivers the importance of these techniques, which can be followed at home to prevent the spread of disease.

Cleaning, Disinfection, and Sterilization

Not all infection control methods are equal—there are different levels of control. From least to greatest, the three main levels of infection control are:

- cleaning or sanitization
- disinfection
- sterilization

Cleaning

The lowest level of infection control is cleaning, or sanitization. This involves the use of soap or detergent to thoroughly clean items and surfaces. Sanitization reduces the total number of microorganisms on an object, such as a medical instrument, to a level that is considered safe for some uses. Most instruments in a health care facility must be sanitized regularly. This typically involves scrubbing the item using warm, soapy water to remove organic matter and other residue. Cleaning or sanitizing must be done before disinfection or sterilization.

Disinfection

Even when an item or surface has been thoroughly cleaned or sanitized, a higher level of infection control, called disinfection, may be needed. Disinfection involves the use of a disinfectant agent to destroy many pathogens. Respiratory therapy and anesthesia equipment are examples of items that are disinfected. Disinfection does not destroy all microorganisms and bacterial spores, although high levels of disinfection are nearly as effective as sterilization (the highest level of infection control, described below). Antiseptics, agents commonly used to disinfect wounds or cuts, are bacteriostatic, which means that they inhibit the growth of microorganisms but do not kill them. Table 18-2 (following page) has more details on disinfection.

Sterilization

The highest level of infection control is sterilization, the method by which all forms of microorganisms, including spores, are destroyed on inanimate objects and surfaces. Infection control methods that kill microorganisms are called bactericidal, or germicidal.

Articles can be sterilized by exposure to any of four conditions:

- steam under pressure in an autoclave
- specific gases, such as ethylene oxide
- dry heat ovens
- immersion in an approved chemical sterilization agent

Any instrument or device that penetrates the skin or comes into contact with a sterile area of the body must be sterilized using one of these methods. Surgical instruments, for example, are all sterilized before surgery. To save time, many health care facilities use disposable sterile supplies and equipment. This eliminates the need for manual sterilization.

PROCEDURE Hand Washing for Medical Asepsis

1. Remove all rings and your wristwatch.

   WHY? *Rings and watches may harbor pathogens that may not be easily washed away. Ideally, rings should not be worn when working with material that may be infectious.*

2. Stand close to the sink without touching it.

   WHY? *The sink is considered contaminated, and standing too close may contaminate your clothing.*

3. Turn on the faucet and adjust the temperature of the water to warm.

   WHY? *Water that is too hot or too cold will crack or chap the skin on the hands, which will break the natural protective barrier that prevents infection.*

4. Wet your hands and wrists under the warm running water, apply liquid soap, and work the soap into a lather by rubbing your palms together and rubbing the soap between your fingers at least 10 times.

   WHY? *This motion dislodges microorganisms from between the fingers and removes the organisms.*

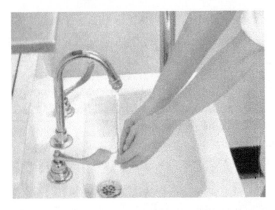

5. Scrub the palm of one hand with the fingertips of the other hand to work the soap under the nails of that hand; then reverse the procedure and scrub the other hand. Also scrub each wrist.

   WHY? *Friction helps remove microorganisms.*

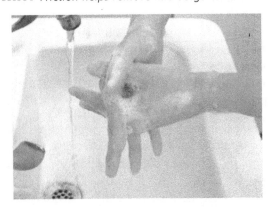

6. Rinse hands and wrists thoroughly under warm running water, holding hands lower than elbows; do not touch the inside of the sink.

WHY? *Holding the hands lower than the elbows and wrists allows microorganisms to flow off the hands and fingers rather than back up the arms.*

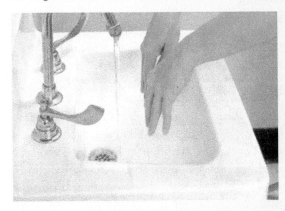

7. Using an orangewood manicure stick, clean under each nail on both hands.

   WHY? *Nails may harbor microorganisms. Metal files and pointed instruments may break the skin and make an opening for microorganisms. This step may be done at the beginning of the day, before leaving for the day, or after coming into contact with potentially infectious material.*

8. Reapply liquid soap and rewash hands and wrists.

   WHY? *Rewashing the hands after using the orangewood stick washes away any microorganisms that may have been removed with the stick.*

9. Rinse hands thoroughly again, while holding hands lower than wrists and elbows.

10. Gently dry hands with a paper towel. Discard the paper towel and the used orangewood stick when finished.

    WHY? *Hands must be dried thoroughly and completely to prevent drying and cracking.*

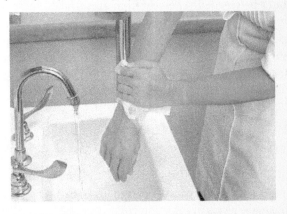

11. Use a dry paper towel to turn off the faucets, and discard the paper towel.

    WHY? *Your hands are clean and should not touch the contaminated faucet handles.*

Table 18-2 Levels of Disinfection and Procedures

Level	Procedures	When to Use	Effect
Low	Commercial products without tuberculocidal properties	Routine cleaning; to clean objects or surfaces with no visible blood or body fluids	Destroys many bacteria and some viruses; does NOT destroy *M. tuberculosis* or bacterial spores
Intermediate	Commercial germicides that kill *M. tuberculosis;* solutions containing 1:10 dilution of household bleach (2 oz. of chlorine bleach per quart of tap water)	To clean instruments that have touched unbroken skin, such as blood pressure cuffs, stethoscopes, and splints	Destroys many viruses, fungi, and some bacteria, including *M. tuberculosis;* does NOT destroy bacterial spores
High	Immersion in approved disinfecting chemical for 45 minutes or according to guidelines on label; immersion in boiling water for 30 minutes (rarely used)	To clean reusable instruments that contact body cavities with mucous membranes, such as the vagina and rectum, that are not considered sterile	Destroys most microorganisms except certain bacterial spores

Personal Protective Equipment

By using personal protective equipment, health care professionals help protect not only themselves from the spread of disease, but also patients, coworkers, and anyone else they may come in contact with. Health care professionals who might be exposed to biohazardous materials at work must have access to:

- gloves
- masks
- gowns
- eye protection

Masks, gowns, and eye protection should be worn in any areas where splashing or splattering of airborne particles may occur. Health care workers should assume that all blood and body fluids are contaminated with pathogens and should always wear gloves when handling specimens or if there is a chance that they might come into contact with contaminated material. For example, gloves should always be worn in these situations:

- drawing blood specimens
- disposing of biohazardous waste
- touching contaminated surfaces
- handling contaminated equipment
- giving injections

Wearing gloves does not replace hand washing, however. In fact, hands should be washed before putting gloves on. After a procedure, all personal protective equipment should be removed and hands should be washed again.

ON LOCATION

Infection Control Actions

Mary, a respiratory therapist at a large regional hospital, is working in the hospital's busy emergency department. When she arrives at the hospital, Mary goes straight to her department, where she puts on a new pair of gloves. She then proceeds to administer a breathing treatment to her first patient. After the treatment is complete, Mary hurriedly removes her gloves and begins taking her next patient's blood pressure. Once the blood pressure reading is complete, Mary administers a breathing treatment to the same patient.

- What, if any, infection control procedures did Mary fail to follow?
- How might similar infection control breaches be avoided in the future?

Disposing of Infectious Waste

Nearly all health care facilities generate some infectious waste. This waste poses health risks and must be disposed of carefully. Federal regulations from the Environmental Protection Agency (EPA) and OSHA set the policies and guidelines for disposing of hazardous materials, and individual states determine policies based on these guidelines.

Many medical offices are considered small generators, meaning they produce less than 50 pounds of waste each month. Hospitals and larger clinics that produce more than 50 pounds of waste each month are considered large generators. Large generators must obtain a certificate of registration from the EPA and keep records of the quantity of waste and their disposal procedures.

Regular Waste Container

Health care facilities provide separate containers for disposing of different kinds of waste. The regular waste

PROCEDURE Removing Contaminated Gloves

1. Choose the appropriate size gloves for your hands and put them on.

   WHY? *Gloves should fit comfortably, not too loose and not too tight. Good glove fit enhances safe manipulation.*

2. To remove gloves, grasp the glove of your nondominant hand at the palm and pull the glove away.

   WHY? *To avoid transferring contaminants to the skin of the wrist, be sure not to grasp the glove at the wrist.*

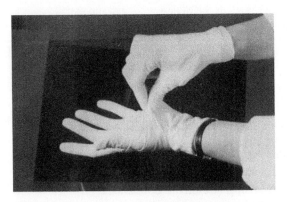

3. Slide your hand out of the glove, rolling the glove into the palm of your gloved dominant hand.

   WHY? *You should avoid touching either glove with your ungloved hand.*

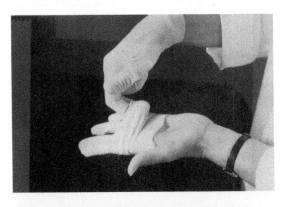

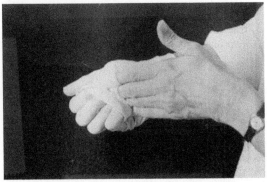

4. Holding the soiled glove in the palm of your gloved hand, slip your ungloved fingers under the cuff of the glove you are still wearing, being careful not to touch the outside of the glove.

   WHY? *Skin should touch skin but never the soiled part of the glove. (The back of your fingers touch the inside of the glove, but it is not soiled.)*

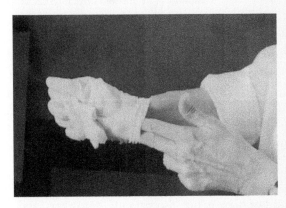

5. Stretch the glove of the dominant hand up and away from your hand while turning it inside out, with the removed first glove balled up inside.

   WHY? *Turning the glove inside out ensures that the soiled surfaces of the gloves are enclosed.*

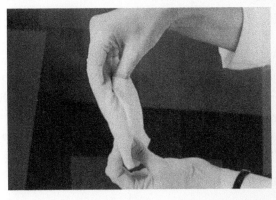

6. Both gloves are now removed, with the first glove inside the second glove and the second glove inside out.

7. Discard both gloves as one unit into a biohazard waste receptacle.

8. Wash your hands.

   WHY? *Wearing gloves is NOT a substitute for washing your hands!*

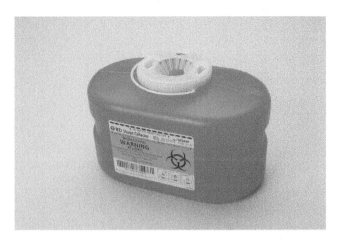

Figure 18-4 Used needles are disposed of in a sharps container.

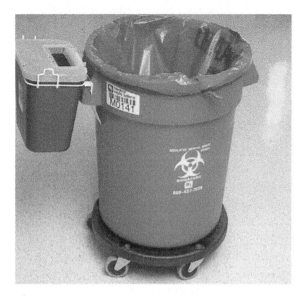

The biohazard waste container is used only for waste contaminated with blood or body fluids.

container is used only for waste that's not contaminated. Some examples include:

- paper
- plastic
- disposable tray wrappers
- packaging material

Most non-biohazardous liquids should be discarded in a sink or other washbasin, not in the plastic bag inside the regular waste container. This step ensures that the liquids will not leak and cause mess inside the waste container.

Sharps Waste Container

The sharps waste container is used only for sharp objects that may puncture or injure someone. These include needles, microscope slides, used ampules, and razors. Never put any sharps in regular waste containers or plastic bags. They need to go in an approved, puncture-resistant container for safety reasons, as shown in Figure 18-4.

Biohazard Waste Container

The biohazard waste container is used only for waste contaminated with blood or body fluids. The following kinds of waste belong in a biohazard waste container:

- soiled dressings and bandages
- soiled examination gloves
- soiled examination table paper
- cotton balls and applications that have been used on the body

Bags in the waste container should not be filled to capacity. When the plastic bag is about two-thirds full, it should be removed from the waste container, with the top edges brought together and secured by tying or with a twist tie. The bag should be placed in a secure, designated area for pick up by an infectious waste service.

Reporting an Exposure

Biohazards, such as viruses, bacteria, fungi, and toxins, present a health risk to humans. These materials are commonly found in many health care settings. If you think you or a patient has been exposed to a biohazard, you'll need to complete an incident report or exposure report in which you describe how the exposure occurred. These reports help health care facilities amend their policies to prevent future exposures.

Exposure to a biohazard must be reported to OSHA if one or more of the following criteria are met. (Employers normally take care of this task.)

- The exposure was work-related and required medical treatment beyond first aid (such as medication or vaccination).
- The employee lost consciousness or had to be medically removed.
- The employee lost days at work or needed to transfer to another job.
- An accident involved an injury from a needle or a sharp object that was contaminated with another person's blood or another possibly infectious material.
- The exposure involved a known case of tuberculosis (TB) and resulted in a positive skin test for TB or a diagnosis of TB by a physician.
- A negative blood test for a contagious disease changed to a positive test after the exposure.

CHECK POINT

7 What is medical asepsis?

8 Identify and briefly explain the highest level of infection control.

Chapter Wrap-Up

Don't forget to visit the Point companion website for additional study resources!

CHAPTER HIGHLIGHTS

- The Occupational Safety and Health Administration and the Centers for Disease Control and Prevention are regulatory agencies that provide safety rules and regulations for health care facilities
- Health care workers should be familiar with safety precautions and preventive actions for a variety of situations, including patient interactions, fires, electrical hazards, oxygen use, chemical hazards, radiation, and workplace violence.
- To avoid confusion or misunderstandings during an emergency, all health care facility employees should know emergency procedures
- Diseases can lead to infection when pathogens, or microorganisms like bacteria or viruses, pass from one person to another. The chain of infection includes a reservoir, an exit from the reservoir, a vehicle of transmission, a portal of entry, and a susceptible host for the pathogen.
- *Standard precautions* are a set of procedures recognized by the CDC to reduce the transmission of microorganisms in any health care setting. Health care workers need to use standard precautions when touching blood, body fluids, damaged skin, or mucous membranes.
- Medical asepsis refers to the measures taken to control and reduce the number of pathogens present on an object or in an area. Cleaning is the lowest level of infection control, followed by disinfection. Sterilization is the highest level.
- Hand washing, wearing personal protective equipment, and properly disposing of hazardous waste are ways that health care professionals can help stop the spread of infectious disease.

REVIEW QUESTIONS

Matching

1. _____ First link in the chain of infection—the person who carries the pathogen
2. _____ Substances that inhibit the growth of microorganisms but don't kill them
3. _____ Third link in the chain of infection—the way by which the pathogen leaves the reservoir and spreads through the environment
4. _____ Bacteria that require oxygen to live and grow
5. _____ Bacteria that can live without oxygen

   a. anaerobic **b.** antiseptics **c.** aerobic **d.** reservoir **e.** vehicle of transmission

Multiple Choice

6. Infection control methods that kill bacteria are referred to as
   a. bacterialotic   **c.** bacteriostatic
   b. bacteriosol   **d.** bactericidal

7. The most significant and most commonly observed infection-causing agent in health care institutions is
   a. bacteria   **c.** fungi
   b. viruses   **d.** mucous

8. The highest level of infection control is
   a. asepsis   **c.** disinfection
   b. cleaning   **d.** sterilization

9. Which of the following is NOT an airborne illness?
   a. common cold
   b. HIV
   c. measles
   d. tuberculosis

10. Special detection badges are used to signal exposure to
    a. airborne diseases
    b. blood-borne diseases
    c. infection
    d. radiation

Completion

11. _____ diseases are spread from person to person when an infected person's blood or certain other body fluids come into contact with the mucous membranes or bloodstream of an uninfected person.

12. _____ diseases are often spread from person to person when an infected person coughs, releasing droplets in the air.

13. The smallest of all microorganisms, _____ are visible only with an electronic microscope.

14. The person infected with a pathogen is also known as the _____ of the disease.

15. When contact is made between the infected reservoir host and a susceptible host, _____ transmission occurs.

Short Answer

16. Briefly explain how health care needs and safety risks change as a person ages. Provide some examples.

   _____

   _____

17. What are some factors that increase the risk of injury in the workplace? What steps can health care workers take to reduce their risk of injury?

   _____

   _____

18. How can fatigue affect a person's safety?

   _____

   _____

19. According to OSHA requirements, what should an emergency action plan contain?

   _____

   _____

20. What are some preventive measures that health care workers can take to reduce the risk of spreading infection?

   _____

   _____

INVESTIGATE IT

1. The Occupational and Safety Health Administration provides not only rules and regulations for the health care industry but also a wealth of information and training resources. Visit the OSHA web site at http://osha.gov, click on the Training tab, and search for available training classes related to safety in the health care industry. Locate and review informational resources related to health care.

2. A great resource for information about safety and infection control is the Centers for Disease Control and Prevention web site at http://cdc.gov. Navigate to the CDC web site and click on the link for Public Health Professionals, found toward the bottom of the page in the "CDC for You" section. If the link is not available, use the following address: http://www.cdc.gov/CDCForYou/public_health_professionals.html. Browse through some of the information provided on this web site, such as the Nationally Notifiable Infectious Diseases page. This page provides annual lists of the infectious diseases health care professionals are asked to report to the CDC.

RECOMMENDED READING

Centers for Disease Control and Prevention. Patient Safety. Available at: http://www.cdc.gov/Features/PatientSafety.

Safe Care Campaign. Preventing Health Care and Community Acquired Infections. Available at: http://www.safecarecampaign.org.

U.S. Department of Health and Human Services. HHS Action Plan to Prevent Healthcare-Associated Infections. Available at: http://www.hhs.gov/ash/initiatives/hai/actionplan/index.html.

U.S. Department of Labor, Occupational Safety and Health Administration. How to Plan for Workplace Emergencies and Evacuations. Available at: http://www.osha.gov/Publications/osha3088.pdf.

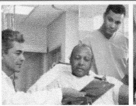
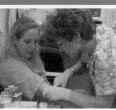
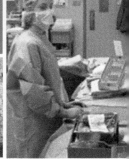

Health Care Economics

19 CHAPTER

CHAPTER OBJECTIVES

After careful study of this chapter, you should be able to:

* Recognize the importance of health care economics.
* Identify the various types of health care institutions.
* Define the most common health care payment methods.

* Characterize the significance of managed care.
* Identify the purpose of cost containment measures.
* Explain the importance of resource management.

KEY TERMS

co-insurance
co-pay
deductible
diagnostic related groups (DRGs)
direct payment
flexible spending account (FSA)
gatekeeper

government institution
government plan
health care cost containment
health maintenance organization (HMO) plan
health savings account (HSA)
in-network provider

managed care
Medicaid
Medicare
out-of-network provider
point-of-service (POS) plan
preferred provider organization (PPO) plan
premium

private insurance
proprietary institution
prospective payment system
resource utilization
TRICARE
utilization review
voluntary nonprofit institution

The costs of health care are a growing concern for all Americans, consumers and providers alike. Rising drug, technology, and professional costs, along with an aging population, are major factors contributing to rising costs.

There's an ongoing discussion in the U.S. about what measures are needed to rein in the cost of health care. Patients, health care providers, insurance carriers, employers, and politicians are all active participants in this continuing debate. Measures designed to lower health care costs, or health care cost containment, aim to create an affordable health care system for all Americans.

All health care professionals should understand the basic economic aspects of health care and how these impact patients. This helps health care providers stay aware of how finances affect each patient's experience. Health care workers can then make conscious and practical decisions that promote affordable, quality care for every patient.

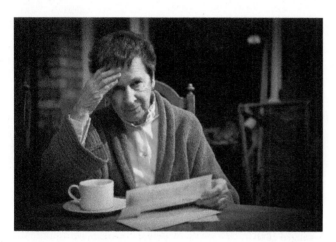

Many Americans experience first-hand the rising cost of health care.

DIFFERENCES AMONG HEALTH CARE INSTITUTIONS

As discussed in Chapter 1, "Today's Health Care System," there are many different kinds of health care facilities—from hospitals to assisted-living facilities to rehabilitation centers. These facilities can be grouped into three categories, depending on how they are funded. The three categories (voluntary nonprofit institutions, proprietary institutions, and government institutions) will be described later in this section.

Regardless of their funding, many of these facilities provide a wide range of community services. These services may include:
- emergency room treatment
- community health education classes and materials
- health screening services
- clinical services
- medical education for physicians, nurses, and other health professionals

ZOOM IN

The Rise in U.S. Health Care Costs

According to the Centers for Medicare and Medicaid Services (CMS), U.S. health care spending for the ten-year period from 2008–2018 is projected to grow by 6.2 percent annually. This is 2.1 percent faster than the country's average annual growth in gross domestic product (GDP)—the value of all goods and services produced in the U.S. each year. By 2018, CMM projects that health care spending will reach $4.4 trillion—roughly 20.3 percent of the nation's GDP.

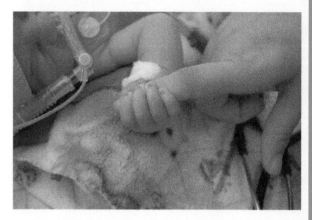

In 2006, the U.S. infant mortality rate was ranked 33rd in the world by the United Nations.

U.S. health care costs are among the highest in the world, averaging just over $2,600 per person in 2006. However, these higher costs don't always mean better care. For example, the United Nations ranked the U.S. infant mortality rate at 33rd in the world in 2006. The infant mortality rate is commonly used to assess a country's overall level of health. The U.S. infant mortality rate was higher than that of many other developed nations with lower health care costs, including the United Kingdom, France, and Germany.

- financial contributions to community organizations
- coordination of events and donations—such as food, clothing, and meeting room space—for community organizations

Voluntary Nonprofit Institutions

A voluntary nonprofit institution is a community facility that receives federal, state, and local tax exemptions in exchange for providing a community benefit, such as services to Medicaid patients and those who are unable to pay. These institutions typically receive other advantages, such as donations that are tax-deductible for donors. To qualify for federal tax-exempt status, an institution must show that it is operated for a charitable purpose. No part of the institution's net earnings may benefit private shareholders or individuals.

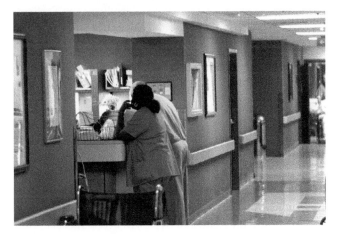

Some hospitals are voluntarily nonprofit, while others are private, for-profit institutions.

Proprietary Institutions

A proprietary institution is a for-profit health care facility usually owned by a corporation. Health care corporations often control a chain of facilities that include hospitals, nursing homes, outpatient facilities, and other health care facilities in several states. These institutions are run just like any other corporation and must pay local, state, and federal taxes.

Government Institutions

A government institution is a public health care facility that receives most of its funding from local, state, or federal sources. These facilities include:

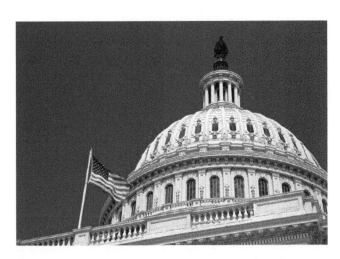

Some health care facilities receive most of their funding from the government.

- Military treatment facilities
- Veterans Affairs (VA) hospitals
- Public or government-funded hospitals
- State mental hospitals
- State rehabilitation facilities

CHECK POINT

1 List major factors causing a rise in health care costs.

2 What are some major differences among the three types of health care institutions (voluntary nonprofit, proprietary, and government) found in the U.S.?

HEALTH CARE PAYMENT METHODS

In the U.S., health care is paid for by one or more of the following three methods:
- private insurance
- direct payment
- government plans

Most patients rely on employer-provided health insurance coverage to pay for most of their medical bills. However, a growing number of Americans pay for their health care costs directly, while others rely on government assistance to cover their medical payments.

Whether health care is provided at a voluntary nonprofit, proprietary, or government institution, the facility must still seek some type of payment for services rendered. Health care professionals should be familiar with the basics of each health care payment method.

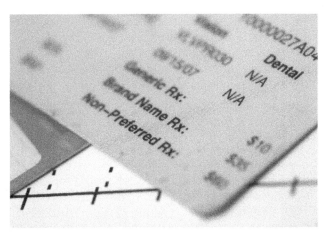

Health care payment methods vary, though many American rely on health insurance rather than direct pay.

Private Insurance

Private insurance in the U.S. is primarily an employment-based health insurance system. This means that most Americans obtain health insurance through their place of employment. Because employers (or other organizations such as unions or professional associations) buy insurance for a group of people, they can get better rates from insurance companies than an individual can. Insurance companies benefit from offering this group insurance because they collect payments from everyone in the group, even though not all people in the group may incur health care expenses covered by the insurance plan.

To lower their own costs, many companies are placing more of the financial responsibility on the insured (the employees covered under the health insurance policy) in the form of premiums, deductibles, co-insurance, and co-pays. A premium is the monthly amount paid to an insurance company for health insurance coverage. In the past, this amount was often paid by employers as part of an employee's benefits package. Today, however, most employees are responsible for paying a portion, and sometimes all, of their monthly premium through pre-tax payroll deductions. In exchange for this monthly premium, the insurance company pays for eligible health care expenses.

A deductible is the money a person pays before the insurance policy provides benefits. For example, if an

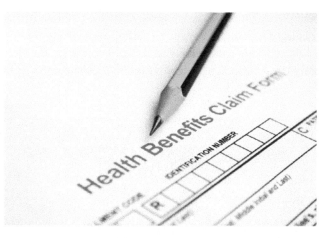

For patients with private health insurance, claims may go directly from the provider to the insurance company.

insured person (the insured) has a $1,500 deductible for hospital or surgical insurance coverage, the insured must pay the hospital for the first $1,500 of hospital costs. After the insured has "met the deductible," the insurance company will pay the remainder of the costs in accordance with the terms of the insurance policy. Deductibles are

A Move Toward Consumer-Driven Health Care

Although employer-provided health insurance has been a tradition in the U.S. health care system, many economists and health care experts agree that Americans can no longer depend on this approach to meet their medical costs. In an attempt to cut costs and boost profits, many companies are paying less of the cost for employee health insurance coverage. Other businesses have eliminated health insurance benefits altogether. These trends, coupled with rising health care costs, are putting a heavy financial burden on American health care consumers.

Many experts believe that giving individuals more control over their own health care funds will reduce health care-related spending. One way to do this is through health-related savings accounts, which provide consumers with the means to control their own health care spending.

A flexible spending account (FSA) is offered through an employer and is usually paired with a traditional health insurance policy. It is the most common medical savings account option. Money is put into an FSA through payroll deductions, before it is taxed. Funds can be withdrawn for qualified medical expenses, such as prescriptions, co-payments, or medical services not covered by the insurance policy. However, employees need to plan carefully before deciding how much money

to put into an FSA, because any funds remaining at the end of the year are forfeited. The plan is called a flexible "spending" account because the money must be spent each year.

A health savings account (HSA) is commonly paired with a high-deductible health insurance plan—a plan that offers low monthly premiums, but requires the insured person to pay a high deductible. An HSA may be offered through an employer's benefits program or arranged by an individual. People pay for their qualified medical care using tax-free HSA dollars, until they meet their deductible. Once the deductible is met, the health insurance company pays for most or all medical costs for the remainder of the year. Unlike an FSA, any funds remaining in an HSA are rolled over at the end of the year. This plan is called a health "savings" account because leftover funds can be saved for future use.

Money accumulated in an HSA can be invested and used to pay for qualified medical expenses later in life. When a person reaches age 65 (or becomes disabled), this money can be withdrawn for any purpose without penalty. Individuals who have high-deductible insurance policies and HSA accounts often are more involved in their health care decisions. They may be less likely to make unnecessary doctor visits or undergo excessive medical tests, because payment for those services comes out of their savings accounts.

one way for an insured person to control health insurance costs—health insurance policies that have high deductibles generally have lower monthly premiums.

Once the insurance plan's deductible has been met, the patient may still have to pay a portion of the medical costs if the insurance plan is a co-insurance plan. **Co-insurance** (which stands for cooperative insurance) is the term used to describe plans that require the insured to share a portion of the costs for health care services (usually 10 to 30 percent). The primary purpose of co-insurance is to lower monthly premiums.

Many health insurance plans also require patients to pay a flat fee, called a co-pay, each time they receive a health care service. For example, an insurance company may require patients to pay $25 for each physician visit or $10 for each prescription filled. Co-pays are paid directly to the service provider, such as a physician or pharmacy.

There are a variety of private insurance plans. Depending on their plan, people often must choose a provider network and other managed care options to reduce their premiums and health care costs. (These different plans are discussed later in this chapter.) Because health insurance plans differ greatly, health care professionals need to know which services a patient is eligible for before the services are provided.

Direct Payment

When patients pay for their health care with their own money, this is known as direct payment. People use direct payment when private insurance doesn't cover all their health care costs, when they don't have private insurance, or when they don't qualify for a government plan.

Some health care economists believe that when people are responsible for paying their own medical expenses, they're more likely to make health care decisions that take costs into account. For example, if people know that they will have to pay all of their primary physician costs

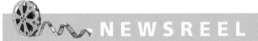

NEWSREEL

Health Care Reform in the U.S.

The U.S. currently spends over $7,000 per person on health care, nearly twice as much as any other industrialized nation. Yet in 2009, nearly 47 million Americans didn't have health care coverage, and millions more had inadequate coverage. When President Obama took office in 2009, he called the U.S. health care system one of the nation's "greatest challenges" and pledged to reduce costs while expanding coverage. Since then, Congress has taken steps toward health care reform, beginning with the passage of the Affordable Care Act that was signed into law on March 23, 2010.

This law puts into place health insurance reforms that are designed to make insurance companies more accountable. The reforms also are intended to lower health care costs, guarantee more health care choices, and improve the quality of health care for all Americans. The Act will not be implemented all at once. Portions of the law have already taken effect, such as giving tax credits to small businesses to help them provide health insurance to their workers. However, other, more significant changes will not be put into effect until 2014 and beyond.

One of those significant changes is the formation of Exchanges—competitive insurance marketplaces where individuals and small businesses can buy affordable, quality health insurance plans. Starting in 2014, if an employer doesn't offer insurance, employees will be able to buy insurance directly through an exchange. Exchanges will offer a choice of health plans that meet certain benefit and cost standards.

As of this writing, one aspect of health care reform that Congress continues to debate is the "public option." While the exact definition changes with each debate, the *public option* is broadly defined as a government-sponsored health insurance plan that would compete with private insurance plans in the exchanges. The goal of a public option is to provide more competition and choice, especially in those places where only a few insurers—and sometimes only one—dominate the marketplace. Individuals and businesses would not be required to purchase or use the public option, but could continue to purchase insurance through private insurers.

In order to compete fairly with private insurers, the public option would be required to operate on a "level playing field" with other insurers. This means that it would have to meet the same benefit requirements and follow the same rules and regulations as private plans. The public option also would have to be financially self-sustaining. In other words, it would not be supported by taxpayer dollars.

Many people wonder how a public option would be able to compete successfully with private insurers. Supporters of the public option believe it would be more cost effective than private plans because it would not have to make a profit, would have lower administrative costs, and would not have excessive executive salaries. These cost savings would make public option insurance plans more affordable for consumers. This, in turn, would pressure private insurers to become more efficient and lower premiums to attract and keep customers.

themselves, they're more likely to shop around and find a care provider who charges less. This "shopping around" by health care consumers creates competition that drives down health care prices.

On the other hand, placing more of the responsibility for health care costs on individuals can have devastating results. According to a study published in the August 2009 issue of *The American Journal of Medicine*, 62 percent of all bankruptcies filed in 2007 were linked to medical costs, and 75 percent of those individuals had health insurance.

Government Plans

A government plan is a health care plan funded by a government agency. Government plans are available for active military personnel and their dependents. Veterans are also covered under government health care plans. However, the two main government-funded health care programs are Medicaid and Medicare, which provide health care coverage to low-income and older Americans. In 2007, nearly 28 percent of Americans were covered under Medicare or Medicaid.

Medicare

The federally-funded health care program for older Americans is called Medicare. This program was established by amendments to the Social Security Act in 1965 to provide health care coverage for Americans aged 65 or older, regardless of income or wealth. Within a decade, nearly all eligible citizens had Medicare insurance for hospital care, extended care, and home health care.

Over the years, several amendments were made to the Medicare program. In 1972, Medicare was expanded to include permanently disabled workers who qualify for Social Security, as well as their dependents.

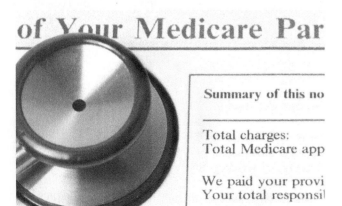

Medicare is a federally-funded health care program established in 1965 to provide coverage for Americans aged 65 or older.

In an effort to control rising health care costs, Medicare converted to a prospective payment system in 1983. This system pays the provider a fixed amount that is based on the medical diagnosis or specific procedure, rather than on the actual cost of hospitalization or care. If the actual cost for care is greater than the fixed amount, the provider must absorb the additional expense.

Most Americans aren't required to pay a monthly premium for Medicare Part A, a program that covers most inpatient care costs. The premium for this program has already been paid through payroll taxes. Medicare Part B, which is voluntary, charges a monthly premium. Medicare Part B covers most outpatient costs, such as physician visits, medications, and home health services. Because Medicare doesn't cover the total cost of all services, people often choose to purchase a supplemental insurance policy offered by a private insurance company.

Two additional plan types are offered to supplement Medicare, both with additional monthly premiums. Medicare Advantage Plans are Medicare-approved plans offered by private insurance companies. Sometimes called Medicare Part C, these plans provide coverage for Part A and Part B services, but generally have extra benefits and lower co-payments than the regular Medicare program. Prescription drug coverage is available under Medicare Part D.

Medicaid

A government program that offers health insurance to many low-income and disabled people is known as Medicaid. Like Medicare, this program was established in 1965 as part of the Social Security Act. Medicaid provides assistance for people of any age who have low incomes. The program also offers health coverage to blind, older, and disabled citizens who receive Supplemental Security Income (SSI) benefits.

Prior to 1996, people who received Aid to Families with Dependent Children (AFDC) were also covered under Medicaid. The AFDC program was replaced by the Personal Responsibility and Work Opportunity Reconciliation Act (PRWORA) of 1996. This act provides states with block grants that can be used to provide cash and services to low-income families with children. Health care coverage under PRWORA depends on individual state regulations.

Government Plans for Military Personnel

Government health care plans are also available for military personnel and their families. The U.S. Department of Defense administers TRICARE, a system that provides medical coverage for active and retired service personnel and their dependents.

New Government Programs

The State Children's Health Insurance Program (SCHIP), established in 1997, provided states with matching funds to help expand health care coverage to over 6 million uninsured children. This program became the center of a national debate when it was set to expire in 2007. Legislation that would have expanded the program by nearly $35 billion passed the House and Senate, but was vetoed by former President George W. Bush. However, in 2009, the Children's Health Insurance Program Reauthorization Act (CHIRPA) was passed by Congress and signed into law by President Barack Obama. CHIRPA added $33 billion in federal funds for children's coverage through 2013.

CHECK POINT

3 How is health care paid for in the U.S.?
4 How do most Americans obtain health insurance?

MANAGED CARE

Health care costs in the U.S. have grown at nearly twice the rate of inflation. The U.S. spends more for health care services than any other industrialized nation, both as a percentage of gross domestic product (GDP) and per person. One response to the rapid escalation in health care costs is managed care, which puts health care providers in the position of managing a patient's use of health care. There are many types of managed care, but most plans fall within one of the following three categories:

- **Health maintenance organization (HMO) plan.** This plan provides coverage only if the care is delivered by a member of its hospital, physician, or pharmacy panel.
- **Preferred provider organization (PPO) plan.** This plan allows patients to receive care from a non-plan provider, but requires them to pay a higher out-of-pocket price if they do so.
- **Point-of-service (POS) plan.** This is a physician-coordinated plan that combines characteristics of both HMO and PPO plans.

All three types of managed care plans have contracts with health care providers, like doctors and hospitals, with predetermined rates for services. Providers in the plan are called in-network providers. Providers who are not in the plan are called out-of-network providers. Typically, the cost of care from an in-network provider is less than from an out-of-network provider.

Managed care plans have a few important characteristics that make them different from other forms of private insurance:
- They consist of a select group of primary care providers.
- They provide a broad range of services, generally emphasizing primary and preventive care.
- They eliminate duplicate services.
- They encourage cost containment.
- They provide a profit for both health care providers and insurance companies.
- They include utilization review.

Utilization review is a process in which an insurer reviews decisions by physicians and other providers about how much care to provide. In many plans, the primary care provider serves as a gatekeeper. A gatekeeper is a physician who not only delivers primary care services but also makes referrals for specialty care.

Managed care plans generally put more emphasis on preventive care. A study published in *The American Journal of Managed Care* found that managed care patients were more likely to receive preventive services, including blood pressure checks, cholesterol screenings, and mammograms.

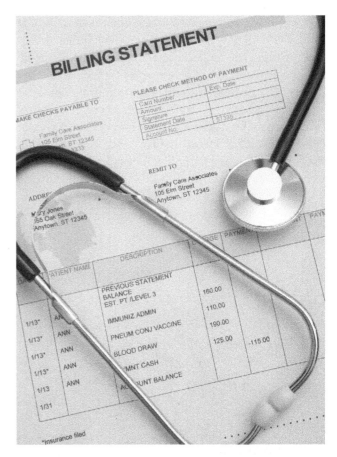

All three types of managed care plans have contracts with health care providers, like doctors and hospitals, with predetermined rates for services.

However, the study also found that health care professionals spent on average two minutes less with managed care patients than other patients. Nonetheless, managed care remains the leading form of health care coverage for Americans, with just over 50 percent of all insurance coverage provided by managed care plans.

✓ **CHECK POINT**

5 What is managed care?

6 How do managed care plans differ from other forms of private insurance?

COST CONTAINMENT MEASURES

A driving force behind the effort to contain health care costs is the diagnostic related group (DRG) classification system, used by Medicare and Medicaid to determine payment for health services. Patients with similar medical conditions are assigned to a DRG. Payment amounts for the DRG are based on the average costs for patients in the group. Patients are assigned to a DRG based on their diagnosis, surgical procedures, age, and other information. Hospitals provide this information on their bills, and Medicare uses this information to decide how much to pay the hospitals. With this type of payment system, patients' diagnoses, treatments, surgical procedures, and any follow-up care are paid in standard fees, regardless of the actual cost of care. For example, all hospitals are paid the same for patients who have their gallbladder removed. The results of DRGs have been dramatic. If the hospital incurs greater cost for the care of the patient than provided by the DRG, the hospital must bear the cost. If the hospital provides care to the patient for less than the DRG payment, the hospital still receives the full payment. As a result, DRGs offer an incentive for hospitals to operate more efficiently.

Since the introduction of DRGs as part of Medicare and Medicaid, other health care plans have begun adopting DRGs as a method of payment. Shorter hospital stays, more outpatient services, and a focus on early intervention and prevention services are just a few of the results of DRGs.

UTILIZING RESOURCES EFFICIENTLY

Health care facilities, both for-profit and nonprofit, are businesses and must operate efficiently to continue to exist. As a result, they expect the health care professionals they employ to make efforts to cut costs. All health care workers need to ask themselves how they can best use health care resources. This is called resource utilization.

One way professionals can better use resources is through conscientious time management. For example, rather than allowing a patient to wait idly in an empty exam room, it is more efficient for a health professional, such as a physician's assistant, to begin a basic patient evaluation before the primary care provider becomes available.

Information technology is another resource utilization tool used by health care professionals. Electronic documentation of patient records and other files not only reduces the amount of time a provider spends searching for and relaying information, but it also reduces the risk of human error. Prescription refills sent electronically save health care workers from having to make multiple phone calls to pharmacies. Test results are analyzed more quickly and accurately by a computer.

✓ **CHECK POINT**

7 What are DRGs? How do they affect the amount paid to providers for health care services?

8 Why should health care workers practice resource utilization?

Chapter Wrap-Up

Don't forget to visit thePoint companion website for additional study resources!

CHAPTER HIGHLIGHTS

- The U.S. health care system is composed of voluntary nonprofit, proprietary, and government institutions. Voluntary nonprofit institutions must provide community benefits in order to retain their nonprofit status and tax exemption. Proprietary institutions are for-profit health care facilities, usually owned by corporations. Government institutions receive most of their funding from local, state, or federal agencies.
- The most common health care payment methods in the U.S. are private insurance, direct payment, and government plans. Most private insurance in the U.S. is obtained through employers. Medicare and Medicaid are the two main government plans.
- Managed care provides coverage for health care through a select group of providers, with predetermined rates for services, and is usually less costly than traditional insurance coverage systems. Health maintenance organizations (HMOs), preferred provider organizations (PPOs), and point-of-service (POS) plans are all managed care plans.
- Diagnostic related groups (DRGs) are a classification system used by Medicare and Medicaid to determine payment for health services based on diagnosis, regardless of the actual cost of care.
- Resource utilization tools that can help health care professionals cut costs include careful time management and information technology.

REVIEW QUESTIONS

Matching

1. _____ Measures to control health care costs and create an affordable health care system.

2. _____ A for-profit health care facility, usually owned by a corporation.

3. _____ A type of insurance plan that requires the insured to share a portion of the costs for health care services even after a deductible has been met.

4. _____ Provides health care coverage to active and retired military personnel and their dependents.

5. _____ A fixed amount that is predetermined by the medical diagnosis or specific procedure.

a. co-insurance   **b.** health care cost containment   **c.** TRICARE   **d.** proprietary institution
e. prospective payment

Multiple Choice

6. Medicare, Medicaid, and TRICARE are all
   - **a.** private insurance plans
   - **b.** managed care plans
   - **c.** government plans
   - **d.** direct payment plans

7. The monthly amount paid to a private insurance company for health insurance coverage.
   - **a.** deductible
   - **b.** premium
   - **c.** co-insurance
   - **d.** co-payment

8. A flat fee paid by the patient directly to the service provider each time the patient receives a health care service.

    a. deductible   **c.** co-insurance

    b. premium   **d.** co-pay

9. The money a patient must pay before an insurance policy provides benefits.

    a. deductible   **c.** co-insurance

    b. premium   **d.** co-pay

10. People use this type of payment when their insurance doesn't cover all health care costs, when they don't have health insurance, or when they don't qualify for a government plan.

    a. prospective payment   **c.** payroll deduction

    b. direct payment   **d.** co-insurance

Completion

11. In return for federal, state, and local tax exemptions, _____ institutions must provide community benefits.

12. The federally-funded health care program designed for older Americans is called _____.

13. The system used by Medicare and Medicaid to determine payment for health services based on diagnosis is the _____ classification system.

14. The government program that provides health insurance for low-income and disabled people is known as _____.

15. A _____ system provides coverage for health care through a select group of providers, with predetermined rates for services.

Short Answer

16. What types of health care providers are in the category of government institutions?

    _____

    _____

17. Why do health care professionals need to understand the economics of health care?

    _____

    _____

18. Name two resource utilization tools that can help health care professionals cut costs.

    _____

    _____

19. Insurance in the U.S. is primarily an employment-based health insurance system. What does this mean?

    _____

    _____

20. Briefly explain the differences between HMO, PPO, and POS managed care plans.

    _____

    _____

INVESTIGATE IT

1. This chapter discussed the benefits of pairing a health savings account (HSA) with a high-deductible health insurance plan. Using the Internet and other available resources, investigate high-deductible health insurance plans that are available for individuals or families. How can an HSA help reduce monthly health insurance premiums? Use search terms such as *health savings account* or *HSA* and *high-deductible health plan* for your Internet search.

2. The Children's Health Insurance Program Reauthorization Act (CHIRPA) passed in early 2009 was hotly debated. Using the Internet and other resources, investigate other prominent pieces of health care legislation. Debate the points made by those in support of each piece of legislation, as well as those opposed. For your Internet search, use the phrase *health care legislation*.

RECOMMENDED READING

Agency for Healthcare Research and Quality. *Questions and Answers About Health Insurance.* Available at http://www.ahrq.gov/consumer/insuranceqa/insuranceqa.pdf.

U.S. Census Bureau. *Income, Poverty, and Health Insurance Coverage in the United States: 2007.* Available at http://www.census.gov/prod/2008pubs/p60-235.pdf.

U.S. Department of Health and Human Services. *Understanding the Affordable Care Act.* Available at http://www.healthcare.gov/law/introduction/index.html.

U.S. Government Accountability Office (2005). *Nonprofit, For-Profit, and Government Hospitals; Uncompensated Care and Other Community Benefits.* Available at: http://www.gao.gov/new.items/d05743t.pdf.

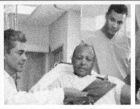
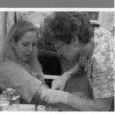
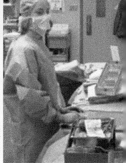
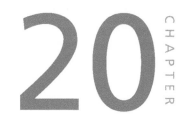

Computers and Other Technology

CHAPTER OBJECTIVES

After careful study of this chapter, you should be able to:

* Discuss the roles of computers and technologies in health care.

* Recognize basic computer hardware components and their operations.

* List general rules for electronic mail, correspondence, research, and document transmission.

* Explain the importance of computer security.

* Identify the most common uses of computers in health care.

* Define key technological advances in health care.

* Describe the trends toward health care globalization and outsourcing.

* Summarize the value of continuing education and self-directed studies to learn about new trends in health care technology.

KEY TERMS

clinical decision support system (CDSS)

computerized physician/ provider order entry system (CPOE)

electronic medical record (EMR)

encryption (en-KRIP-shən)

health informatics

medical coding

medical informatics

patient monitoring systems

reporting systems

telemedicine

tele-monitoring

telesurgery

For nearly all Americans, personal computers are a part of everyday life. Most industries have relied on computers for decades to help them operate more efficiently and cost effectively. Computerization has had the same impact in health care. From administrators to laboratory technicians, virtually all health care workers now rely on computers as key tools.

Technological advances in recent decades have drastically changed how most health care professionals perform their duties. While these developments have enhanced patient care, they also have imposed new responsibilities on providers, who need to have an understanding of computers and related technologies. This chapter discusses the various ways that computers are used throughout the health care system.

COMPUTERS IN HEALTH CARE

Computers were initially used in health care in much the same way as in other businesses, with administrators being among the first to use them. Electronic billing statements and patient invoices greatly reduce the amount of paperwork medical offices have to fill out and track. Medical software programs speed the work by filling out the billing and medical coding entries automatically. Medical coding is the set of symbols and numbers used to communicate specific treatments and diagnoses between a care facility and the payment provider.

Computers were also adopted for scheduling patient appointments and tracking inventory. The switch from written records made scheduling more streamlined and less complicated, minimized human errors and oversights, and allowed for seamless scheduling across multiple offices. Tracking medical supplies and other inventory items through a computer is also more efficient and reliable than doing the same work by hand, which helps the organization reduce costs.

While the administrative advantages gained from using computers are considerable, the benefits of computers in direct patient care are still unfolding. Other areas that benefit from computers include:

- medical data storage and access
- clinical problem solving
- data reporting
- patient monitoring
- home health monitoring
- medication dispensing
- provider and patient communication
- diagnostic testing and imaging
- laboratory testing and data analysis
- education
- time management

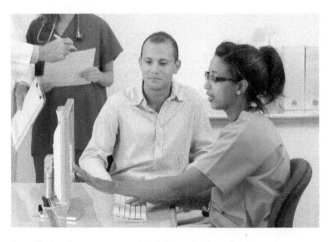

A medical assistant enters patient information into the computer system.

General Uses of Computers

Today, in health care facilities of every type, computers are used for clinical as well as administrative purposes. Among many other uses, computer software analyzes laboratory and radiology reports and helps providers select the best medications to prescribe. Computers promote communication among health care professionals and provide information about new treatment options. Because computers have become so widespread, professionals need a basic understanding of computer hardware components, no matter what area of health care they work in. In addition, they need to understand common office applications, such as email and word processing. They often learn specific applications in on-the-job training once they're employed.

Hardware

The most commonly used computer hardware components are described in Table 20-1. With desktop computers, the CPU, RAM, hard drive, and CD or DVD drive are usually housed in the same unit, although other components are separate. With laptops, the keyboard, touchpad, and monitor are also part of the computer unit.

When computers first came onto the health care scene, most professionals used desktop or laptop machines. While those are still widely used, handheld devices, or personal

Table 20-1 Major Hardware Components of a Computer System

Component	Description
Central processing unit (CPU)	The central processing unit (CPU), or microprocessor, is the circuitry imprinted on a silicon chip that processes information. The CPU consists of a variety of electronic and magnetic cells that read, analyze, and process data. The cells process the operating system and software that instruct the computer to perform operations.
Random access memory (RAM)	This component, in the form of small modules that plug into the main circuit board, stores programs and data temporarily until the information is written for long-term storage on a permanent storage device. If data in RAM is not saved to such a device, it will be lost when the computer is turned off.
Hard drive	A computer's hard drive provides storage for programs, data, and files. The capacity of a hard drive, or the amount of data that it can store, is currently measured in gigabytes and terabytes.
Input devices 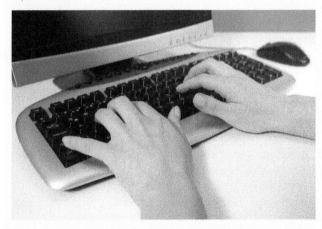 You might not think of it this way, but the keyboard is an "input" device.	The keyboard is the primary means by which information is entered into most computers. Besides the typical letter and number keys, special function keys, such as Alt, Ctrl, Insert, and Esc, provide increased capabilities. Ergonomically designed keyboards, with sculpted or contoured shapes, help avoid injury to the wrists from repetitive stress. Wireless keyboards provide the freedom to use the keyboard away from the computer. Several input devices allow the user to move objects displayed on the screen or to select from menu options. The most common type is a mouse that uses optical sensors to detect the motion of the ball on its underside. Similar devices include the trackball and the touchpad, often found on laptop computers because they are compact. The trackball is like a mouse, with a ball moved with a finger or thumb. A touch pad is a flat surface that works as a mouse, transferring movement from fingers or thumbs to the screen. A pen or stylus is an input device that can be used to make selections on screens or to write directly onto a tablet PC. The handwriting is then converted to typed text. With these devices, health care workers can draw diagrams or make annotations directly within the patient's medical record. A touch screen allows users to touch an area of the computer screen with a finger to choose an object. A special type of monitor is needed for touch screen capabilities. Tablet PCs, iPads, and many smartphones have this sort of screen. On many of these, a touch screen keyboard can be called up for traditional input. A microphone paired with speech recognition software allows health care workers to input information by speaking. Improvements in the accuracy and ease of use of speech recognition software allow a person's voice to do most of the work instead of a keyboard and mouse.

(Continued)

Table 20-1 Major Hardware Components of a Computer System (*continued*)

	Scanner and barcode readers, often associated with retail checkout lanes, are also commonly used in health care. To help reduce medication errors, the Food and Drug Administration (FDA) requires that certain drug and biological product labels contain a linear barcode, which is then scanned, or read, by a barcode reader. Test results and other information also can be added to a patient's medical file using a scanner. Barcode readers and scanners often use Bluetooth®, a technology that provides wireless connections between a variety of devices.
Monitor	The television-like device that displays text and images is a monitor. Monitors come in a variety of sizes and degrees of quality. Flat-panel liquid crystal display (LCD) monitors are popular and provide some protection from unauthorized viewing because of limited viewing angles.
Printer	Printers use various technologies, have a wide range of speeds, and print in either black only or color. Health care workers use printers to generate invoices and bills, correspondence, schedules, laboratory orders and results, forms for insurance companies, and prescriptions.
Secondary storage systems	Nearly all computers have multiple methods for saving data. A compact disk (CD) or digital video disk (DVD) contains digitally encoded data. Computer programs often come on these disks before they are installed on the computer. A disk is typically inserted into a disk drive built into the computer, which reads the information. A memory stick is a removable memory card that comes in various shapes and sizes. It is used to transfer information from a device, such as a camera, to a computer. A flash drive is a portable storage device that plugs directly into a computer's universal serial bus (USB) port, allowing the user to carry data easily from one computer to another. An external hard drive is a portable storage device that is often used to create a file backup from a computer's hard drive. This device can then be stored in a safe location (preferably in a separate place from the original files) to allow data retrieval in case the original hard drive is damaged or destroyed. Online and centralized network storage provide larger facilities with expanded storage space for a large number of medical records.

digital assistants (PDAs), have also become an extremely useful tool in the health care setting. At a minimum, these devices come loaded with the following software:

• address book
• calendar
• email
• word processing

Health care providers can send information back and forth between a PDA and a desktop computer via the Internet, a direct connection, or Bluetooth. PDA software allows health care providers to perform several important tasks, including:

• accessing patients' charts
• using pharmacy and formulary dosing tools
• accessing Micromedex (a drug information/toxicology database)
• downloading and viewing health books and journals
• viewing procedures that they may not perform routinely

- setting up virtual offices
- viewing financial information

PDAs can also be used in place of bedside charts, so that patient charts can't be viewed by visitors or unauthorized personnel. Patients themselves can use handheld devices to monitor their own vital signs or test for blood sugar levels.

Electronic Mail

Commonly called email, electronic mail allows users to send and receive messages and transmit computer files. Email provides many benefits to the health care system. It enhances communication, promotes teamwork, eliminates phone tag, and provides written documentation of messages. However, professionals must take reasonable steps to ensure compliance with the HIPAA Privacy Rule when handling emails containing patient information. (See Chapter 11, "Law, Ethics, and Professionalism in Health Care," for more information on HIPAA.)

All professionals, regardless of their field, should keep these general rules in mind when using email:

- An office email address should only be used to send work-related messages. An office email account shouldn't be used to send personal messages.
- Chain letters or other inappropriate emails should never be forwarded from an office email account.
- All email messages should be professional. A good rule of thumb is not to write anything you wouldn't want your mother or boss to read.
- An email's encryption feature should always remain active to ensure that all messages are scrambled and can't be read by anyone other than the intended recipient.

Word Processing

Word processing refers to the electronic creation and editing of documents on a computer. As with other written communications, health care professionals should ensure that their electronically generated messages are clear and accurate. Whether you are corresponding with patients or recording test results, your communications should always be professional.

Proper spelling is extremely important. One wrong or incorrectly placed letter could alter the entire meaning of a medical term. Inaccurate information in a document can lead to the injury of a patient, the prospect of legal action, and possible harm to the health care practice. For assistance with terminology, medical dictionary software can be added to most word processing programs. This helps ensure accuracy by checking for the correct spelling and use of common medical terms and abbreviations. A word of caution: Verify that the spellchecker's suggested spelling of the word is correct. The spelling of one medical term is often only one or two letters different from another term.

Any patient information contained in a medical document falls within the guidelines of the HIPAA Privacy Rule governing medical correspondence. (See Chapter 11 for more information on HIPAA.) Documents can be attached to an email or printed out to be delivered. Either way, steps should be taken to ensure that all communications are kept secure.

Research

The Internet contains an abundance of health-related information. To ensure that the information is legitimate and valid, only web sites from trusted sources should be used when researching online. The National Library of Medicine, presented by the U.S. National Institutes of Health, offers current health information, library catalog services, research and technology resources, training and outreach assistance, and much more.

Several medical search engines are also available through the Internet. A search engine allows users to find sites that contain relevant information. While there are a number of general search engines, such as Google, Yahoo, and Dogpile, health care search engines are preferable for professional needs because they are more likely to return web sites containing the most relevant information. PubMed and OmniMedicalSearch are examples of two such medical search engines.

After accessing a reliable search engine, users enter keywords relating to the desired subject in the site's search box. These keywords should be focused to limit the number of responses, or hits, the user receives. For example, when searching for information about the signs

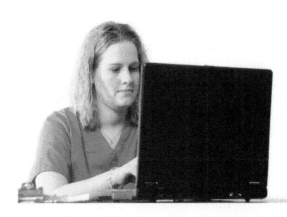

Health professionals often use computers to search the internet.

ZOOM IN

Guidelines for Selecting Safe Web Sites

Health care professionals should remember these points when searching the Internet for health-related information:

- Use web sites run by trusted sources, such as those with ".gov," ".edu," or ".org" in the address. These sites, set up by government agencies, universities, hospitals, or other organizations like the American Heart Association, will have reliable information.
- Beware of sites using words and phrases like *breakthrough*, *medical miracle*, and *secret formula*.
- Avoid sites that advertise that they have cured a disease.
- Use caution when the phrase *ancient remedy* is found.
- Be cautious with information from web sites that contain advertising or those that are operated by businesses, which typically have ".com" in their address. While some ".com" sites contain legitimate information, others are guided by purely commercial interests.

and symptoms of juvenile diabetes, the words *"juvenile diabetes," signs*, and *symptoms* may be entered, with a space between each word. This will result in web sites that contain information with all four search words. Placing the words *juvenile* and *diabetes* in quotes limits search results to sites that refer specifically to that disease. Otherwise, the search might yield documents about gestational diabetes or type 2 diabetes that also contain the word *juvenile* somewhere in the text.

Document Transmission

Computers provide a wealth of resources, services, and support for busy health care professionals. From medical research to patient records, providers count on technology to share sensitive medical information rapidly and securely. The Internet provides a safe avenue for sending and receiving this information when general safety guidelines are followed.

It is extremely important to use only secure sites when transferring patient information electronically. Be sure to use the security method employed at your facility to ensure that the information is read only by the intended recipient.

Computer Security

Computers are a must in all physicians' offices. These machines make many elements of health care more

streamlined and effective. However, their use can also lead more easily to the invasion of patients' privacy, to unethical behavior, and even to loss of information. To avoid these problems, health care professionals should keep these points in mind:

- Never give passwords or access codes to anyone, including another health care professional. Health care workers often must enter unique passwords or codes to verify that they have the right to access patient data, such as health records and laboratory reports. Protecting these identifying codes helps preserve privacy of information.
- Do not leave a computer terminal unattended after having logged on. Always ensure that you are logged off and that any patient information is closed before leaving a computer terminal.
- Never create, change, or delete records unless given specific authority to do so.
- Regularly back up files containing records. If part of a record is inadvertently deleted, the information can be restored from backup copies. Follow the protocol used at your institution.
- Internet access at the office should be used only for work-related tasks. It is inappropriate to surf the Internet for personal reasons while at work.

ZOOM IN

Guidelines for Creating and Using Passwords

Most health care practices establish written policies for the assignment and use of passwords in order to protect both patient and practice information. Those policies should be adhered to at all times. Even if a practice does not have a formal password policy, health care professionals can ensure that passwords are secure by following these basic guidelines:

- Passwords should be unique and include both letters and numbers.
- Initials, birthdates, and phone numbers should never be used as passwords.
- System-wide passwords that allow computer access should be changed as soon as an employee leaves a practice.
- Professionals should never, under any circumstances, share their passwords with colleagues.
- Written notes containing passwords shouldn't be taped to computer monitors or left lying around on desktops.
- Additional password verification should be established for certain secure sites, such as those with access to laboratory test results.

• Test results should only be accessed for patients currently being treated by the health care professional's practice. It is illegal and unethical to obtain test results for other patients.

The increasing use of computerized patient information systems to store and analyze patient data has prompted most health care practices to develop policies and procedures that ensure the privacy and confidentiality of patient information. These policies should specify what types of patient information can be retrieved, by whom, and for what purpose. Patient consent is necessary for the use and release of any information that can be linked to the patient.

Uses of Computers in Health Care

Health care professionals must collect data to ensure the delivery of appropriate patient care. Hospitals, insurers, and regional health care alliances are promoting the electronic collection and management of health-related information. Computers are essential to this process, which improves the quality, safety, efficiency, and cost effectiveness of health care.

Health Informatics

Health care professionals regularly share files containing information vital to patient care, such as medical records, test results, prescription history, billing details, and health insurance coverage. The area of health informatics, sometimes called medical informatics, integrates information technology and health care to optimize the process used to obtain, store, and use health care information for patient care and public health purposes. Computers are the gateway by which this information is passed quickly, efficiently, and—as long as proper measures are taken—securely.

With computer-based records, health data can be easily distributed to other systems, as long as each system stores records in the same standard format. This ease of sharing allows health care professionals to evaluate an individual patient's progress, as well as the progress of groups of patients with similar diagnoses. The collection and analysis of this information leads to better and more efficient health care delivery.

Electronic Medical Record

The collection, analysis, and sharing of a patient's information are all made possible because of the electronic medical

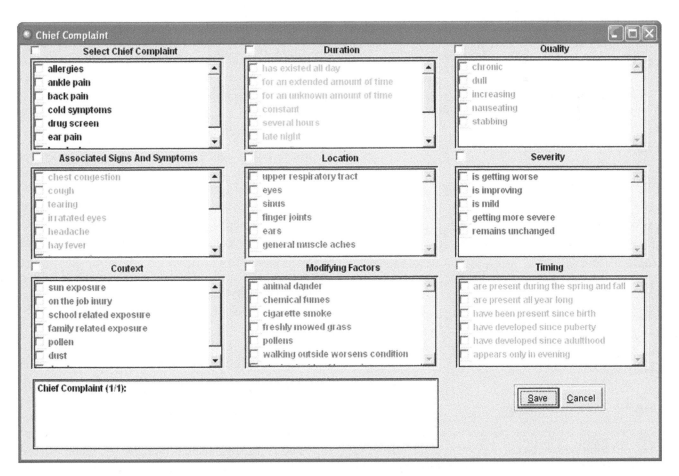

Example of electronic medical record input screen.

record (EMR), also known as the electronic health record, which contains several kinds of patient health information gathered from different sources:

● patient identification data
● clinic and inpatient notes
● preventive care delivery
● laboratory data
● radiology data
● pharmacy data
● surgical procedures performed
● emergency department visits
● billing information

Clinical Decision Support System (CDSS)

Information contained in an EMR is easily retrieved and analyzed by a computerized expert system. An expert system is a customized program that assists health care professionals in making diagnosis and treatment determinations. One such system, a clinical decision support system (CDSS), provides administrative, clinical, cost control, and decision support for several activities in a health care institution, including:

● promoting use of best practices
● preventive care
● diagnosis and treatment plans
● condition-specific guidelines
● monitoring of medication orders
● procedure authorization
● avoidance of duplicate or unnecessary tests
● ensuring patients stay on therapy protocols
● referrals and referral follow-up
● coding and documentation
● population-based management

Computerized Physician Order Entry System (CPOE)

Although CDSSs can be used independently, they're often integrated with another type of computer system, a computerized physician/provider order entry system (CPOE). This system allows certain licensed health care professionals (physicians, nurse practitioners, and physician assistants) to enter medical orders. The fact that licensed professionals input the orders directly, rather than leaving the work to someone else, reduces the possibility of an error occurring.

Health Care Education

Computers and technology are also extremely important tools for educating health care professionals and patients. A wealth of information, such as signs and symptoms, disease descriptions, recent research studies, and government health regulations, is readily available online or through software applications and databases. This information is accessed quickly and easily through the use of handheld devices and computers. However, it is very important that patients and health care workers make sure they're relying on legitimate and trusted sources when obtaining medical information.

Reporting Systems

Health care reporting systems collect various types of data pertaining to patient care. This data can then be shared with government agencies for regulatory compliance purposes and with other providers. Information obtained through a health care reporting system can also be used to assist in treating patients. For example, if a hospital admits a patient with symptoms of a rare disease, this information can be shared with other health care facilities through a reporting system. If other facilities admit patients with similar symptoms, the number of reports could indicate an outbreak. Without the reporting system information, each case might be viewed as an isolated instance. In situations like this, complete, accurate, and up-to-date medical data becomes a powerful tool to help diagnose, treat, and stop the spread of disease.

Medical facilities also use reporting systems to capture and track information such as medication errors, patient accidents or falls, patient misidentification, and post-surgical infections. These systems play a large role in health care quality improvement initiatives, in which data are analyzed to find areas where patient care can be improved.

Patient Monitoring

Health care providers use patient monitoring systems to keep a constant electronic watch over a patient's physical status and vital signs. The monitors for several patients are then linked to a central location, such as a nurses' station, where they're constantly monitored.

Computer-controlled medication dispensing systems use technology to give patients predetermined amounts of medication at proper intervals. These systems may have a patient control that allows the patient to choose when medication is dispensed, but there are limits set within the machine.

Patient home health monitoring, often called telemonitoring, collects data on patients' health from their homes. These systems are generally programmed to ask patients brief questions about their health status. The systems can also be set to display medication reminders. Wireless devices can monitor a patient's blood pressure, pulse rate, oxygen intake, weight, and blood glucose levels. Once the data is collected, it is transferred over a

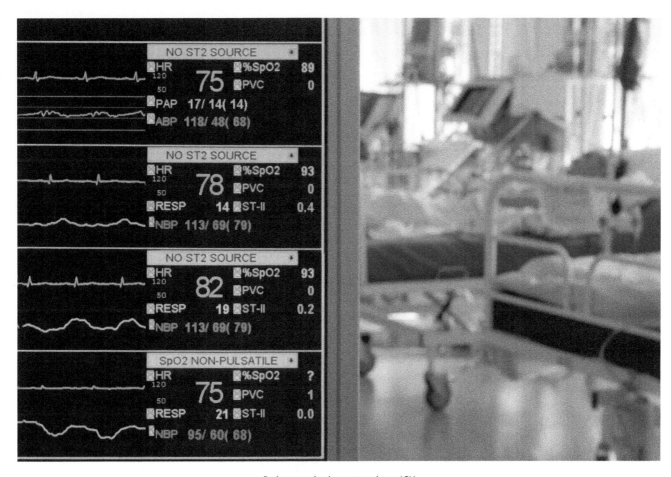

Patient monitoring system in an ICU.

phone line or Internet connection to a secure web site or directly to a provider's office. Health care workers can also use phone systems to verify that a patient's pacemaker is functioning correctly. These systems are especially useful for monitoring disabled or older patients who are unable to manage their own conditions.

Diagnostics

Several therapies, diagnostic procedures, and imaging systems also use computer technology. In electroconvulsion therapy (ECT), electronic signals are sent through a portion of the brain to control depression and seizures. In computerized tomography scan (CT scan), where an X-ray technician produces images of a patient's body, computers are vital to performing the scans and analyzing the data. Other diagnostic procedures also employ computer technology, including magnetic resonance imaging (MRI), positron emission tomography scan (PET scan), and ultrasound.

Laboratory Tests and Data Analysis

Today, many routine laboratory tests are performed using computers. For example, the results of a complete blood count (CBC) are determined quickly through computer analysis of a patient's blood sample. Computers are also used for other types of health data analysis, such as analysis of bodily fluids to reveal the level of electrolytes in a patient's system.

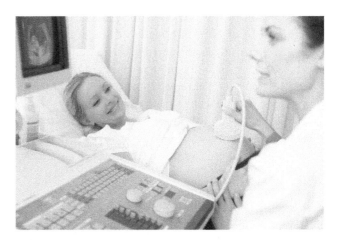

Diagnostic imaging is one example of computer use in health care. As the technologist performs the ultrasound, the images appear on a computer monitor.

1 What benefits have computers and technology brought to health care?

2 In addition to administration, what areas of health care have been improved by technological advances?

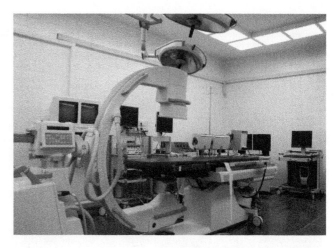

Operating rooms today are filled with sophisticated computer equipment.

OTHER TECHNOLOGY IN HEALTH CARE

Health care continues to evolve as technology advances. Computerized health records, increased managed care, and streamlined diagnostic plans all rely on computers to store and access information. Without a doubt, technology will continue to impact the future of medical research, development, diagnosis, treatment, and management.

Key Technological Advances

Technological advances continue to save lives, extend patient life spans, and enhance quality of life. Digital imaging technology has improved the quality of X rays, mammograms, and other diagnostic procedures. These improvements have led to more precise and earlier disease detection and treatment.

Improvements in noninvasive and robotic surgical skills have led to more widespread use of these techniques. These techniques reduce recovery time and lower infection rates compared to traditional surgery. For example, non-invasive extracorporeal shock wave lithotripsy (ESWL) uses shock waves to shatter kidney stones into smaller pieces that can travel through the urinary tract more easily. Robotic-assisted radical prostatectomy, a surgery that treats prostate cancer, results in reduced blood loss, less pain, and shorter hospital stays compared to traditional methods.

Telemedicine is a branch of medicine that involves the transfer of medical information through interactive visual media to enable consultation among physicians at a distance. It can include remote medical exams or procedures. Telesurgery combines multimedia, telecommunications, and robotic technologies to provide surgical care from a distance. With this type of technology, less experienced surgeons in remote areas of the world can receive training in advanced surgical techniques from experts located hundreds or thousands of miles away.

Scientific progress in genetic testing and mapping is dramatically reducing the cost of this type of analysis. Researchers are working on the development of a computer chip that could allow doctors to tailor treatment to a patient's unique genetic makeup. Scientists believe this technology also will lead to the mapping of genes linked to specific diseases and more efficient identification of new viruses and disease outbreaks.

Researchers in the area of rehabilitation are working to develop an interface between brain and machine that would allow the brain to control prosthetic limbs. Engineers are creating robotic hands with the ability to instantly decode and interpret brain signals. If these advances are achieved, patients with prosthetic limbs would have the ability to move more naturally.

Globalization and Outsourcing of Health Care

A somewhat controversial consequence of the spread of new technologies in health care is a movement toward the outsourcing of health care-related jobs. Modern communication and transmission technology means that billing, coding, transcription, and other data-related tasks are just as easily, and more cost effectively, performed by someone living in another country. With an increased emphasis on cost reduction in recent years, many in the health care industry are sending these tasks overseas, despite the loss of jobs in the U.S.

3 How have technological advances improved overall patient care?

4 How is tele-surgery used to benefit patients?

STAYING CURRENT IN TECHNOLOGY

With such emphasis on technological advances, continuing education is a necessity for all health care professionals. A person must be properly trained in order to get the maximum benefit from any computer or software package. Because technology and software continually change and evolve, health care professionals must commit to life-long learning to stay current with advances.

Continuing Education Courses

Continuing education courses are required for recertification in many health care careers, but they can also help professionals stay up to date with new technologies. Classes, seminars, and other educational opportunities offered through professional organizations are great resources for learning about technological trends. Many organizations also offer online learning resources or professional publications that feature articles on the latest research studies and developments in health care.

Employers often provide in-service educational opportunities to their employees. These types of opportunities are beneficial to employees not only because of the training received, but also because they are free and typically take place during the employee's normal work schedule.

Health care professionals also should check with local higher education institutions to learn about seminars or other continuing education opportunities they may offer.

By attending a professional conference or a health care-related lecture, professionals can gather valuable information about the newest technologies.

Self-Directed Study

Most software applications come packaged with a tutorial. This is a short on-screen course on how to use the software. A user's manual is also a standard feature of most software programs although more and more software packages are providing such information only online. Help screens in the software also give support for many questions and issues. Professional journals often provide online resources for health care professionals. It is important for health care providers to search for and read articles related to the latest technological trends in health care.

CHECK POINT

5 Why is continuing education about technology so important for health care professionals?

6 By what methods can health care professionals keep up with new technologies in their areas?

Chapter Wrap-Up

Don't forget to visit thePoint companion website for additional study resources!

CHAPTER HIGHLIGHTS

- Computers are used to improve the quality and effectiveness of patient care, reduce errors, and lower costs.
- An abundance of health-related information is found on the Internet, but only trusted web sites should be used.
- Established policies for the assignment and use of passwords should be adhered to at all times to keep confidential health care information secure.
- The area of health or medical informatics integrates information technology and health care to optimize the processes used to obtain, store, and use health care information for patient care and public health.
- Health care organizations use systems such as electronic medical records (EMR), clinical decision support systems (CDSS), and computerized physician/provider order entry systems (CPOE) to store patient health information. These systems also provide administrative, clinical, cost control, and decision support and allow health care professionals to enter medical orders electronically.
- Computer technology has made possible the use of reporting systems, monitoring systems, and diagnostic and imaging systems in health care.
- Because of technology, many data-related health care tasks are just as easily, and more cost effectively, performed by people living in other countries, so many of these tasks are being outsourced.

REVIEW QUESTIONS

Matching

1. _____ Set of symbols and numbers used to communicate specific treatments and diagnoses between a care facility and a payment provider

2. _____ Type of program used to locate information on the Internet

3. _____ Identifiers added to drug labels to reduce medication errors

4. _____ Handheld device that has simple computer functions but can also provide access to health data

5. _____ Identifier that permits access to secure health information

   a. search engine   **b.** PDA   **c.** medical coding   **d.** password   **e.** barcodes

Multiple Choice

6. What is the name for the computerized health information system health care professionals use to monitor referrals, treatment plans, and tests?
   - **a.** electronic health record
   - **b.** electronic medical record
   - **c.** clinical decision support system
   - **d.** computerized physician order entry system

7. Which of the following is the main reason for outsourcing health care jobs?
   - **a.** to take advantage of better computer systems
   - **b.** to access better trained health care professionals
   - **c.** to replace lost workers at home
   - **d.** to control costs

8. Which of the following is NOT a potential danger of a computerized health information system?

    a. potential for invasion of patients' privacy
    b. quick access to up-to-date information
    c. possibility of unethical behavior
    d. chance of information loss

9. This monitoring system collects and reports data about patients' health from their homes.
    a. DSL monitoring   **c.** tele-monitoring
    b. tele-commuting   **d.** digital monitoring

10. Which of the following is *least* likely to indicate a web site that contains reliable health information for professional uses?
    a. .com   **c.** .gov
    b. .edu   **d.** .org

Completion

11. For assistance with terminology, _____ can be added to most word processing programs.

12. An email's _____ feature should always remain active, to ensure that all messages are scrambled and can't be read by anyone other than the intended recipient.

13. A health care _____ is more likely to return web sites containing the most relevant health information.

14. Thanks to advances in _____ patient life spans are extended, lives are saved, and the overall quality of life is enhanced.

Short Answer

15. Briefly describe a health care-related situation in which a medical reporting system would prove beneficial.

_____

_____

16. What is tele surgical monitoring?

_____

_____

17. How has the use of computers in health care paralleled the use of computers in the world in general?

_____

_____

18. What are computer-controlled medication dispensing systems, and how do they work?

_____

_____

19. What type of information may be contained in an electronic medical record (EMR)?

_____

_____

INVESTIGATE IT

1. Health care-related computer systems are among the most rapidly growing technologies. Using the Internet and other available resources, learn more about health care-related computer systems and how they might help improve both provider and patient care experiences. Also consider the potential drawbacks of these systems. One web site that offers a wealth of information in this area is http://www.microsoft.com/industry/healthcare/default.mspx.

2. Quick and effective Internet searches can yield valuable information. When searching for web sites that contain accurate health-related information, a medical search engine should be used. Use the search term *medical search engines* to find and learn about the most popular medical search engines. Practice searching for health-related topics using one or two of these specialized search engines and a general search engine. How do the results, or hits, returned by a medical search engine compare to the hits returned by a general search engine?

RECOMMENDED READING

Hamal, A.K.; Menon, M. Henry Ford Health Institute. *Laparoscopy, Robot, Telesurgery and Urology: Future Perspective*. Available at http://jpgmonline.com/article.asp?issn=0022-3859;year=2002; volume=48;issue=1;spage=39;epage=41;aulast=Hemal.

Hewlett Packard. *The Case for the Tablet PC in Health Care*. Available at http://www.hp.com/sbso/solutions/healthcare/hp_tablet_whitepaper.pdf.

Home Healthcare Hospice and Community Services. *Home Telemonitoring*. Available at http://www.hcsservices.org/services/vna/home_telemonitoring.php.

McGee, Marianne Kolbasuk. Information Week. *Wal-Mart Rolls Out E-Health Records To All Employees*. Available at http://www.informationweek.com/news/software/database/showArticle.jhtml;jsessionid=QM2XHC1RV5Q0AQSNDLPSKH0CJUNN2JVN?articleID=210605059.

Nemko, Marty. U.S. News and World Report. *Ahead of the Curve: Health Informatics Specialist*. Available at http://www.usnews.com/articles/business/best-careers/2008/12/11/ahead-of-the-curve-health-informatics-specialist-2009.html.

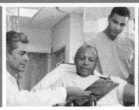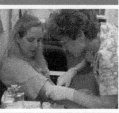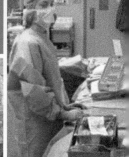

Advocacy

21 CHAPTER

CHAPTER OBJECTIVES

At the end of this chapter, the student should be able to:

* Define patient advocacy, workplace advocacy, and professional advocacy.
* Identify opportunities to advocate for patients.
* Understand the nursing profession's obligation to advocate.
* Describe actions the nurse could take in advocating for patients.

* Give an example of how the nursing profession advocates for patients.
* Give examples of how the nursing profession advocates for its workplace environment.

KEY TERMS

Advocacy for patients	Autonomy	Decision-making capacity	Moral courage
Advocacy for the profession	Code of ethics	Empowerment	Moral distress
	Competency	Incompetent	Therapeutic relationships

Members of every health care profession believe they have a responsibility to act as a patient advocate. No single profession "owns" the role as advocate, but nursing has promoted this role as integral to good nursing care. What does it mean to be a patient advocate? This chapter focuses on the nurse's role as patient advocate, as well as the broader concept of advocacy in nursing. Advocacy is one of the four common ethical themes in nursing practice that will be expanded on in each of the chapters of Unit 3: Clinical Ethical Issues.

WHAT IS ADVOCACY?

Imagine that you travel to a foreign land where you do not know the culture or language. How do you get your needs met? You can attempt to communicate through gestures or using pictures, but you cannot be sure that you are being understood. It would certainly help if you had an advocate, someone who knows the country's culture, language, and the system in which you are attempting to interact. The health care system is analogous to a foreign land for many patients. This language is full of jargon, abbreviations, and colloquialisms. Most health care institutions have a hierarchy, policies, procedures, standards, routines, and rituals that seem mysterious to patients, families, visitors, and students learning to be health care professionals. As nursing students become familiar with health systems, they become insiders. As insiders, health care professionals have an obligation to assist patients to navigate the health care system to get their needs met. However, the nursing student first needs to learn the role of the professional nurse, how the nursing process is enacted, and how nursing care is delivered in the specific health care setting.

Along with understanding the disease process, diagnostic procedures, treatments, symptom management, and psychosocial implications of health promotion, maintenance, and restoration, nurses need to learn the system in which patient care occurs. In some systems, such as the ambulatory setting, healthy individuals seek preventative activities like screening tests. Patients with symptoms seek diagnostic tests, and diagnosed patients seek treatment. As part of the nursing process, the nurse learns the reason for and the patient's expectations of the visit. Nursing assessment begins at the first interaction with the patient and continues through the entire patient contact period. Patient education, clarification, and reinforcement of information occur, along with an assessment of the patient's understanding. A patient may be prepared for an examination or educated on medication administration. The nurse may help a patient to understand information given by another professional. In this setting, the nurse acts an advocate by helping meet the patient's expectations of this outpatient visit. The word advocacy comes from Latin *advocare*, meaning "to call to one's aid." To advocate on behalf of a patient is to come to his or her aid or to give voice to his or her concerns. Providing information to the patient and keeping him or her informed aids the patient in the encounter with the health care system.

There are numerous mentions of advocacy in the American Nurses Association (ANA) (2001) Code of Ethics for Nurses With Interpretive Statements. In the Canadian Nurses Association (CNA) (2002) Code of Ethics for Registered Nurses, eight values are described that are key to nursing practice. To effectuate many of those values, the nurse must advocate for the patient. In both codes, the nurse is expected to advocate for the rights of patients for safe, humane, and culturally competent nursing care. Advocacy in this example might mean that the nurse should contact a medical translator for a patient whose first language is not English. The ANA code also uses the term "advocates" in discussing the nurse's duty to protect the patient's privacy, ensure that the patient and important others have a voice in decision-making, and protect the patient from incompetent, unethical, illegal, or impaired practice of any health care provider.

Advocating for institutional change on behalf of all patients is also included in the ANA code. The Canadian code beckons nurses to "advocate for practice environments that have the organizational structures and resources necessary to ensure safety, support and respect for all persons in the work setting" (CNA, 2002, p. 8).

THE CALL TO ADVOCACY

Myra Levine (1989), one of the earliest nurse ethicists, described every interaction between a nurse and patient as a moral interaction. Meeting a patient, taking a history, being present during the examination, and performing an examination are profoundly moral interactions and need to be conducted with respect and competency. Patients often are vulnerable and depend on health care providers to instruct them on what to expect, explain findings, explain options, and give advice, when appropriate. Although there is a hierarchy of professionals in terms of power and authority in the health care setting, the nurse has power over the patient in many encounters because of the special knowledge the nurse has. The nurse is usually in control of the situation, with patients being told where to go and what to do. The nurse often has information that the patient does not have, such as how to navigate the health care system. Even the most sophisticated patients may not know the particular nuances of the health care setting that can affect their care. The nurse can "run interference" for the patient by educating him or her and removing barriers so the patient can achieve the desired goals.

Whose Goals to Promote?

The goals might be negotiated between the patient and health care provider or might be articulated by the patient but not endorsed by the health care team. Conflict can occur if the goals of the patient and the professionals are not the same and are even incompatible. Does the nurse advocate for what the patient wants against the nurse's better judgment? For example, a patient with breast cancer wants to use only homeopathy and diet to combat the cancer. Her oncologist recommends a lumpectomy, radiation treatments, and oral chemotherapy. Does the nurse advocate for the patient by supporting her decision to forgo traditional treatment or does he or she try to educate the patient to accept the traditional treatment? If the patient has not discussed her preferences with the oncologist, the nurse can facilitate a discussion between them. In addition, the nurse can assist the patient to obtain information about the pros and cons of the various types of treatment the patient is considering. While respecting the patient's right to make a decision consistent with her values, the health care team is also expected to offer their recommendations based on their experiences and knowledge of the state-of-the-art techniques relating to the particular condition. Ultimately the decision is the patient's.

THE STRENGTH TO ADVOCATE

Nurses with less experience may hesitate to assume an advocacy role. Working in health care requires humility in light of the growing amount of medical information. A nurse may feel that he or she does not know enough to question a physician or fellow nurse. It is very appropriate for the nurse to ask for information about a decision or course of action. The nurse may also do some research through the library, Internet, or personal contacts. Knowing standards of care, policies and procedures, and professional position or policy statements are helpful in advocating. Knowing the patient's wishes and communicating with the patient, family (if appropriate), and the health care team are also very helpful in advocating. A nurse can advocate for the patient by providing the patient with necessary information or facilitating decision-making by talking with the patient. Allowing the patient to speculate, think out loud, and use the nurse as a sounding board is part of the therapeutic relationship. As nurses experience more opportunities to advocate, they will become more comfortable with the role.

At a minimum, nurses advocate for patients by avoiding preventable harms. The nurse can do this in several ways: maintaining competence in the area of nursing in which he or she practices, applying critical thinking skills when implementing the treatment plan, and acting to promote the health and safety of patients while they are in his or her care. Individual acts of the nurse, as well as participation in groups designed to avert iatrogenic illnesses and injuries (those caused by the medical treatment or health care staff) for the patient population, are acts of advocacy. For example, as a nurse is reviewing newly written physician orders, she notices that the new medication may interact with a current medication the patient is receiving. Instead of assuming that the physician was aware of all the medications taken by the patient or that the pharmacy will identify the potential drug interaction as the order is filled, the nurse contacts the physician to discuss the order. Doing so prevents a potential harm to the patient. In another example, the nurses on a particular unit observe that there has been an increase in patient falls. The nurses on that unit come together to examine the root cause for the falls and devise a plan to reduce their incidence. Advocacy, based on the ethical principles of autonomy of the patient, beneficence, and non-maleficence, is an ethical obligation of the nurse.

CASE STUDY 21-1

Nurse Anchor is assigned to a 73-year-old woman with a wound on her foot. Dressing changes have been very uncomfortable, and Nurse Anchor suggests that he give the patient pain medication prior to changing the dressing. The surgeon, Dr. Carney, arrives on the unit earlier than expected and begins to change the dressing. Nurse Anchor comes into the room and asks Dr. Carney to wait until he can medicate the patient. The surgeon says to the patient, "You do not mind if I get this over with, do you? I'll hurry so it will not hurt as much." The patient hesitates for a moment, and says, "I suppose so." How can the nurse advocate for this patient?

Possible response. Nurse Anchor says to his patient, "If you want, I can give you your pain medication now like we discussed and we can ask Dr. Carney to return in 15 minutes. Would you prefer that?" Nurse Anchor realizes that many patients, especially elderly patients, do not question physician authority, and the nurse believes the patient would prefer not to experience pain during the dressing change. The nurse said what he thought the patient wanted to say; he "gave her a voice."

CASE STUDY 21-2

During her pediatric rotation, Student Nurse Baker is with a 3-year-old boy in the playroom. The policy on the pediatric unit is that all procedures are performed in the procedure room and not in the playroom because the playroom is considered a safe place. A medical student comes in and says to the child, "There you are, I have been looking for you. I need to take a quick look at you," and begins to examine the child.

Possible response. Student Nurse Baker informs the medical student that the playroom is an "exam-free zone" and she will bring the child to the procedure room so that the medical student can complete her examination. The medical student agrees and stops examining the child until they have all moved to the procedure room.

Suppose the medical student insists on completing her exam in the playroom and says she will not do anything to hurt the child. The student nurse responds with, "He needs to know that this is a safe place and he can come here to play. If you need to do the exam now, I will bring him to the procedure room for you." The student nurse has advocated for the child, who cannot speak for himself. The medical student was prioritizing her need to complete the exam over the child's need to feel safe in the playroom.

Now suppose that the child experienced acute respiratory distress while in the playroom. The student nurse would act immediately to save the child's life, prioritizing his need to breathe over his need to feel safe in the playroom. Advocacy requires analyzing the situation and deciding what actions will give the patient a voice and will advance his or her interests.

RELATIONSHIPS BETWEEN HEALTH CARE PROFESSIONALS

The Doctor–Nurse Game

Much has been written about the "doctor–nurse game" since the phrase was coined by Stein (1967). The communication style signified by this "game" represents deference on behalf of the nurse to the authority of the physician. In this sort of relationship, the nurse identifies the patient's needs or problems and makes recommendations to the physician, but in a passive way so that it appears the physician is arriving at the recommendations on his own. The use of the male pronoun is intentional because most physicians were men and nurses women in 1967. Savage (1995) found that this type of communication style persisted because nurses found it was effective when they advocated for their patients. For example, an experienced nurse on a bone marrow transplant unit notices a patient may be having beginning signs of graft-versus-host disease. She contacts the physician, a first-year resident, and describes the patient's signs and symptoms. The physician thanks her for telling him and starts to hang up. She adds, "Is there anything you want me to do . . . any medication to order or blood to have drawn?" She is expecting him to proceed in the usual way that graft-versus-host disease is managed, and because he did not, she attempts to elicit the expected response without openly telling him what should be done. As part of the resident's education, the nurse could be asking in a Socratic fashion what should be done next, but it is more likely that she has found that leading the resident to the expected response will result in getting the orders that she believes is best for her patient. However, the interaction seems to perpetuate the "doctor–nurse game."

The doctor–nurse game, issues involving physician–nurse relationships, and fear of physicians have been reported in the United States (Mason, 2002), the United Kingdom (Radcliffe, 2000), Mexico (Hojat et al., 2001), Australia (Ahern & McDonald, 2002), and Canada (Boychuk Duchscher, 2001). It also has been found that patient outcomes, as well as nurses' job satisfaction, are greatly affected by the quality of the nurse–physician relationship (Aiken, Havens, & Sloane, 2000; Longo, Young, Mehr, Lindbloom, & Salerno, 2002; Rosenstein, 2002). Furthermore, new graduates have described interacting with physicians as a major source of anxiety (Boychuk Duchscher, 2001). Why are these facts important in advocacy? When the nurse must challenge the status quo on behalf of the patient, moral courage is required, and the doctor–nurse game only makes this more challenging.

Handling Conflict Between Team Members

In the foregoing case examples of advocacy, the nurse (and student nurse) had to interact with a physician (and medical student) to advocate for their patients. In both cases, the nurses questioned the physicians' actions. It is quite possible that the physicians could have reacted angrily and become verbally abusive toward the nurses; fearing that outcome, the nurses might not have spoken up. It is also possible that the nurses could be concerned about their ongoing relationship with the physicians; thus they might have thought that the lesser of two evils would be to allow the physicians to continue. Speaking up on behalf of patients requires moral courage. If, in either case, the nurse did not get the outcome she desired, she would need to decide what to do next. Within a health care system, she could follow the chain of command in the nursing structure. She could notify the charge nurse. The student nurse could have contacted her instructor or the staff nurse assigned to her patient. Although these scenarios describe what seem like minor issues, they represent fundamental ethical issues for nurses. The nurses are acting to prevent harm (principle of non-maleficence) to their patients and to promote patient well-being (beneficence).

Relationships among nurses, student nurses, physicians, and medical students directly affect patient care. As with all human interactions, there are complex issues involving hierarchy, gender, personalities, and other intangible factors. Sometimes the intensity of the work of health care is used as an excuse for a lack of civility in interactions in the health care setting. Use of respectful language, professional decorum, and diplomacy when necessary should ensure effective communication and functional relationships among health care professionals.

CASE STUDY 21-3

Nurse Ash observes an orthopedic resident going into her patient's room, so she follows him in. He removes the patient's dressing and opens the sterile dressing he intends to apply. As he is donning his sterile gloves, the tips of the fingers of the glove brush up against the patient's bedside table, but he continues. What should the nurse do if she believes the physician has contaminated his glove? Because the physician proceeds with changing the dressing, the nurse might assume that he was unaware of the contamination. It is possible, though, that the physician was aware, and was anxious to complete the dressing change even though he risks infecting his patient.

Possible response: Nurse Ash begins to open another package of sterile gloves for the physician and says, "Let me open these for you. I notice you just contaminated your right glove." The nurse is stating the observation she made and offering assistance to the physician to avoid possible harm to the patient.

Suppose the physician responds, "No, I did not contaminate my glove." What should the nurse do if she is certain the glove has been contaminated? The interaction with the physician may feel uncomfortable for the nurse, yet the duty to prevent harm to the patient is paramount. The nurse says, "Because it's possible that you did contaminate your glove, even though you do not think you did, the safest course of action to avoid possibly infecting the wound is to change your gloves. I have another pair here for you." Again, the nurse states objectively what is known, and offers an option that is in the patient's best interests.

UNCERTAINTY, DILEMMA, AND DISTRESS

Ethical issues are often embedded in the clinical context, where there are sociopolitical forces of power, institutional culture, and professional codes. The "right" course of action is often not clear, hence the frequent reference to an issue being gray rather than black and white. Jameton (1984) used the language of uncertainty, dilemma, and distress (p. 131). There can be ethical uncertainty, a question of whether the problem is an ethics problem. There are ethical dilemmas when a choice must be made between two equally unpleasant alternatives. An example of a dilemma might be the decision to amputate a gangrenous limb. The patient does not want to lose a limb, but does not want to die of septicemia.

Even if the nurse clearly identifies what he or she believes is the right course of action, there may be resistance to that course. To challenge the status quo once again requires the courage to speak up on behalf of a specific patient or a population of patients. Nurses may experience moral distress as they analyze a situation; they may not always be able to articulate the ethical components but will describe feeling that something "is not right." In advocating for patients, nurses decide what is the "right" thing to do. Here are additional examples of situations in which a nurse could advocate for a patient. Think of different courses of action the nurse could take and a rationale for those actions.

CASE STUDY 21-4

Nurse Hunt works in home health care nursing. She visits a gentleman, Mr. Dash, who had a stroke. His son and daughter check on him and run errands for him, but he lives alone and eats frozen microwave dinners. His appearance and his home are unkempt and disheveled. When checking his medication, Nurse Hunt discovers that he has nearly full bottles of antihypertensive and anticoagulant medications. He said he sometimes forgets whether he has taken them and figures it is better to skip them than take a double dose. Despite pillboxes, schedules, and other reminders, he does not regularly take his medication. His blood pressure is 230/150. Nurse Hunt begins to call the physician to report her findings and Mr. Dash asks her not to, saying he does not want any more medication, hospitalization, or therapy. He wants to be left alone.

Possible actions. The nurse believes that she needs to act quickly. Does she comply with the patient's wishes to be left alone, or does she contact the physician and seek medical input? She considers whether she knows the patient well enough to accept his refusal of treatment, or if she has the time to assess his decision-making capacity. She is concerned that if she does not act quickly, the patient could experience another stroke. She explains to Mr. Dash that she thinks he could be in imminent danger of having another stroke, and should that happen while she is there, she would call an ambulance. She also tells him that he could be experiencing depression, which is interfering with his ability to make decisions. She would like the three of them, Mr. Dash, the physician, and herself, to make a plan on what to do about his blood pressure. He has the right to refuse treatment, but she would like to make sure he is fully capable of making the decision to forgo life-sustaining treatment.

In this scenario, Nurse Hunt does not know Mr. Dash very well, and because there is not such a relationship to draw on, she hesitates to act on his request at the cost of his health. She thinks his present condition could negatively affect his ability to make decisions. This may appear to be the antithesis of advocacy, yet it is not. The nurse respects the autonomy of the patient. For the patient to exercise autonomy, he must first be competent and have decision-making capacity. Competence is decided by a court of law, and he has not been declared incompetent, so he is presumed to be competent. Decision-making capacity, however, is not a legal condition; it is a "real-life" state and can be transient. Depending on the current situation, a patient may or may not have decision-making capacity. In light of the lack of time to assess the patient's capacity, the nurse is acting to preserve life.

Now suppose that Nurse Hunt knew Mr. Dash quite well, knew of his desire to forgo further treatment, knew of his family's agreement to honor Mr. Dash's wishes, and believed he had decision-making capacity in his decision to forgo treatment. His current request not to have his hypertension treated is consistent with their previous discussions. Nurse Hunt explains to Mr. Dash that his hypertension may precipitate another stroke, and it may be further disabling but it may not cause his death. She encourages him to complete an advance directive so a surrogate can make decisions for him if he is incapacitated. Nurse Hunt may have suggested to Mr. Dash and his physician that a "Do Not Resuscitate" order be written so that any health professional in the home at the time of an arrest will not be legally compelled to resuscitate him. Although Nurse Hunt may have strong feelings that Mr. Dash should accept treatment, she is advocating for what he, as a competent adult who has decision-making capacity, wants.

CASE STUDY 21-5

Nurse Gorrell works on a medical unit. He is caring for an 82-year-old man who had a myocardial infarction and is experiencing left heart failure. Consistent with his advance directives, and with his family's agreement, a "Do Not Resuscitate" order was written. He is receiving palliative care. In the morning a phlebotomist prepares to draw blood. Nurse Gorrell checks the orders and discovers that the order for routine laboratory tests was not canceled. He calls the intern to get an order to cancel the blood work, but the intern says he still wants it. The intern says the attending will ask him what the patient's potassium is and he'll have to have an answer for him. Nurse Gorrell then asks what the intern intends to do if the potassium result is abnormal, and he replies, "Nothing. That's not the point. The point is, I have to have the information if I am asked."

Possible response. Nurse Gorrell is not convinced that the patient should endure the discomfort and expense of a blood test that will not alter his course of treatment. He advises the intern that he is going to ask the phlebotomist to wait until he speaks to the attending physician. Once he reaches the attending, he asks whether it is necessary to obtain the potassium level, and the attending agrees it is not necessary.

Suppose the attending said that he is curious to see whether the potassium level has changed, but that knowing the level will not persuade him to change any treatment. Nurse Gorrell then suggests that the patient be asked if he will agree to a test that is not for his benefit but for the physician's knowledge. Or the nurse may ask the physician if he believes the value of knowing the results outweighs the discomfort and cost to the patient. The nurse may not be able to prevent the blood from being drawn even if he believes there is no justifiable reason to do so; however, he should bring the issue of unnecessary tests on dying patients to the appropriate group within the institution. There may be a continuous quality improvement (CQI) committee or a committee addressing palliative or comfort care for dying patients. In the process of developing a unit or department policy, dialogue can occur between professional groups so that there will be an understanding of each group's perspective and a mutually agreeable policy can be enacted.

LEARNING HOW TO ADVOCATE

In a bibliometric analysis of articles on patient advocacy, Mallik and Rafferty (2000) concluded that advocacy by U.S. nurses has become "more contentious and militant as nurses seek to empower themselves with the advocacy role" (p. 8). Foley, Minick, and Kee (2002) found that nurses learn advocacy in a haphazard manner that is dependent on situations. They identified three ways that nurses learn advocacy. In the first, the nurse identifies how he or she learned to "stand up for others" in the past. Standing up for one's siblings against a bully is an example of how a nurse may have experienced advocacy prior to coming into the profession. Learning by watching how other nurses advocate is the second way. The third is by gaining confidence through experience, validation, and mentoring. As nurses are socialized into the profession, they should be alert for opportunities to share their inside knowledge of the health care system and advocate for patients by helping them to navigate it.

ADVOCACY FOR THE PROFESSION

The American Nurses Association in the United States, the Canadian Nurses Association in Canada, and other associations in the United States and elsewhere exist for a number of reasons. One major purpose is to advocate for the health and welfare of their citizens or special patient populations and for the advancement of the nursing profession. The 1991 ANA Code of Ethics for Nurses

With Interpretative Statements (ANA, 2001) represents the profession's expectations of its members. Most of the provisions in the 2001 ANA code pertain to client–patient interests, whereas some address workplace issues. All codes provide the ethical impetus for advocacy.

Workplace Advocacy

Having a work environment that is conducive to optimal performance is a goal of nursing. Staffing and workload determinations are critical to the nurse's performance. The nurse prioritizes and delegate tasks. Having too many patients or patients who are acutely ill requires the nurse to shift time and attention to those patients. Although it may be idealistic to expect nurses to deliver the highest quality care every day, nurses do strive to achieve this. On those days that they believe they will not be able to devote the amount of time and attention to patients who need it the most, they advise their managers and negotiate for the optimal assignments. If this type of workload dilemma occurs chronically, the nurses must advocate for a change, such as increasing the number of nurses on their unit, decreasing the patient census, or referring more acute patients to better-staffed units. This type of negotiation is part of workplace advocacy. The nurses may be part of a collective bargaining unit of their professional organization, such as the UAN (United American Nurses, AFL-CIO) of the American Nurses Association, or may have a structure within their nursing division like shared governance through which they can negotiate change with the organization's administrators.

Nurses often work through their professional association to advocate for better working conditions. Staffing, workload, and delegation are key issues that immediately affect patient care. Other workplace issues include nurse safety and health. Workplace violence, such as may occur in the emergency department or on a psychiatric unit, threatens the health of nurses, patients, other employees, and visitors. Nurses advocate for security measures that provide for safe delivery of care. Other environmental workplace issues include freedom from sexual harassment and avoidance of hazardous materials or situations conducive to workplace injury.

Mandatory overtime, especially in times of nursing shortages, is a source of conflict between nurses and administrators. Fatigue can lead to errors, and nurses who want to prevent the possibility of harm to patients may resist mandatory overtime. The conundrum that occurs with the "proof" that mandatory overtime risks patient safety is that nurses will risk their own health to avoid harm to patients. Many nurses have stories of a near-miss of patient harm that occurred when they were working overtime but that they did not report for various reasons.

In a nurse's estimation, for example, the fatigue from overtime contributed to the likelihood of error. The operative issue is that nurses judge whether they are capable of safely providing several hours of patient care beyond the end of their shift; with mandatory overtime, their judgment about the safety of care is irrelevant. They are ordered to remain on the unit and take care of patients until they are relieved; if they leave at the end of their shift without reporting off to another nurse, they could be accused of patient abandonment. Each institution should have a definition of patient abandonment, and the nurses should have input into the definition and procedure for safely transferring care. The principle of non-maleficence, or preventing harm, holds for the prevention of harm to the nurse and others who deliver care, as well as for prevention of harm to the patients. Identifying unsafe situations, either for patients or staff, is an ethical obligation of health care providers.

To attract people into the profession of nursing, the work life of nurses needs to be continuously evaluated. Educational preparation, entry level for practice, and socialization into the profession are important issues for discussion. Workplace issues, in addition to those described earlier, include the use of needle-less intravenous systems, latex allergy management, and work-related disability benefits, and should be addressed in every facility employing nurses. Ongoing education through in-services, formal education with tuition reimbursement, and paid release time to attend conferences also should be the focus of advocacy. On a broader societal scale, nursing, through professional organizations, advocates by disseminating position statements on important issues for patients and families and for nurses. At the end of 2005, the ANA has 84 position statements including those pertaining to blood-borne and airborne diseases; ethics and human rights issues; social causes and health care; drug and alcohol abuse; nursing education, practice, and research; consumer advocacy and workplace advocacy; and the use of unlicensed assistive personnel. They have also issued joint statements with other professional and consumer groups. Practicing nurses can aid in the efforts to improve their profession by participating in their association's advocacy activities.

SUMMARY

For nursing to thrive, nurses need to advocate for the profession. This differs somewhat from patient advocacy, but patients benefit from successful advocacy for the profession. Advocacy, based on the principles of autonomy of the patient, beneficence, and nonmaleficence, is an ethical obligation of the nurse.

Don't forget to visit thePoint companion website for additional study resources!

CHAPTER HIGHLIGHTS

- Identify how your patient might benefit by your advocacy today.
- Review the ANA (2001) Code of Ethics for Nurses With Interpretive Statements for provisions related to patient advocacy. What specific assistance does the code provide for the situation you identified in Clinical Exercise 1?
- Find policies and procedures in your current clinical setting that reflect workplace advocacy. Suppose you have a latex allergy. Is there a policy that addresses how you are to observe standard precautions in light of this?
- Discuss with a staff nurse in your clinical setting how he or she assesses the decision-making capacity of patients.

REVIEW QUESTIONS

- Observe the consent process with one of the patients in your clinical setting.
- How was the patient's decision-making capacity assessed?
- Was there any information you thought should have been given to the patient but was not? What would you have done differently?
- What was the nurse's role in the consent process? Would you do anything differently than what the nurse in this case did? If so, what would you do and why?
- Your patient has been diagnosed with a terminal illness. His family asks that he not be told his diagnosis, and the physician agrees not to tell him at this time. During his morning care, he tells you that he thinks he is not being told everything.
- What do you say to him, and why?
- Do you believe he has a right to know?
- Do you believe his family is making decisions for him in his best interests?
- Ask a staff nurse in your clinical setting how he or she would handle a situation like this.
- The family of your patient with a brain tumor in intensive care wishes to bring in a reflexologist—someone who attempts to heal through applying pressure to specific areas of the patient's feet and hands.
- How should you advocate for your patient and family in this case?
- What criteria would you consider to determine whether this intervention is in your patient's best interests?
- Who ultimately decides whether this intervention can be performed for your patient?
- What alternative could you propose to balance the patient's values with his medical needs?
- You are caring for a patient who has no family. The patient recently underwent surgery for removal of a cancerous tumor of the bowel. The insurance company authorized 6 days of hospitalization, and you believe the patient will not be ready for discharge by the sixth day.
- How do you advocate for the patient?
- What resources are available to you to advocate for the patient?

RECOMMENDED READING

American Nurses Association Commission on Workplace Advocacy. Information on ANA activities regarding appropriate staffing, health and safety issues, patient safety and advocacy, workplace rights, and other resources for nurses is available at www.nursingworld.org/wpa/infolnks.htm

Canadian Nurses Association. (2002). Code of ethics for Registered Nurses. Available at http://cna-aiic.ca/CNA/practice/ethics/code/default_e.aspx

Federal Citizen Information Center. Support group and consumer information is available at www.pueblo.gsa.gov

Library of Congress. Legislative information and links for tracking bills in Congress are available at http://thomas.loc.gov/

United American Nurses, AFL-CIO. Information is available at http://nursingworld.org/uan

REFERENCES

Ahern, K., & McDonald, S. (2002). The beliefs of nurses who were involved in a whistleblowing event. *Journal of Advanced Nursing, 38*(3), 303–309.

Aiken, L. H., Havens, D. S., & Sloane, D. M. (2000). The Magnet Nursing Services Recognition Program: A comparison of two groups of Magnet hospitals. *American Journal of Nursing, 100*(3), 26–36.

American Nurses Association. (2001). *Code of ethics for nurses with interpretive statements*. Washington, DC: Author.

Boychuk Duchscher, J. (2001). Out in the real world: Newly graduated nurses in acute-care speak out. *Journal of Nursing Administration, 31*(9), 426–439.

Canadian Nurses Association. (2002). Code of ethics for Registered Nurses. Available at http://cnaaiic.ca/CNA/practice/ethics/code/default_e.aspx

Foley, B. J., Minick, M. P., & Kee, C. C. (2002). How nurses learn advocacy. *Journal of Nursing Scholarship, 34*(2), 181–186.

Hojat, M., Nasca, T. J., Cohen, M. J. M., Fields, S. K., Rattner, S. L., Griffiths, M., et al. (2001). Attitudes toward physician–nurse collaboration: A cross-cultural study of male and female physician and nurses in the United States and Mexico. *Nursing Research, 50*(2), 123–128.

Jameton, A. (1984). *Nursing practice: The ethical issues*. Englewood Cliffs, NJ: Prentice Hall.

Levine, M. E. (1989). Ethical issues in cancer care: Beyond dilemma. *Seminars in Oncology Nursing, 5*(2), 124–128.

Longo, D. R., Young, J., Mehr, D., Lindbloom, E., & Salerno, L. D. (2002). Barriers to timely care of acute infections in nursing homes: A preliminary qualitative study. *Journal of the American Medical Directors Association, 3*(6), 360–365.

Mallik, M., & Rafferty, A. M. (2000). Diffusion of the concept of patient advocacy [Electronic version]. *Journal of Nursing Scholarship, 32*(4), 399–404.

Mason, D. J. (2002). MD–RN: A tired old dance. *American Journal of Nursing, 102*(6), 7.

Radcliffe, M. (2000). Doctors and nurses: New game, same result. *BMJ, 320*(7241), 1085.

Rosenstein, A. H. (2002). Nurse–physician relationships: Impact on nurse satisfaction and retention. *American Journal of Nursing, 102*(6), 26–34.

Savage, T. A. (1995). Nurses' negotiation processes in facilitating ethical decision-making in patient care. *Dissertation Abstracts International, 56*(12), 6675B.

Stein, L. I. (1967). The doctor–nurse game. *Archives of General Psychiatry, 16*, 699–703.

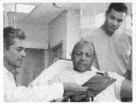
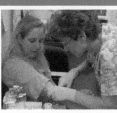
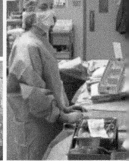

The Nursing Profession and the Community

LEARNING OUTCOMES

After completing this chapter, you should be able to:

* Outline how moving care into the community will affect nursing practice.

* Analyze the philosophy behind community-based care to determine how that relates to your own philosophy of nursing.

* Explain approaches to patient/client empowerment.

* Differentiate primary, secondary, and tertiary prevention and how these concepts can be applied in different nursing settings.

* Outline the various components of disease management and how those provide for health promotion.

* Discuss how Healthy People 2020 priority areas and leading health indicators relate to the goals of Healthy People 2020.

* Explain the nurse's role in disaster response in the community.

* Differentiate the major categories of complementary/alternative healthcare medicine.

* Discuss major issues that surround the use of complementary/alternative medicine.

* Describe ways in which you could use your knowledge of complementary/alternative therapies when working with clients.

KEY TERMS

Alternative healthcare
Biologically based practices
Community-based nursing
Complementary healthcare
Continuity of care
Disaster management

Disease management
Energy medicine
Health disparities
Healthy People 2020
Herbal medicine
Homeopathy

Integrative medicine
Manipulative and body-based practices
Medication reconciliation
Mind–body medicine
Naturopathy

Primary prevention
Secondary prevention
Tertiary prevention
Transition planning
Triage

The emphasis in healthcare has increasingly moved out of the institutional setting and into the community. Individuals are treated in ambulatory centers or even in workplaces and return to their homes or perhaps to work. This has both financial and health advantages. Care in a hospital in-patient setting is the most expensive type of care. While the high-technology care and constant surveillance are essential for the seriously ill, for the less seriously ill, that environment poses a myriad of hazards such as infection, medication errors, and lack of rest. In the home, family members must become caregivers, and healthcare workers have a new relationship with patients and families. In all settings, healthcare has moved to a promotion and prevention model and goals are broader than simply curing illness. This whole movement has impacted nursing in many ways.

UNDERSTANDING COMMUNITY-BASED NURSING

The nursing profession has unique privileges that include a trusted relationship with patients and families, access to individuals when they are most vulnerable, and legal status as a profession. In response, as the community's needs change, the nursing profession has an obligation to expand its knowledge base for practice, enlarge its repertoire of skills and abilities, and commit to meeting newly identified needs in innovative and creative ways.

Community-based nursing refers to the wide variety of settings other than in-patient institutions in which nursing is practiced. Public health, home health, ambulatory care, occupational health, and school nursing all reflect community-based practice. From the inception of modern nursing, community-based care has been part of the nursing profession. Graduate nurses of the first hospital training schools worked in homes nursing the sick. In the early part of the 20th century, the public health nurses working in settlement houses in the immigrant neighborhoods of New York and other large cities brought health education, direct care, and advocacy skills to bear on the many health problems confronting the community. As more aspects of healthcare moved into hospitals and other institutional settings, more nursing took place in those environments. However, public health and home care continued the long tradition of nursing in the community.

Care in the community is cost-effective and often more acceptable to the client because it causes less disruption in life. New opportunities arise as the understanding of care in the community enlarges. The principles of community-based care include an emphasis on advocating for patients, promoting patient education and self-care, focusing on health promotion and disease prevention, and recognizing the importance of family, culture, and the community.

Community-based care requires effective communication and collaboration. The key in all of these community settings is that the patient/client is in charge. The client decides to work with the nurse, to accept or reject advice and suggestions, and to enter and leave care. The nurse serves as an educator, a guide, a resource person, and an advocate, but health action is taken by the client and family. In addition to those who see themselves as working in a community-based setting, all nurses need to be aware of the community in which the client resides and be able to provide care that fits within the scope of the person's life rather than simply an "episode" of illness. Care must be family-centered and culturally competent. Nurses working in all environments must be aware of community health organizations, knowledgeable about availability and accessibility of services and supplies, and familiar with the location and specialty of healthcare providers. An interdisciplinary team approach in which the nurse may serve as a collaborator and coordinator takes on new meaning. As all nurses become more community-focused, the boundaries between the institutional nurse and the community-based nurse blur. All need an understanding of how the client functions in each setting, and each setting must adapt to facilitate transitions from one care environment to another.

CLIENT EMPOWERMENT

A community-based philosophy rests on a fundamental belief in the right of the client to control his or her life, including situations related to healthcare. Giving over control to clients removes healthcare professionals from a position of power over others and requires instead that they participate by empowering clients and families. It requires a partnership or alliance between the nurse and the individual and family that is much different from the traditional hierarchical nurse/patient relationship.

Empowering others requires possessing knowledge of the alternatives available, the ability to teach based on that knowledge, and the skills to help others make decisions and take appropriate action based on their decisions. Nurses can empower others when they assure that those people have the information necessary to make choices within their lives and when they enable patients and families to make their own choices and manage their own health.

Clients are often fearful of making healthcare decisions because so much is unknown. In addition, not everyone has the same interest in decision making. While some patients want to make decisions and need the information to do that, others do not want the burden of decision making. Nurses must navigate these difficult situations and recognize that the patient's decision to NOT have information or to not be burdened with certain types of decisions also represents the patient's autonomy. In such situations, determining what type of information and the depth of information a client wishes to receive is an important aspect of providing care. The nurse then has the additional responsibility of determining to whom the patient has delegated decision making.

Empowerment supports patients/clients in remaining who they are, not in remaking them into some ideal of a person. The elderly woman who asks that her son make decisions for her is empowered when caregivers respect her enough to allow her to live her life as she chooses. Trying to persuade this woman to change who she is and become the model of an independent person does a disservice to her and increases the distance between her and her caregivers when she most needs to be able to trust in them (Fig. 22.1).

HEALTH PROMOTION AND DISEASE PREVENTION SERVICES

Health promotion and disease prevention have long been the major focus of public health nurses, who concentrate on entire populations. This same focus on health promotion and disease prevention is now expanding to nursing in every setting. By recognizing that the determinants of health lie outside of the institution and are found in the community, nurses in the acute care setting enlarge their practice to make it more community-based in philosophy.

The various levels of prevention can be addressed wherever the nurse practices.

Primary Prevention

Primary prevention involves the efforts to prevent disease from ever occurring. Primary prevention can be aimed at stopping the cause of disease. On a community-wide level, water treatment and sanitation prevent the spread of communicable diseases by eliminating their sources for the entire population. Helping individuals to be more successful in resisting disease and maintaining health represents another aim of primary prevention. Generalized efforts to educate people regarding healthy diets are aimed at this type of primary prevention. Some efforts involve the individual client and family as the primary focus, although they may benefit the entire community. Immunizations prevent disease not only in the people immunized but also in others by lowering the overall existence of communicable disease throughout the community. Smoking cessation campaigns are aimed at primary prevention and help the individual who quits smoking, but also benefit those who might otherwise be subject to second-hand smoke.

Primary prevention can be a focus of nurses in acute and long-term care settings as well as those who work in the community. Nurses need to think in terms of life span development and identify the common preventable diseases and disorders that occur at any point in life. For example, when the patient must stop smoking to have surgery and remain in the hospital, the impetus may exist to stop smoking for good. Nurses may help

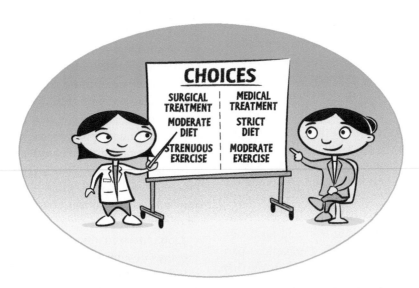

FIGURE 22–1 Teaching people to manage their own health, giving them the information to make choices within their lives, and helping them to carry out those choices empower them.

patients to examine their options, consult with physicians for medications to manage withdrawal, point out available smoking cessation programs, and in other ways help the patient to quit smoking. Some facilities focus on each contact with a patient as an opportunity to review immunization history and encourage updating of immunizations before leaving the hospital. This is particularly important in ensuring that the elderly have pneumococcal pneumonia immunization or flu vaccine. When planning for discharge, nurses can build in teaching regarding better dietary practices and help patients understand how those will help in long-term health as well as recovery from the current episode of illness.

Long-term care environments have steadily increased their emphasis on health promotion for even the most disabled individuals. Immunizations, fall prevention through strengthening and balance exercises, and activity programs to prevent social isolation and the accompanying depression serve as primary prevention interventions. Nurses are typically the professionals championing these programs, teaching clients and their families, and increasing public awareness of the concerns.

Secondary Prevention

Secondary prevention involves early identification of health problems through screening and the prevention of complications and adverse consequences of illness. Nurses in ambulatory settings help clients to identify screening tests that are important for them and facilitate scheduling those tests. When admission histories are obtained, the nurse in the acute care setting can attend to information about screenings that are needed and encourage the patient to value that activity. To do this effectively, the nurse must understand the current recommendation for screening in specific groups within the population. Asking about screening emphasizes its importance to clients and reinforces other information they may have. It may also create an opportunity for clients to gather additional information. Similarly, in the long-term setting, it is important that nurses continue their focus on prevention activities among the residents. Screening of the elderly population includes different priorities based on the incidence of problems in that age group and the potential years left.

Complications of illness greatly increase morbidity and mortality. Nurses in both acute and long-term care focus on preventing complications as a consistent part of their practice. Careful assessment and timely nursing intervention can prevent the formation of pressure ulcers, falls, and hypostatic pneumonia. These are only a sample of the many secondary prevention actions taken in the institutional care environment.

Tertiary Prevention

Tertiary prevention focuses on preventing long-term disability and restoring functional capacity. Rehabilitation efforts often have been singled out as the major place where tertiary prevention occurs. However, long-term care has a regulatory mandate to prevent deterioration of elderly individuals. Although some argue that decreased functional status is a realistic process that happens at the end of life, the increased emphasis on maintenance of function has revealed that even the extremely debilitated elderly may be helped to avoid the complications of dependency and to maintain functional independence in the face of disability longer than was previously thought.

Disease Management

One approach to increasingly sophisticated and targeted prevention services is found in disease management programs. **Disease management** focuses on providing the best evidence-based care for an individual with a specific chronic illness, such as diabetes. These programs are often instituted by health plans or clinics that recognize that failure to manage chronic illnesses knowledgeably results in increased rates of hospitalization, increased demand on the system for high-cost care, and increased incidence of potentially life-altering complications.

By targeting high-impact diseases such as diabetes for special attention, the aim is for both secondary and tertiary prevention. The person with diabetes who is enrolled in such a program receives comprehensive nutrition education, teaching regarding the management of blood glucose through medication and activity, and regular diagnostic evaluations that include hemoglobin A1c and blood glucose measurements to monitor blood sugar control over time, urine analysis to identify renal function, regular eye examinations to identify and treat retinal complications, and regular foot exams to prevent and treat lesions that might progress to gangrene and amputation. While the intensive involvement in prevention services is costly, the process saves overall through the lowered incidence of hospitalization, blindness, renal failure, and amputations, not to mention the cost of human suffering all of which have monetary costs as well.

Computerized documentation systems facilitate the activities of nurses who are charged with tracking individuals enrolled in a disease management program. They alert the nurse to contact the person through telephone calls, e-mails, or letters when screening services are needed. This same nurse meets with the person to discuss test results. By providing a consistent contact person, the patient feels more comfortable asking questions and is more motivated to maintain needed health practices and lifestyle changes.

HEALTHY PEOPLE 2020

The nation has been addressing health objectives for the whole population through a series of efforts that began with its first set of goals published in 1980 as Healthy People 1990. These have been updated at 10-year intervals and **Healthy People 2020** was released in January of 2010 (US-DHHS, 2010). While the goals of each campaign have not been reached, attention has been focused on them and strategies to work toward them are being refined.

Vision, Mission, and Goals of Healthy People 2020

Display 22.1 presents the statements of vision, mission, and goals for the Healthy People 2020 campaign. The vision provides a single comprehensive statement that defines the entire Healthy People effort. The mission points to actions that will be needed to achieve the goals. The overarching goals provide a framework in which outcomes can be developed.

Achieving these goals will require a policy focus at all levels of government. Healthcare providers, both individual and institutional, will need to examine their processes and policies. In addition to the roles they have in patient teaching, health professionals must recognize the importance of motivation in taking action to improve health. Exploring motivation and the structures that support positive health behaviors will facilitate the engagement of individuals in health promotion activities. To achieve the goals of Healthy People 2020 individuals must become aware of their own responsibility for their health. They need to be knowledgeable about what promotes health and what interferes with health. They must make informed choices that lead toward greater health.

Priority Areas of Healthy People 2020

The priority areas for action under the Healthy People 2020 plan include promotion of healthy behaviors, promotion of a healthy and safe community, improvement in the systems for personal and public health that will provide access and eliminate **health disparities**, and the prevention or reduction of major diseases and disorders that account for a large proportion of the healthcare problems in society. All of these areas for action will help to achieve the four overall goals.

Healthy behaviors are easy to identify and hard to put into practice. These include adding physical activity to life, managing nutrition well, avoiding being overweight and obese, ceasing tobacco use, practicing safe sexual behaviors, being judicious in the use of alcohol, reducing injury and violence, and maintaining a healthy environment. These are primary prevention behaviors that nurses in all settings can address. The challenges of behavioral change on a large scale have led to increased use of media, such as television advertisements, to impart to individuals information regarding healthy behavior. However, behavioral change is a complex phenomenon and whether these broad strategies are effective is not clear.

 DISPLAY 22.1 Healthy People 2010–2020 Vision, Mission, and Goals

VISION: A society in which all people live long, healthy lives.

MISSION: To improve health through strengthening policy and practice, Healthy People will
- Identify nationwide health improvement priorities
- Increase public awareness and understanding of the determinants of health, disease, and disability and the opportunities for progress
- Provide measurable objectives and goals that can be used at the national, state, and local levels
- Engage multiple sectors to take actions that are driven by the best available evidence and knowledge
- Identify critical research and data collection needs

GOALS
- Eliminate preventable disease, disability, injury, and premature death
- Achieve health equity, eliminate disparities, and improve the health of all groups
- Create social and physical environments that promote good health for all
- Promote healthy development and healthy behaviors across every stage of life

(USDHHS, Healthy People 2010, *www.healthypeople.gov/hp2020/advisory/PhaseI/summary.htm*)

Promoting healthy and safe communities has long been considered the province of public health departments. As our understanding of safe communities broadens, the role of domestic violence as a health problem has become more prominent. Many agencies promote awareness of what constitutes domestic violence through posters in public rest rooms, through television spots that highlight resources for help for those facing this problem, and by adding routine assessment for abuse to health histories.

Addressing individual behavior is only successful when the systems of the community support it. Access to health services is essential for people to obtain the screenings and preventive care they need. For example, family planning services contribute to the health of both mothers and infants. Medical products must be safe and a public health infrastructure must be in place to support a healthy community. Nurses recognize that many individuals never visit a dentist and that assessment of oral health can be part of physical assessment done in other settings, with referral to dental professionals when obvious problems are identified.

While the number of different diseases and conditions fills volumes of books, there are a limited number of conditions that account for the majority of illness and disability. The successful identification and treatment of these diseases create a substantial move toward greater health and quality of life for millions.

Leading Health Indicators for Healthy People Initiatives

Leading health indicators are classifications for measurement to determine the success of the Healthy People initiatives (Display 22.2). Measures for each category have been devised and are being tracked to determine trends and to evaluate specific strategies for targeted groups. Some are indicators for which a decrease indicates

progress—such as tobacco use. For others an increase indicates success—such as access to healthcare. Specific measurements that will reveal prevalence in the population must be devised for each indicator.

Nurses' Roles in Supporting Healthy Communities

While many nurses work professionally in the community, all nurses can support personally the health of their communities. One personal role is as a supporter and advocate for political measures that would improve the health of the community. This might include contacting representatives at local, state, or national levels and advocating for passage of important health-related laws or projects.

Another personal role includes being active as a community service volunteer in a homeless shelter, school, or other community agency. Blood drives, blood pressure screening events, and educational programs may all seek the services of nurses as community volunteers. Within a neighborhood, church, or other setting, nurses are often asked to be a resource person for health-related questions. While nurses need to be careful not to give medical advice or make recommendations without adequate information, they can advise healthy behaviors, suggest health-related screening, help identify that a problem exists, suggest seeing a healthcare provider for a problem presented, help individuals understand the directions given to them by their physician, or teach people about their medications. Some have suggested that nurses can also be role models of healthy lifestyles for those around them. Although many nurses reject the idea that their lives should be lived with this in mind, others recognize that actions often speak to others much louder than words. The nurse who persists in smoking has less credibility when suggesting healthy lifestyle behaviors

DISPLAY 22.2   The Leading Health Indicators

- Physical activity
- Overweight and obesity
- Tobacco use
- Substance abuse
- Responsible sexual behavior
- Mental health
- Injury and violence
- Environmental quality
- Immunization
- Access to healthcare

USDHHS, Healthy People 2020

COMMUNICATION IN ACTION

Talking With a Neighbor About Health Concerns

Joe Reynolds is a nurse who works on the surgical unit of a local community hospital. While he works in his yard, a neighbor approaches him and begins to chat. After a few minutes of talking about yard maintenance, the neighbor says, "Uh—Joe, do you know much about these PSA tests?" Joe replies, "A bit. Do you have a question about them?" "Well, I went in to see my doctor. He did some tests and said my PSA is too high and I should go see a urologist. What the heck is it anyway and why should I see another doctor?" Joe asks, "What explanation did the doctor give you?" The neighbor replies, "Well, he talked about numbers and said something about cancer and then I don't remember what else he said." Knowing that even hearing the word cancer can cause enough stress that a person might not hear the remainder of the doctor's explanation, Joe decides to do some simple teaching. He explains, "Well, the test means that something is going on in your prostate. It is an important test, but the results can be positive even when you don't have cancer; other things can cause the readings to be high. However, it really should be checked out so that you get the proper treatment. A urologist specializes in this kind of problem and will do more tests to find out exactly what is going on and then talk to you about whether you need treatment." The neighbor says, "Thanks, Joe. Guess I should make that appointment." Joe replies, "Yes, I think you should. Let me know if there is anything I can help with."

to others. Some nurses have used this situation to illustrate their understanding of the difficulty of undertaking lifestyle changes and have entered into groups that work together on healthier living.

MAINTAINING CONTINUITY OF CARE

Continuity of care for the individual means that there is an uninterrupted process across settings in which a person seeks care. In an ideal world, there would never be a duplicated test, a failure to account for medications currently prescribed, or a lack of information upon which the care provider could make decisions. However, the current system is far from ideal. When a mother with young children goes to the emergency room and does not have immunization information, this may affect the care provided. When a person leaves the hospital and does not understand the discharge instructions, that person's health is compromised. When an elderly resident moves from the nursing home to the hospital and information on medications for chronic illnesses does not accompany that person, serious complications may result. The Joint Commission requires that the institutions it accredits study this problem and establish effective policies and procedures to ensure continuity of care.

Transition Planning

Transitions are the movement of the patient from one care environment to another, such as from home care to

hospital, from hospital to nursing home, or from one unit in a hospital (such as the intensive care unit [ICU]) to another (such as the general medical unit) as needs for care change. **Transition planning** refers to the planning process that takes place to assure that the patient's well-being is maintained throughout the time of transition. The actual actions of healthcare providers during the transition are often termed the "Handoff." Many facilities are establishing policies and protocols on exactly what actions must be taken during a handoff. Medication reconciliation, discussed below, is a critical part of the handoff.

The transition to a new care environment has been identified as a time in which the potential for error rises. Whether moving from home to an outpatient setting or between units in the same facility, transition planning is critical to effective care. While physicians usually have the authority to prescribe the move, the nurses are the ones who usually serve as the coordinators of transitions.

Discharge Planning

Planning for a transition often begins when a decision is made for the patient's care to be moved to another setting. Some transitions can be predicted before the decision about timing is made. For most patients, discharge from a hospital is an expected event; therefore, planning for discharge begins immediately upon admission, if possible. Upon admission to a hospital, a projected timeline for care may contain specific outcomes to be met along a care pathway. A discharge coordinator may be charged with following the patient to assure that planning is accomplished in a timely manner. The discharge coordinator may be a nurse or may be a social worker. This person works with the family to arrange the appropriate setting for postdischarge care.

All nurses assume responsibility for ensuring that medical orders and nursing plans move with the patient to the next location. Written materials that document these orders and plans are essential for accuracy. Teaching is incorporated throughout the process. When discharge is to a nursing home or rehabilitation setting, the goal is that the receiving setting is prepared to provide the care needed. When the person is going home, the nurse is often responsible for ensuring that needed referrals have been arranged and for providing discharge teaching. Patients going home also need written materials to refer to in relationship to self-care. Family members, when available, are integrated into the planning for discharge. The nurse in the institutional setting may follow up with the patient after discharge to ensure that the patient's healthcare needs are being met in the new environment and that communication has been clear. Appropriate documentation of this process is essential.

Transfers

Whether an individual moves from one unit within an institution to another or from the hospital to a nursing home, a careful plan is still needed. While some transfers occur because of sudden changes in a patient's condition or because the demand for beds has accelerated transfers out of a particular unit, most are part of the ongoing therapeutic plan. For a patient admitted for surgery, this might include an admitting unit, the surgical suite, the postanesthesia care unit, the surgical unit, before discharge to home or a rehabilitation setting.

Many facilities now have a separate transfer form that is initiated by the nurse in the unit where the patient's care begins. This form identifies all the key transition information. During the handoff the transferring professional and the receiving professional can quickly review the key information, assess the patient, and enter the receiving assessment and acknowledgment of the information on the form. This same process also might be used for the aid car personnel handing off to the nurse in the emergency department or the nurse handing off to a nurse in a nursing home (although this latter process might occur over the telephone with written documentation by fax). The advantage of this process is that the receiving nurse does not need to spend a lengthy time trying to find the most important information in a voluminous medical record. Both people are accountable for ensuring that the key information is identified and acted upon.

Medication Reconciliation

One of the major areas of concern for patient safety at the time of any transition is the continuity of medications that the patient has been taking for the successful management of health problems. The recognition of the importance of this with regard to patient safety has resulted in the process called **medication reconciliation**, which occurs after a person is admitted to a care facility. This process is the result of recommendations by The Joint Commission Patient Safety Goals and the Institute for Safe Medication Practices (The Joint Commission, 2010).

Medication reconciliation at admission involves carefully documenting all the medications and their dosages, including prescribed medications, over-the-counter medications, vitamin/mineral supplements, and herbal products the person was taking before admission to the care setting. These are then compared to what has been ordered for current care. Any differences are brought to the attention of the medical care provider in order for the best care decision to be made.

This same process is used at all times of transition. Medications change when a person leaves an ICU. Nurses on a surgical unit must be aware of the medications a patient received while in the operating room. When a patient is admitted through an emergency room, the medication given there will affect ongoing care. If additional medications are ordered in that setting, the nurses must know whether they were given or must still be given after the patient comes to the care unit.

Facilities develop a standardized form on which medication reconciliation is documented. These records become part of the patient record and are also used to document quality improvement in maintaining safe medication administration by ensuring appropriate continuity of medication orders across transitions.

Critical Thinking Activity

A charge nurse in a nursing home is planning for the transfer to the hospital of an 87-year-old resident who fell and fractured her hip. This resident has a history of congestive heart failure, osteoarthritis, and osteoporosis, but had been ambulatory using a cane and cognitively intact before the fall. What concerns should be addressed before the transfer occurs? What are the issues that will be of concern during the transfer? What information will the receiving nursing unit need in order to provide effective care?

Continuity of Care Documentation

Historically medical records for any individual may be scattered among the various offices of a primary care physician, a number of specialty physicians, one or more pharmacies, a physical therapist's office, and a hospital. If an individual has geographically moved more than once, these healthcare record sites are multiplied by the number of cities or areas in which the person lived. This may result in discontinuity in care. Clients may not remember exactly what tests were done or their exact results. They may find it difficult to pinpoint whether a particular episode of symptoms occurred 3 or 5 years ago. Although everyone is encouraged to keep a current list of prescription medications and their dosages with them, how many actually carry through with this? When seeking past records is too cumbersome, tests may be redone; there may be no baseline against which to compare results, or significant problems may be overlooked.

The hurricanes of 2005 that saw tens of thousands of individuals displaced from the Gulf Coast region of the United States brought these concerns to the forefront. Cancer patients were evacuated but needed to continue treatment; however, their records remained in flooded hospitals. Individuals with chronic illnesses ran out of prescriptions and were unable to get needed medications. These and many other problems occurred because health records were no longer accessible.

While electronic health records (EHR) that encompass the documentation of a particular health system, including both inpatient and outpatient settings, are becoming more common, many people still receive care where these are not available. Even an excellent EHR will not be available outside of the system. Two computer programs for solving this problem have emerged. They are the Continuity of Care Record (ASTM International, 2005) and the Continuity of Care Document (Corepoint Health, 2009).

The purpose of these computer programs is the creation of an electronic document that "provides a core data set of the most relevant administrative, demographic, and clinical information facts about a patient's healthcare, covering one or more healthcare encounters. (It) includes a summary of the patient's health status (eg, problems, medications, allergies) and basic information about insurance, advance directives, care documentation, and the patient's care plan" (ASTM International, 2005). The Continuity of Care Document is structured to coordinate with additional healthcare documentation standards and to be more compatible with a wide variety of EHR systems. Either would provide the ability to place the patient's information on some type of media or transfer it electronically to another system to facilitate continuity of care. (Fig. 22.2).

While these computer programs are not in widespread use, they have great potential for alleviating the problems involved in patient transitions. As individuals and healthcare agencies become more familiar with these options, the expectation is that there will be increased use of them and nurses will be required to access and use the information contained in this record.

DISASTER RESPONSE IN THE COMMUNITY

Potential disasters have always been a concern in communities, but they have become a greater focus of attention since the 9/11 collapse of the Twin Towers in New York City, Hurricane Katrina in New Orleans, and the 2010 earthquake in Haiti. Display 22.3 lists the 11 major causes of community disasters. Some disasters, such as a fire, may occur in any community; others, such as an earthquake or a hurricane, occur more frequently in one part of the country than in another. **Disaster management** refers to the plans that are in place designating the community's response to a disaster.

Volunteers in Disaster Response

Many communities have plans in place to mobilize volunteers for some roles in a disaster. For example, in areas with earthquake potential, community planning focuses at the neighborhood level, with volunteers responding to neighbors. Basic first aid and management of food, water, and shelter cannot wait for professional rescuers to arrive in the event of widespread damage to roads, power, and other infrastructure. Nurses might take a leadership role in their own neighborhoods because they understand issues of both public health and disease management. Their ability to respond to people's emotional needs as well as physical concerns provides a foundation for effective leadership. There are federal government resources available to help individuals and families to make personal disaster plans. In most disasters, personal advanced planning can make an enormous difference. See the Disaster Planning and Federal Emergency Management Administration (FEMA) Web sites listed for help in individual planning (*www.ready.gov/; www.fema.gov/*).

Disaster response volunteers may include Red Cross workers. The Red Cross is designated by the federal government as the key disaster response voluntary agency. Although there is a central paid staff, the majority of Red Cross workers are volunteers. The Red Cross provides training and organization for both healthcare professionals and others who are willing to respond to disasters. It manages shelters and serves as a conduit for donated

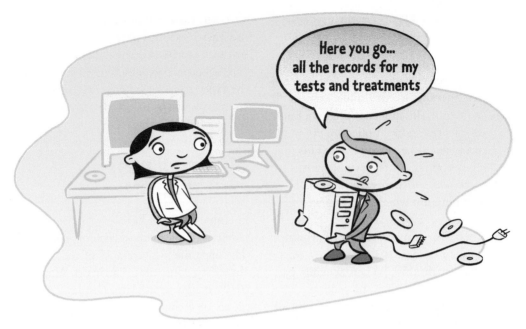

FIGURE 22.2   In an ideal healthcare system, every person would have a "Care Continuity Record."

DISPLAY 22.3   Types of Community Disasters

- Acts of terror
- Disease—especially epidemic disease
- Drought
- Earthquake
- Fire
- Flood
- Food contamination
- Hazmat (hazardous material spill)
- Hurricane
- Power outages
- Tornado

funds, services, and government assistance to help those who are victims of disaster. They have also produced, in conjunction with FEMA, publications with information regarding disaster preparedness for many types of disasters (American Red Cross, 2009).

Other voluntary and nonprofit organizations also respond to disasters. One of the largest and most widely known is the Salvation Army, a Christian group that provides a wide array of social services at all times. During disasters, Salvation Army workers are active in setting up shelters, providing meals, and helping affected individuals to rebuild their lives. Other religious and disaster response organizations may also be mobilized depending on the size of the disaster.

Institution and Agency Disaster Response

Firefighters, police officers, ambulance drivers, the National Guard, and health professionals are all part of response plans. Most of these individuals are trained for disaster response by their employers.

Firefighters are often the frontline responders to those injured in a disaster. They provide the rescue and emergency medical response skills to save lives. As first responders, firefighters risk the potential for serious injury, smoke or dust inhalation, carbon monoxide poisoning, and heat-related illness from the wearing of protective gear in hot environments. Nurses working in triage must be cognizant of this risk to emergency workers.

Hospitals often serve a pivotal role in managing injuries or illness related to a disaster. Each hospital has plans in place for both internal disasters (such as a fire in one wing of the hospital) and external disasters (such as a tornado in the community). In communities with multiple hospitals, coordination in disaster planning and preparation is essential. Based on their locations and services, each might be designated for a different role.

Learning about their agency's disaster plans should be part of the orientation of all employees. Nurses in hospitals have major roles in responding to disasters. Current patients will be discharged as quickly as possible to open up beds for disaster victims or may have to be moved if the institution is located in an affected area, Units will be reorganized to enable the acceptance and treatment of multiple victims. Nurses may be asked to move to emergency departments to be part of teams that will provide triage. **Triage** involves the initial screening of victims for the purpose of prioritizing treatment and making the most effective and efficient use of both human and material resources. When major triage is no longer needed, nurses may then return to units for patient care.

Part of a disaster plan for any agency is a call-in system. This system is a planned process for notifying staff not on duty that there is a disaster and they should report for work. Building such a call-in list is usually the responsibility of the manager of each unit. There may be a telephone tree with people designated to call others within their neighborhood or geographic area, in order for everyone to be notified more quickly. Healthcare professionals sometimes face an ethical dilemma regarding being called in for a disaster. Their own families and neighborhoods may need them, but the hospital is treating the most seriously injured or ill and needs everyone.

Specific Disaster Concerns

Hurricane Katrina on the Gulf Coast pointed out the tremendous challenges of managing a widespread disaster when the local resources for response are destroyed. Without hospitals, fire departments, and other agencies, all help had to come from outside the community. Transportation and communication were identified as major problems. Moving large numbers of people, arranging for shelters, and communicating among those trying to provide emergency help all became more than the system was prepared to manage. The total resulting effect on people's lives and health is still not known. As a consequence of this situation, communities are looking more closely at their disaster planning and requesting that both the federal and state governments develop better contingency plans. The federal government operates a Web site that is an entry point for learning about the federal government's disaster planning and services (*www.ready.gov/.*)

Communicable diseases that strike large numbers of individuals in a community are considered *epidemics* while those that strike large numbers around the world are termed *pandemics*. Influenza is considered a pandemic when a new strain arises to which most people are susceptible and cases arise in large numbers in multiple countries such as occurred with the H1N1 strain in 2009. Nurses need to become knowledgeable about transmission methods for communicable diseases and the role of immunizations. They must be prepared to give accurate information to those who express concerns. They also need to understand their personal role in any institutional plan for response to an epidemic.

Terrorism, which was most visible in the United States in the 9/11 attacks on the United States, remains a concern. The subway and bus bombings in London in 2005 demonstrated the vulnerability of large cities to the concerted efforts of a few terrorists. A great deal of the federal government's support for disaster planning is focused on terrorism. Part of the disaster planning of every urban community relates to terrorism response. Whole communities may be involved in disaster response drills, and people may be recruited to play the part of victims. A simulated disaster is staged, and all the plans of the various community agencies are activated. A disaster drill provides a mechanism to find out what works and to plan more effectively.

COMPLEMENTARY AND ALTERNATIVE HEALTHCARE

The National Center for Complementary and Alternative Medicine (NCCAM) has defined this field as "a group of diverse medical and healthcare systems, practices, and products that are not generally considered to be part of conventional medicine" (NCCAM, 2010, Defining CAM). Conventional medicine may also be referred to as allopathy, Western, mainstream, orthodox, regular medicine, and biomedicine. This definition of complementary and alternative medicine (CAM) focuses more on what alternative care is *not* than what it *is*, because of the broad range of healthcare practices included in this category. Common among these practices are acupuncture, homeopathy, naturopathy, music therapy, and herbal medicine. NCCAM includes prayer for health reasons as a therapy practice. The list of healthcare practices considered complementary and alternative shifts constantly as some are proven safe and effective, others are proven of little value or even harmful and fade from use, and still others emerge. According to its 2007 survey (NCCAM, 2008),

39.3% of adults in the United States use some form of CAM. Overall, CAM use is greater among women and people with higher education levels. Survey results indicated that CAM is most often used to treat and/or prevent musculoskeletal conditions or other conditions that involve chronic or recurring pain.

These healthcare approaches are considered *alternative* when they are used in place of conventional medical care. The same approaches are considered *complementary* when they are used along with conventional medicine. **Integrative medicine**, as defined by NCCAM, "combines mainstream medical therapies and CAM therapies for which there is some high-quality scientific evidence of safety and effectiveness" (NCCAM, 2010). Thus, integrative medicine supports the higher standard of research evidence for effectiveness.

NCCAM provides training for researchers in the area of CAM, funds grants for research into the effectiveness of all types of alternative care, and disseminates research findings about CAM to both professionals and the public. The National Library of Medicine maintains a database, CAM on PUBMED, which allows for research in relationship to specific diseases, conditions, and therapies (see end of chapter Web sites).

CAM takes place almost entirely within the community, and the client often serves as its primary controlling factor, as opposed to conventional medicine, in which the official healthcare provider controls access to care through ordering diagnostics, prescribing treatments, and determining admission to and discharge from a care facility. As **complementary** and **alternative healthcare** practices remain popular with the public, healthcare providers are challenged to understand these diverse approaches and to work effectively with clients who choose those resources. There is also a need to assist in client education so that choices are made wisely and with sound information.

Major Types of Complementary and Alternative Medicine

NCCAM has categorized CAM into four domains for the purpose of discussion and study. These domains include mind–body medicine, biologically based practices, manipulative and body-based practices, and energy medicine (Tables 22.1 and 22.2). Additionally, CAM studies alternative whole medical systems that cut across many of the domains.

Specific alternative care providers may use more than one type of treatment in their practice. Additionally, there are many areas of overlap between conventional medical practice and CAM. The major types of alternative care available are described briefly in the following sections.

Table 22-1 Alternative Whole Medical Systems

System	Examples
Traditional indigenous systems	Traditional oriental medicine Qi gong Acupuncture Herbal medicine Oriental massage Ayurvedic medicine Native American medicine Other folk medicine systems (Mexican, South American, etc.)expansion or dilation blood condition formation or presence of inflammation tumor falling or downward displacement
Unconventional Western systems	Homeopathy Naturopathy

Table 22-2 Types of Complementary and Alternative Practices

Classifications	Specific Therapies
Mind–body medicine	Relaxation exercises Hypnosis Meditation Dance Prayer Visualization Biofeedback
Biologically based practices	Herbal medicines Special diets Food supplements Vitamin therapy Biologic substances, such as bovine and shark cartilage
Manipulative and body-based practices	Chiropractic Massage therapy Reflexology
Energy medicine	BEM applications to the body Radiofrequency hyperthermia Radiofrequency diathermy Magnets Nerve stimulators Biofields—manipulations of energy fields originating within the body: Reiki, therapeutic touch

Whole Medical Systems

Whole medical systems represent complete systems of theory and practice that approach healthcare differently than the traditional Western biomedical approach. NCCAM has identified two approaches to entire systems of healthcare that differ from Western medicine: traditional indigenous systems and unconventional Western systems of medicine (NCCAM, 2010). Each system uses a variety of specific therapies.

Traditional Indigenous Systems. In indigenous medicine, there are complete systems of explanation for health and illness, and therapies are chosen based on these theoretic systems of belief.

Some indigenous systems are quite formal in approach, with individuals studying and serving apprenticeships before practice. These include traditional Asian medicine and ayurvedic medicine from India. Traditional Asian medicine may include the use of qi gong (a form of energy therapy), oriental massage, acupuncture, and herbs. Ayurvedic medicine, a traditional system from India, has existed for more than 5,000 years and has a specific theoretic and therapeutic focus on imbalance in the individual's consciousness. Lifestyle interventions are the major form of ayurvedic preventive and therapeutic treatment. As the popularity of Ayurvedic treatment has grown, a number of medical centers, retreats, and spas provide these treatments in the United States.

Informal approaches are often termed *folk medicine*; these traditions usually are handed down by word of mouth and are used by individuals and families to treat common health problems. Indigenous medicine practitioners use a variety of approaches to healthcare, often combining herbs, food, and traditional ceremonies. Little is understood about many of the herbs used, but some have demonstrated therapeutic effects while others may be questionable.

In a given ethnic group, certain people may be designated as healers or as having special knowledge and ability regarding illness. They may have had a period of apprenticeship, but it is informal in nature and not mandated by any outside authority. The advice of the indigenous healer may be sought instead of the advice of a physician. Native American cultures may use a *shaman*, or medicine man/woman. Mexican Americans may use the services of a *curandero*, or healer. A system of understanding hot and cold disorders and foods that help to balance heat and cold in the body is part of many of these folk traditions. NCCAM points out that "other traditional medical systems have been developed by Native American, Australian Aboriginal, African, Middle Eastern, Tibetan, Central and South American cultures" (NCCAM, 2010). To work most effectively with a client who uses folk medicine, you need to learn about the specific beliefs and resources that the client is using.

Unconventional Western Systems of Medicine. Unconventional Western systems of medicine originated in Western society but did not find general support. Some individuals continue to practice in the theoretic precepts of these systems and have reemerged as the public looks for alternatives to conventional medical care.

Perhaps the most common of these unconventional Western systems is homeopathy. **Homeopathy** is based on the belief that exposure to extremely small quantities of either the substance causing an illness or a related substance will stimulate a cure. Of course, this principle is also the basis for immunization and allergy desensitization. The application of this principle to other diseases, however, has not been accepted by the medical community. The dilutions used in many homeopathic remedies are so great that a dosage may contain only a few molecules of a substance. Homeopathy was popular in the early 20th century but fell into disrepute as standard medical research advanced. There is currently a resurgence of interest in this approach to therapy, and new research is being done. Homeopathic practitioners once again are offering an alternative to standard medical care.

Naturopathy gets its name from the natural agents used in treating disease, such as food, exercise, air, water, and sunshine. The naturopathic physician treats people by recommending changes in lifestyle, diet, and exercise, and promoting the use of vitamins and herbs. For many, lifestyle and dietary changes are a successful form of treatment. Naturopathic physicians follow a prescribed course of study that includes clinical experiences with clients and results in the doctor of naturopathy degree. Currently, 15 states, the District of Columbia, and the United States territories of Puerto Rico and the United States Virgin Islands have licensing laws for naturopathic doctors (The National Association of Naturopathic Physicians, 2010). However, questions have been raised about the use of naturopathic physicians in primary care, especially regarding the adequacy of their training in the recognition and treatment of more serious illnesses and the concern that many of the herbal remedies prescribed by naturopathic physicians are untested and unregulated.

Mind–Body Medicine

Mind–body medicine seeks to control physical processes through the mind's capacities. In addition, it treats emotional concerns. Increasingly, mind–body interventions are being incorporated into standard healthcare practice. Traditional psychotherapy, a well-established part of standard healthcare, is a mind–body approach to health. The use of prayer, support groups, yoga, meditation, relaxation, biofeedback, and visualization are all mind–body therapies.

Relaxation exercises, breathing techniques, meditation, and visualization are used to reduce anxiety, reduce blood pressure, and lessen the body's response to stressors. Yoga and other forms of controlled exercise also focus on breathing and mind-calming processes for these same purposes. While yoga originated in Hindu religious practices, most yoga in the United States keeps the techniques but does not include the religious philosophy. These techniques also are designed to prevent stress-related problems from developing; for many people, they are part of a plan to increase health and well-being. These techniques may be suggested for the management of specific health problems such as those causing pain or those related to cardiovascular responses and may be used in conjunction with traditional medical treatment.

Every major religion of the world responds in particular ways to those who are ill. A well-established way for supporting an ill person is through the prayers of others who care. Nurses recognize that spiritual distress has a significant impact on a client's ability to move toward wellness. Supporting the individual's quest for spiritual solace and healing has been a part of the mission of many healthcare agencies that were established by religious bodies. The separation of prayer and spiritual care from other healthcare is a modern phenomenon.

Visualization may be used to help children manage painful medical procedures. Suggestions regarding healing and postoperative recovery are used in the operating room by some anesthesiologists and surgeons. The anesthesiologist may talk to the patient who is still anesthetized, suggesting that pain will be minimal, nausea will not occur, and recovery will be rapid. This is similar to posthypnotic suggestion. Hypnosis has been used in other illnesses for symptom relief (Fig. 22.3).

Biofeedback is a specific mechanism used to assist individuals by altering physiologic responses through mental processes. The machines used for biofeedback provide visual or auditory feedback of physiologic parameters such as blood pressure or galvanic skin response. By observing these parameters, the individual learns to change the underlying physiologic process. Some individuals with migraine headaches use biofeedback control over circulation to abort migraine attacks rather than take medications. Biofeedback is recognized as effective for a variety of processes that are under autonomic nervous system control.

Mind–body interventions in general allow people to participate actively in their own care. People often are changed emotionally and psychologically in the process of treating illness or disease. A big advantage of the mind–body therapies is that they are safe and economical and can be used easily in conjunction with other therapies.

Biologically Based Practices

Biologically based practices include **herbal medicine**, special diets, food supplements, vitamins, and specific biologic substances such as bovine and shark cartilage. Nonvitamin, nonmineral natural products such as fish oil and flax seed are the most commonly used alternative medicine (NCCAM, 2008).

Herbal medicines are plant products that are used to treat illnesses. As research into plant products continues, our understanding of the efficacy of herbs increases. Many in the United States who describe themselves as herbalists received their training in herbs during an apprenticeship with an experienced herbalist. There are educational programs for herbalists, but they are not regulated in every state.

Potential problems in the use of herbs and supplements include unreliable dosage and bioavailability, safety and efficacy, and interactions with prescribed medications. The bioavailability of various herbal preparations may vary widely, making it difficult to stabilize dosage. And because plants grow under different circumstances and with different soil and other conditions, the proportion of active ingredient within the plant may vary considerably. This makes accurate and stable dosage of herbs difficult.

While herbal products are available in tablet form with doses listed on the label, at present, there are no laws regulating the potency or purity of herbs sold in the United States. Many herbs are imported from around the world where accurate labeling and content purity may not be monitored. Because herbs are not considered drugs, there are no regulations regarding testing for efficacy or safety, as there are with products that must be approved by the Food and Drug Administration (FDA). This means that some herbs that are sold may contain contaminants. Serious illnesses and even deaths have been traced to contaminants in herbal medicines.

Some countries, such as Germany, have regulated herbal medications for many years. Canada has a system of regulating "natural health products" that includes regulations for herbal and homeopathic remedies. The Canadian system is based on a phased-in process that addresses products with the highest risk potential first (Natural Health Products Directorate, 2006).

Sometimes the active ingredient in an herb may have potent side effects or interact with medications prescribed. The FDA took action to remove the herb ephedra from the market after severe illness, including stroke and cardiac effects, and death were associated with its use (FDA, 2004).

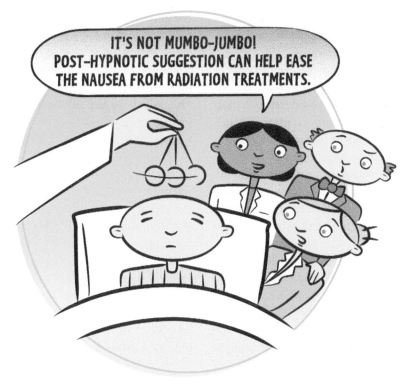

FIGURE 22.3 Alternative healthcare is moving more and more into mainstream practice.

When nurses interview patients regarding their medication history, asking specific questions about vitamins, herbs, supplements, and other therapeutic agents is critical. Patients may not consider these to be "medication" and so may not provide information about these substances being taken. The result may be that the source of an adverse response is missed or a harmful interaction with prescribed medications occurs. With increasing frequency, medical clinics and physicians' offices are asking clients to list on medical histories all over-the-counter medications, vitamins, and herbs as well as those requiring prescriptions.

Biologic treatments include a variety of substances not approved as medical treatment by the FDA. These products have been developed by individuals and organizations and are often sold as food supplements rather than as medicines. Cartilage products from sharks, cattle, sheep, and chickens are being used to treat both cancer and arthritis. Peptide fractions derived from human blood and urine, called antineoplastons, are being used to treat cancer. Coley's toxins are killed cultures of bacteria that have been used for treating cancer. Apitherapy is the use of honeybee venom to treat rheumatic diseases, dermatologic conditions, chronic pain, and cancer. Research

COMMUNICATION IN ACTION

Assisting With Complete Reporting

Maggie Wilson works in an ambulatory clinic. She is reviewing Mabel Wilson's written new patient information. As she speaks with Mrs. Wilson, she says, "I see that you wrote here that you take supplements. Would you please tell me exactly what supplements you are taking?" Mrs. Wilson says, "Oh, I figured those didn't make any difference; they aren't like real medicine or anything, just like food." Maggie replies, "Supplements need to be considered along with medicines because they all have some effect. Sometimes that is a benefit to you, but sometimes they could interfere with drugs that might be prescribed. Whenever you see a doctor, you need to be sure to let the doctor know all the prescribed medicines, over-the-counter medicines, and supplements that you use. Please tell me what you take so I can add them to your record."

on the efficacy of these treatments is costly, and sponsors willing to bear that cost are hard to find. Some small studies are being funded with federal grants.

Medical research is beginning to identify some benefits of using food and vitamins in therapeutic ways. We have long known that many individuals who develop type 2 diabetes may be able to manage their blood sugar through dietary control. The role of antioxidants in decreasing cell damage and the effect of certain phytochemicals contained in cruciferous vegetables in preventing bowel cancer are just two examples of the theoretic benefits of nutrients. Some parents have used strict dietary regulation as a management tool for children with attention deficit hyperactivity disorder.

There are hazards in this approach to healthcare, however. Megadoses of vitamins may prove toxic such as liver toxicity from excessive vitamin A. Some nutrients interact with medications, decreasing their effectiveness. Individuals who choose to avoid all traditional medical care and rely on unsubstantiated claims about the therapeutic effects of nutrients may suffer deterioration in health.

All healthcare professionals need to support and encourage healthy dietary practices. Often it is possible to assist clients who rely on the use of nutrients for healthcare by becoming knowledgeable about the research regarding nutrition, accepting what clients believe helps them (as long as it is not detrimental to their well-being), and keeping an open mind. When we are willing to acknowledge the validity of some aspects of their preferred approach to healthcare, these clients may be willing to combine more conventional medical care along with their nutritional approaches.

Manipulative and Body-Based Practices

Manipulative and body-based practices include the physical manipulation of the body to achieve health goals. Some authors refer to these as "manual healing." Manipulative therapy is found in massage therapy and reflexology. Massage therapy uses both fixed and movable pressure and holding by the hands and sometimes the forearms, elbows, or feet. There is evidence that these techniques affect the musculoskeletal, circulatory–lymphatic, and nervous systems. Reflexology is massage of the feet to activate points on the feet that correspond to other body parts or systems.

Perhaps the most commonly known type of manipulative practice is chiropractic. Chiropractic care is based on the theory that disease is caused by interference with nerve function. It uses manipulation of the body joints, especially the spinal vertebrae, in seeking to restore normal function. The chiropractor also may use other treatments commonly associated with physical therapy, such as massage and exercise. There are definite differences among chiropractors. Some state that there are illnesses that cannot be treated through manual healing and do recommend that certain clients seek conventional medical care. Others believe that all illnesses may be treated by chiropractic methods and do not refer clients for conventional medical care. A major concern is that some clients may have more serious illnesses that may be missed altogether or not recognized in time to be given optimal medical attention. Another problem with chiropractic care is the use of chiropractic treatments on infants and young children in place of immunizations and other well-child services. Many people with joint and muscle strain and tension find that chiropractic treatments relieve discomfort and support effective functioning.

Acupuncture, which is a part of traditional Chinese medicine, is growing in popularity as an alternative care practice. While primarily used for managing musculoskeletal pain where evidence of efficacy is accumulating, acupuncture has also been used to control appetite for weight loss. There are few adverse effects; most, including infection from nonsterile needles and penetration of organs, are associated with unskilled practitioners.

Energy Medicine

The use of **energy medicine** (sometimes referred to bioelectromagnetic [BEM] therapies) is based on the understanding that electrical phenomena are found in all living organisms. There are magnetic fields that extend from the body, which can be measured and may be affected by external forces. The mechanisms by which the electromagnetic fields occur in the body, how these can be changed, and the effects of such changes are under study. Many modalities have been used for years without clear studies of their effectiveness. Some believe that BEM may be a unifying theory explaining why such widely diverse therapies as acupuncture and homeopathy produce results.

Some energy medicine is based on applying external energy to the body. There are thermal applications of BEM therapy in the form of radiofrequency hyperthermia and radiofrequency diathermy. Nonthermal applications include magnets and nerve stimulation. One common application is the use of magnets to relieve musculoskeletal problems. Magnetic insoles for shoes and magnets to be worn on the body are widely available.

There are also methods used to manipulate the interior biofields of the individual. These include therapeutic touch and Reiki. Both of these practices are based on a system of changing the energy fields without applying external energy forces to the body. In therapeutic touch, the practitioner moves hands above the body or touches lightly, perceives energy fields, and modifies them through hand movements. While the originator of therapeutic touch (Krieger, 1979) and some practitioners claim that their research supports this practice, others studying therapeutic touch have not been able to discern either the energy fields or methods of change and find the methodology of those studies reporting effectiveness to be flawed (Bullough & Bullough, 1998; Coursey, n.d.). Therapeutic touch has found acceptance by some within the nursing community, and a nursing diagnosis titled "energy field disturbance" has been included in the NANDA-I taxonomy. This is a matter of controversy, and there are strong objections by some to its inclusion without replicable research support. Nurses interested in therapeutic touch should research it further.

Understanding the Use of Complementary and Alternative Healthcare

According to the 2007 survey by NCAM (2008), the use of alternative and complementary therapies is increasing. For many clients with chronic conditions, mainstream medical care offers few options. Long-term treatments with medications often produce their own iatrogenic (treatment-caused) health problems, some of which are as troubling to the individual as the original disease process. A common response of conventional medicine to these problems has been to add more medications and more treatments, each with its own potential adverse effects. Mainstream healthcare providers often give little attention to the problems of daily living that are of greatest concern to the individual. Stress and anxiety also add to the burden of these clients. For clients with acute health conditions, certain treatments or medications may produce unpleasant or harmful side effects. Clients often are looking for alternative treatment methods that do not appear to have the same potential for harm.

Some alternative therapies have been available for many years, and there are people who believe that they have been helped significantly by these approaches. Unfortunately, traditional healthcare providers often have dismissed these therapies without investigating them thoroughly. On the other hand, few alternative therapies have been formally researched, and proponents often rely on undocumented reports of effectiveness.

Research into alternative therapies now is supported by the federal government but only in a small way compared to other research. The federal government has an Office of Alternative Healthcare, the NCCAM, and a Web page of references (see list of Web sites). More attention is being paid to the responses of individuals. Concern about the role of stress in illness has prompted an increased openness to nonmedical methods of managing stress. The possibility of alternative care practices working in a complementary fashion with traditional medical care is gaining wider acceptance. Often these complementary therapies are used to address the whole person and not simply the disease.

Part of the appeal of alternative healthcare is the caring and personalized response that clients often receive. People who have been intimidated by businesslike clinics and made to feel unimportant by impersonal professionals may find that the warm, concerned, accepting atmosphere of the nonconventional setting meets many personal needs. The fact that stress and anxiety play a major role in any health problem may help explain why many people are helped by therapies that may not be based on sound scientific knowledge. Because of the trust placed in nurses, they are in a unique position to relate with people about the issues that surround alternative and complementary therapy. Gallup polls continue to identify nurses as the most trusted professionals when ethics are considered (Gallup Poll, 2010).

To learn more about any specific therapy, or to research alternative and complementary therapies for any condition, use the CAM Citation Index found on the Web site of the NCCAM (see references). You may also search MEDLINE, the database of the National Library of Medicine, through the free PubMed Web site (*www.nlm.nih.gov/nccam/camonpubmed.html*) to research various therapies.

Assisting Clients Who Choose Alternative Healthcare

Many people who support conventional methods of healthcare have long ignored or repudiated the value of unorthodox healthcare traditions. We must recognize that complementary and alternative healthcare practices persist because people find them to be valuable. Acknowledging healthcare alternatives and working cooperatively with them is usually much more productive than trying to oppose them.

NCCAM suggests a five-step process for the consumer considering a particular complementary or alternative therapy. This process has a heavy emphasis on careful information gathering.

Assess Safety and Effectiveness

The first step is for the individual to assess the safety and effectiveness of the therapy in relationship to his or her own condition. One of the difficulties is finding accurate safety and efficacy data. Web sites and other sources of information require close scrutiny to determine the qualifications and bias of the sponsoring individual or group. The NCCAM Web site (*www.nccam.nih.gov*) contains Fact Sheets regarding specific therapies and additional links to research reports and scientific papers. Research reports may also be found through PubMed, the National Library of Medicine's online access (*www.ncbi.nlm.nih.gov/PubMed*). All complementary and alternative therapies are classified there under the Medical Subject Heading of "complementary therapies." The University of Pittsburgh Health Sciences Library System maintains an Alternative Medicine Homepage (*www.pitt.edu/~cbw/altm.html*) that provides links to additional information sites on the Web.

Examine the Expertise of the Therapy Practitioner

The second step is to examine the expertise of any therapy practitioner. Whether this person is a physician or another type of provider, determine whether there is appropriate education and licensing if that is required. Consumers should be encouraged to ask directly about education and credentials for practice. Some consumer organizations will direct individuals to reliable practitioners in the community. Clients who may be reluctant to ask directly about credentials can check whether credentials are available on a Web site or in printed information from the practitioner.

Investigate Service Delivery

Service delivery is the third aspect the client should investigate. How many patients are seen per day? Where is the therapy available and what barriers does that pose? Are standards for safety, privacy, and confidentiality in place? Remember that alternative providers are not included in the federal Health Insurance Portability and Accountability Act of 1996 legislation that mandates confidentiality in conventional healthcare settings unless they are eligible for reimbursement through Medicare or Medicaid. Most alternative providers are responsible for establishing their own standards and policies without outside oversight.

Research the Cost of Therapy

A fourth consideration is the cost of the therapy. Part of this is investigating what coverage may be obtained from an insurance carrier or whether any is available. Are the costs clear? How are payments made? Some unscrupulous practitioners collect large sums of money before any service and then may not provide what was promised. Some types of alternative care (eg, chiropractic care for an acute back injury) may be reimbursable under a traditional health plan.

Discuss the Treatment with Your Regular Healthcare Provider

The fifth step is to discuss this proposed treatment with a regular healthcare provider. The interaction of any traditional treatment and a complementary or alternative treatment may or may not pose a problem. Many healthcare providers support the use of various complementary therapies.

Things that the healthcare provider must also consider are such issues as client choice, informed consent, and the ethical principles of beneficence and nonmaleficence. As complementary and alternative therapies move into the mainstream, greater accountability to the public is essential.

 Critical Thinking Activity

Identify a specific form of complementary or alternative therapy. Search the health literature regarding this therapy. Review the information available in other sources. Analyze the information to determine whether the data supporting the use of this therapy are weak, moderate, or strong. Provide a rationale for your determination.

Don't forget to visit thePoint companion website for additional study resources!

CHAPTER HIGHLIGHTS

- Community-based nursing emphasizes advocating for patients, promoting self-care, focusing on health promotion and disease prevention, and recognizing the importance of family, culture, and the community.
- Health promotion and prevention of illness and disease are a part of nursing practice in all settings.
- Client empowerment through teaching, explaining options, and supporting decision making is a foundation for community-based care.
- Primary prevention focuses on preventing disease; secondary prevention focuses on early diagnosis through screening and preventing complications; tertiary prevention focuses on preventing long-term disability and restoring functional capacity.
- Disease management strives to promote health through effective treatment of targeted diseases and health conditions.
- Healthy People 2020 is a federal effort that includes overall goals, priority areas, and leading indicators to measure progress in developing healthier communities.
- Maintaining continuity of care requires transition planning, with special emphasis on reconciling medication records from one setting to another.
- Ensuring that healthcare records are available wherever the client seeks care is becoming a possibility through computerization of medical records and the development of transportable records that contain essential information.
- Alternative healthcare encompasses those types of care outside of conventional Western medicine and includes mind–body medicine, biologically based practices, manipulative and body-based practices, and energy medicine as well as alternative whole medical systems.
- Alternative care therapies are considered complementary therapies when used along with traditional medical care. Integrative medicine involves the deliberative planning for using both traditional medical care and alternative care in a coordinated manner.
- Understanding the different types of alternative healthcare services, why people choose alternative healthcare, and how nurses may assist people who seek this care will form a foundation for more effective relationships with clients.
- Alternative and complementary therapies can be evaluated based on a five-step process that includes safety and effectiveness of the therapy, credentials of the provider, service delivery, cost of services, and consultation with the regular healthcare provider.

WEB SITES FOR SELECTED PROFESSIONAL ORGANIZATIONS

Web sites relevant to this chapter can be found at accessed through *http://thePoint.lww.com/activate* and by entering the code found on the inside cover of your text.

RECOMMENDED READING

American Red Cross. (2009). *Preparing and getting trained: preparedness fast facts*. Retrieved January 6, 2011, from http://www.redcross.org/

ASTM International. (2005). ASTM Standard E2369-051. *Continuity of care record (CCR)*. West Conshohocken, PA: Author. Retrieved January 7, 2011, from www.astm.org/Standards/E2369.htm

Bullough, V. L. & Bullough, B. (1998). Should nurses practice therapeutic touch? Should nursing schools teach therapeutic touch? *Journal of Professional Nursing, 14*(4), 254–257.

Corepoint Health. (2009). *The continuity of care document: changing the landscape of healthcare information exchange*. Retrieved January 6, 2011, from http://www.corepointhealth.com/sites/default/files/whitepapers/continuity-of-care-document-ccd.pdf

Coursey, K. (n.d.) Further notes on therapeutic touch. *Quackwatch*. Retrieved January 4, 2011, from http://www.quackwatch.org/01QuackeryRelatedTopics/tt2.html

Food and Drug Administration. (2004). *FDA acts to remove ephedra-containing dietary supplements from market.* Retrieved January 6, 2011, from http://www.fda.gov/NewsEvents/Newsroom/ PressAnnouncements/2004/ucm108379.htm

Gallup Poll. (2010). *Nurses top honesty and ethics list for 11th year, 2010.* Retrieved January 5, 2011, from http://www.gallup.com/poll/145043/Nurses-Top-Honesty-Ethics-List-11-Year.aspx

Joint Commission on Accreditation of Healthcare Organizations. (2010). *National patient safety goal on reconciling medication information.* Retrieved January 5, 2011, from http://www.joint-commission.org/npsg_ reconciling_medication/

Krieger, D. (1979). *Therapeutic touch.* New York, NY: Prentice-Hall.

National Association of Naturopathic Physicians. (2010). *Licensed states & licensing authorities.* Retrieved January 5, 2011 from http://www.naturopathic.org/content.asp?contentid=57

National Center for Complementary and Alternative Medicine. (2008). *The use of complementary and alternative medicine in the United States.* Retrieved January 4, 2011 from http://nccam.nih. gov/news/camsurvey_fs1.htm

National Center for Complementary and Alternative Medicine. (2010). *What is complementary and alternative medicine?* NCCAM Publication No. D347. Retrieved January 6, 2011 from http://nccam.nih.gov/health/whatiscam/

Natural Health Products Directorate. (2006). *National health products master file.* Retrieved January 5, 2011 from http://www.hc-sc.gc.ca/dhp-mps/prodnatur/legislation/docs/master_ file_fichier_principal-eng.php

US Department of Health and Human Services (US-DHHS) (January, 2010) About Healthy People, Washington, DC. Retrieved April 19, 2011 from http://www.healthypeople. gov/2020/about/default.aspx.

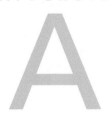

Professional and Government Resource Organizations

Patient Care

American Academy of Physician Assistants. Available at: http://www.aapa.org

American Association of Medical Assistants. Available at: http://www.aama-ntl.org

American Society of Podiatric Medical Assistants. Available at: http://www.aspma.org

American Medical Technologists. Available at: http://www.amt1.com

Association of Surgical Technologists. Available at: http://www.ast.org

National Association of Emergency Medical Technicians. Available at: http://www.naemt.org

American Optometric Association. Available at: http://www.aoa.org

Joint Commission on Allied Health Personnel in Ophthalmology. My Eye Career for Ophthalmic Medical Technicians. Available at: http://www.myeyecareer.org/OMP/OMPSplash.html

Nursing

American Academy of Nurse Practitioners. Available at: http://www.aanp.org

American Association of Nurse Anesthetists. Available at: http://www.aana.com

American College of Nurse-Midwives. Available at: http://www.acnm.org

American Nurses Association. Available at: http://www.nursingworld.org

National Association for Practical Nurse Education and Service, Inc. Available at: http://www.napnes.org

National Association of Health Care Assistants. Available at: http://www.nahcacares.org

National Federation of Licensed Practical Nurses, Inc. Available at: http://www.nflpn.org

Dental

American Dental Assistants Association. Available at: http://www.dentalassistant.org

Dental Assisting National Board. Available at: http://www.danb.org

American Dental Association. Available at: http://www.ada.org

American Dental Hygienists' Association. Available at: http://www.adha.org

Laboratory and Pharmacy Services

Accreditation Council for Pharmacy Education. Available at: http://www.acpe-accredit.org

American Society of Health-System Pharmacists. Available at: http://www.ashpfoundation.org

American Association of Pharmacy Technicians. Available at: http://www.pharmacytechnician.com

National Pharmacy Technician Association. Available at: http://www.pharmacytechnician.org

National Pharmaceutical Association. Available at: http://www.npha.net

American Medical Technologists. Available at: http://www.amt1.com

American Society for Clinical Laboratory Science. Available at: http://www.ascls.org

National Accrediting Agency for Clinical Laboratory Sciences. Available at: http://www.naacls.org

Diagnostic and Imaging Services

Alliance of Cardiovascular Professionals. Available at: http://www.acp-online.org

Cardiovascular Credentialing International. Available at: http://www.acp-online.org

American Medical Technologists. Available at: http://www.amt1.com

American Society for Clinical Pathology. Available at: http://www.ascp.org

American Society of Echocardiography. Available at: http://www.asecho.org

American Society of Radiologic Technologists. Available at: https://www.asrt.org (Visit the Career Center.)

Society of Nuclear Medicine. Available at: http://www.snm.org

Society for Vascular Ultrasound. Available at: http://www.svunet.org

Society of Diagnostic Medical Sonography. Available at: http://www.sdms.org

American Registry for Diagnostic Medical Sonography. Available at: http://www.ardms.org

National Phlebotomy Organization. Available at: http://www.nationalphlebotomy.org

American Registry of Radiologic Technologists. Available at: https://www.arrt.org

American Society of Radiologic Technologists. Available at: https://www.asrt.org

Nuclear Medicine Technology Certification Board. Available at: http://www.nmtcb.org

Therapy and Rehabilitation

American Association for Respiratory Care. Available at: http://www.aarc.org

American Massage Therapy Association. Available at: http://www.amtamassage.org

American Occupational Therapy Association. Available at: http://www.aota.org

American Physical Therapy Association. Available at: http://www.apta.org

Associated Bodywork & Massage Professionals. Available at: http://www.abmp.com

Health Information and Administration

American Academy of Professional Coders. Available at: http://www.aapc.com

American Health Information Management Association. Available at: http://www.ahima.org

Association for Healthcare Documentation Integrity. Available at: http://www.ahdionline.org

The Professional Association of Healthcare Coding Specialists. Available at: http://www.pahcs.org

Other Health Resources

American Institute of Biological Sciences. Careers in the Biological Sciences. Available at: http://www.aibs.org/careers/#1

American Society for Clinical Pathology. The Pathology Profession. Available at: http://www.ascp.org/MainMenu/pathologists/CareerCenter.aspx

American Society for Microbiology. Meet the Scientist with Carl Zimmer. Available at: http://www.microbeworld.org/index.php?option=com_content&view=category&id=37:meet-the-scientist&layout=blog&Itemid=155

Johnson & Johnson Services, Inc. DiscoverNursing.com. Available at: http://www.discovernursing.com

Nemko M. Best Careers 2009: Biomedical Equipment Technician. *U.S. News & World Report* [serial online]. December 11, 2008. Available at: http://www.usnews.com/articles/business/best-careers/2008/12/11/best-careers-2009-biomedical-equipment-technician.html

Smith S. Young leaders in industrial hygiene. *Occupational Hazards*. May 2008;70(5):25–28.

Thilman J. Working backward [biomedical engineering]. *Mechanical Engineering*. July 2008;130(7):30–34.

University of Minnesota. Outbreak at WatersEdge: A Public Health Discovery Game. Available at: http://www.mclph.umn.edu/watersedge/.

Weir K. Body builders [biomedical engineers who design prosthetics and orthotic devices]. *Career World*. January 2008;36(4):24–26.

Preparing for a Successful Interview

Preparing for a successful interview in a health career is in many ways no different from other fields. Job candidates need to present themselves in the best possible light. Some of the most effective ways to do this are described below.

Preparation

- Research:
  - Find out everything you can about the organization with whom you'll be interviewing.
  - Get a grasp of the tasks and responsibilities of the position for which you're interviewing.
  - Look online for examples of typical interview questions as well as the kinds of questions your might face in your particular field.
  - Seek out typical wages and salary ranges for your field and the position for which you're interviewing.
- Prepare:
  - Make notes about specific experiences in your education and work to date and connect them with your understanding of the job's expectations.
  - Rehearse out loud answers to questions you expect to be asked.
  - Articulate your strengths, weaknesses, and the reasons you want to obtain the position.
  - Formulate questions about the organization and about the position.
  - Contact the people you will use as references to ensure they can recommend you, to alert them that your prospective employer may contact them, and to verify their contact information.
  - Find out whatever you can about the interview situation: will you be interviewed by a panel? By several different people in succession?

- If possible, find out the steps in the hiring process; if you do well in your interview, you'll want to understand what's next.

Professionalism

- Appropriate attire:
  - For most interview situations men should wear a suit with a collared shirt and tie, while women should wear a skirt or pantsuit with a modest blouse or sweater underneath.
  - Shoes must be in good repair and clean.
  - Tattoos and body jewelry should not be visible.
  - Women may wear light natural-looking make-up to enhance appearance, but must take care to avoid bright colors.
  - Men should be clean-shaven or facial hair should be carefully groomed.
- Personal hygiene:
  - Ensure that your hair is clean and neat.
  - Fingernails should be clean and trimmed.
  - Your teeth must be clean and your breath fresh.
- Professional behavior:
  - Ensure that your cellular phone and other devices are switched off before you enter the interview site. (For example, you should not be texting or having a personal conversation while you're in the waiting area for the interview.)
  - Do not chew gum.

At the Interview

- Make sure you know the location of the interview site and how to get there, and scout out potential barriers to arriving on time.

- Aim to arrive 10–15 minutes before the scheduled interview time.
- It's natural to feel nervous, but remember your preparation, your training, education, and work experiences, and stay calm.
- Put aside any shyness or timidity you may feel. Speak with confidence.
- Pay attention to your non-verbal communication. Sit up straight, make eye contact, and avoid fidgeting.

- Avoid making any negative comments about previous experiences or employers.
- Send thank you letters within one day of the interview to everyone with whom you interviewed.

Even if you are not offered the position, regard each interview as a learning experience and practice for the next!

C

Metric Conversion Table

Unit	Abbreviation	Metric Equivalent	U.S. Equivalent
Units of length			
kilometer	km	1,000 m	0.62 mi; 1.6 km/mi
meter	m	100 cm; 1,000 mm	39.4 in; 1.1 yds
centimeter	cm	1/100 m; 0.01m	0.39 in; 2/5 cm/in
millimeter	mm	1/1,000 m; 0.001 m	0.039 in; 25 mm/in
micrometer	μm	1/1,000 mm; 0.001 mm	
Units of weight			
kilogram	kg	1,000 g	2.2 lb
gram	g	1,000 mg	0.035 oz; 28.5 g/oz
milligram	mg	1/1,000 g; 0.001 g	
microgram	μg	1/1,000 mg; 0.001 mg	
Units of volume			
liter	L	1,000 mL	1.06 qt
deciliter	dL	1/10 L; 0.1 L	
milliliter	mL	1/1,000 L; 0.001 L	0.034 oz; 29.4 mL/oz
microliter	μL, mcL	1/1,000 mL; 0/001 mL	

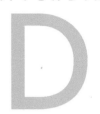

Common Abbreviations and Symbols

Abbreviation	Meaning
$\bar{a}$	before
abd	abdomen
ac	before meals
ADLs	activities of daily living
ad lib	as needed
adm.	admitted, admission
amp.	ampule
ant.	anterior
AP	anterior-posterior
ax.	axillary
b.i.d.	twice a day
BP	blood pressure
BR	bed rest
BRP	bathroom privileges
C	Centigrade
$\bar{c}$	with
caps	capsule
C.C.	chief complaint
cc	cubic centimeters (1 cc = 1 mL)
CVP	central venous pressure
c/o	complaints of
D/C	discontinue
disch; DC	discharge
drsg	dressing
dr	dram
elix	elixir
ext	extract or external
F	Fahrenheit
fx	fracture, fractional
gm	gram

Abbreviation	Meaning
gr	grain
gtt	drop
"H," SC, or sub q	hypodermic or subcutaneous
h	hour
HOB	head of bed
h.s.	bedtime (hour of sleep)
hx	history
I & O	intake & output
IM	intramuscular
IV	intravenous
kg	kilogram
KVO	keep vein open
L	left; liter
lat	lateral
MAE	moves all extremities
mg	milligram
ml, mL	milliliter (1 mL = 1 cc)
NAD	no apparent distress
NG	nasogastric
noc	night
NPO	no apparent distress
os	mouth
OOB	out of bed
oz	ounce
$\bar{p}$	after
p.c.	after meals
post	posterior
prep	preparation
prn	when necessary
$\bar{q}$, q	every

(continued)

Abbreviation	Meaning
$\overline{q}$, 2 (3, 4, etc.) hours	every 2 (3, 4, etc.) hours
qd	every day
qh	every hour
q.i.d.	four times a day
qod	every other day
q.s.	quantity sufficient
R/O	rule out
ROM	range of motion
$\overline{s}$	without
SBA	stand by assistance
SC	subcutaneous
SL	sublingual
SOB	shortness of breath
sol, soln	solution
spec	specimen
S/P	status post
sp. gr.	specific gravity
S.S.E.	soapsuds enema
ss	one half
stat	immediately
tab	tablet
t.i.d.	three times a day
tinct or tr.	tincture
TKO	to keep open
TPN	total parenteral nutrition
TPR	temperature, pulse, respiration
tsp	teaspoon
TO	telephone order
TWE	tap water enema
VO	verbal order
VS	vital signs

Abbreviation	Meaning
VSS	vital signs stable
W/C	wheelchair
WNL	within normal limits
>	greater than
<	less than
=	equal to
~	approximately equal to
≤	equal to or less than
≥	equal to or greater than
↑	increased
↓	decreased
♀	female
♂	male
°	degree
#	number or pound
×	times
@	at
+	positive
−	negative
±	positive or negative
F_1	first filial generation
F_2	second filial generation
PO_2	partial pressure oxygen
PCO_2	partial pressure carbon dioxide
:	ratio
∴	therefore
%	percent
2°	secondary to
Δ	change

Glossary

A

accreditation—an educational institution that is recognized by an outside agency, such as a national board or commission, as having standards that qualify graduates for professional practice

acculturation—a process by which a member of a minority group shifts his or her identity from the minority group to the dominant group and adopts the values, attitudes, and behaviors of the dominant culture; also known as *cultural assimilation*

acronym—a word created from the first letter of each word in a phrase or each item on a list

acrostic—a phrase or sentence created from the first letter of each item on a list

acute care facility—a health care facility that provides care for patients who have extremely serious, severe, or painful conditions that require immediate medical attention

administrative tasks—job duties that usually involve carrying out office procedures

advanced practice nurse—a registered nurse who has more extensive education and training and a broader set of work responsibilities, which may include providing primary care

aerobic—requiring oxygen to live

airborne disease—disease that is spread from person to person through droplets in the air.

altruism—concern for the welfare and well-being of others

anaerobic—does not require oxygen to live

antiseptics—agents commonly used to disinfect wounds or cuts

assault—a threat or attempt to touch someone without that person's permission

assisted-living facility—a facility that generally provides housing, group meals, personal care, support services, and social activities in a community setting

autocratic leadership—a leadership style whereby the leader assumes complete control over the decisions and activities of the group; also known as *directive leadership*

autonomy—the right to self-determination or personal independence

B

bactericidal—an infection control method that kills microorganisms; also known as *germicidal*

bacteriology—the study of bacteria

bacteriostatic—agents that inhibit the growth of microorganisms, but do not kill them

balloon angioplasty—a procedure in which a balloon attached to the end of a catheter is used to clear blockages in blood vessels

battery—an offensive touch or use of force on a nonconsenting person

biotechnology—the manipulation of genetic material in living organisms, or parts of living organisms, to make products and services

blood-borne disease—disease that is spread from person to person when an infected person's blood or certain other body fluids come into contact with the mucous membranes or bloodstream of an uninfected person

body language—nonverbal communication that relays a message without speaking or writing a single word

bridge—an artificial tooth or crown attached to adjoining teeth

bronchoscopy—a procedure in which a flexible tube is inserted into the nose or mouth and through the trachea to view the lungs

C

cardiac catheterization—a procedure in which a tube is inserted into a vein and guided toward the heart to reveal blood vessel blockages

career ladder—a hierarchy of careers in a field. In nearly all cases, a person needs more education or training to move from a lower career on the ladder to a higher one

carrier—a person infected with a pathogen

Centers for Disease Control and Prevention (CDC)—a U.S. government agency dedicated to the prevention and control of disease, injury, and disability

certification—a credential from a professional organization that shows that a health care worker meets the requirements set by the certifying organization to demonstrate mastery of the job

certified nursing assistant (CNA)—a health care professional who performs simple, basic nursing functions and care for patients' personal needs under the direction of an LPN or RN; sometimes known by other titles, such as certified nurse assistant, nursing assistant, or nursing aide

channel of communication—the medium by which a message is sent

charting by exception format—an abbreviated documentation method that makes use of well-defined standards of practice and documents only significant or abnormal findings

chemical burn—a lesion that results when a wet or dry corrosive substance comes into contact with the skin or mucous membranes

chest physiotherapy—a variety of techniques used to eliminate secretions, re-expand lung tissue, and promote efficient use of respiratory muscles

chronological order—an arrangement of items or events in the order of time

chronological organization—a method of organizing information in written communication whereby items are presented in sequence, from the earliest date to the most recent date

civil law—a body of law, sometimes referred to as private law, that focuses on issues between private citizens, such as medical malpractice

civil rights—the rights of personal liberty held by all U.S. citizens and guaranteed by the 13th and 14th amendments to the Constitution and by acts of Congress

clarification—the act of making a message more understandable

clinical decision support system (CDSS)—a computerized expert system that provides administrative, clinical, cost control, and decision support for several activities in a health care institution

clinical tasks—tasks that involve examining and helping treat patients

co-insurance—the portion of the medical costs a patient may still have to pay once an insurance plan's deductible has been met (typically a percentage of the total amount the health care provider charges)

common law—a traditional civil law of an area or region resulting from rulings by judges on individual disputes or cases

communication—the exchange of information

comparison organization—a method of organizing information in written communication whereby two or more pieces of information are compared

competence—the ability to perform specific functions accurately and in a timely manner

complementary therapies—treatment methods that typically promote healing through nutrition, exercise, or relaxation; sometimes referred to as alternative medicine

computerized physician/provider order entry system (CPOE)—a computerized system that allows licensed health care professionals to enter medical orders, resulting in reduced errors

conflict—a disagreement between team members; conflict is to be expected when a variety of personalities are brought together on a team

constitutional rights—the rights afforded to all citizens through the U.S. Constitution

co-pay—a flat fee that many health insurance plans require patients to pay each time they receive a health care service

critical thinking—a systematic way to form and shape one's thinking that functions purposefully and exactingly

crown—a cap for broken or weak teeth

cultural assimilation—a process by which a member of a minority group shifts his or her identity from the minority group to the dominant group and adopts the values, attitudes, and behaviors of the dominant culture; also known as *acculturation*

cultural diversity—a group of people whose members are characterized by a wide range of distinctions, including race, national origin, religion, language, physical size, and gender

culture—a shared system of beliefs, values, and behavioral expectations that provide social structure for daily living

cytology—the study of the structure of cells

D

deductible—the money a person must pay before an insurance policy provides benefits

defamation of character—the act of harming another person's reputation by making false or malicious statements

democratic leadership—a leadership style that promotes a sense of equality between the leader and the other participants by sharing decisions and activities among all members of the team

dental assistant—a trained professional who assists a dentist and performs both clinical and administrative work under a dentist's supervision

dental hygienist—a trained professional who works under a dentist's supervision and provides a wide range of dental services focused on preventing and treating tooth and gum disease and promoting good oral hygiene and health

dentures—dental appliances that replace missing teeth

development—an orderly pattern of changes in structure, thoughts, feelings, or behaviors resulting from maturation, life experiences, and learning

diagnostic related group (DRG)—a classification system used by Medicare and Medicaid to determine payment for health services based on diagnosis, surgical procedures, age, and other information

diagnostic services—health care services that determine the presence, absence, or extent of disease and provide data on the effectiveness of treatment

direct patient care—care that involves hands-on contact with patients

direct payment—the act of paying for health care with one's own money

directive leadership—a leadership style whereby the leader assumes complete control over the decisions and activities of the group; also known as *autocratic leadership*

disinfection—the use of a disinfectant agent to destroy many pathogens; however, it does not destroy all microorganisms and bacterial spores

distress—a type of stress that causes a negative reaction

dominant group—the group within a society that tends to control that society's values

durable power of attorney for health care—a legal document that designates a person to make health care decisions on behalf of a patient in the event the patient becomes incapacitated

E

echocardiography—the use of ultrasound to examine the heart and blood vessels

electrical burn—a lesion that results when skin comes into contact with electricity or lightning

electrocardiogram (EKG or ECG)—a test that records the electrical activity of the heart

electronic medical record (EMR)—an electronic document that contains patient health information, gathered from different sources

electrophysiology—the study of electrical activity in the body

embryo—the developing offspring during the first eight weeks of life

encryption—an electronic security feature that ensures that all email messages are scrambled and can't be read by anyone other than the intended recipient

ethics—sets of guidelines set by professional organizations that determine right or wrong behavior

ethnicity—a sense of identification with a group based on a common heritage

ethnocentrism—the belief or assumption that a particular social or cultural group is superior in some way

exposure report—a document completed by health care providers when a patient or a provider has been exposed to a biohazard; also known as an *incident report*

extended care facility—a facility that provides health care and help with the activities of daily living to people who may be physically or mentally unable to care for themselves; this type of care may last from days to years

F

false imprisonment—an illegal act that occurs when an attempt is made to restrain an individual or restrict the person's freedom

familial—when a disease tends to occur often in a particular family

feedback—in communication, a response that is sent back to the sender

fetus—the developing child in the uterus from the beginning of the third month until birth

flexible spending account (FSA)—a monetary account, offered through an employer, into which money is put through payroll deductions, before it is taxed. Funds can be withdrawn for qualified medical expenses as needed, but the funds must be spent each year

fluoroscopy—a type of test that uses a continuous beam of X rays to observe movement in the body

folk medicine—a form of prevention and treatment that uses old-fashioned remedies and household medicines handed down from generation to generation within a particular culture

G

gatekeeper—a physician who not only delivers primary care services, but also makes referrals for specialty care

general practitioner—a physician who diagnoses and treats a variety of common health problems

germicidal—an infection control method that kills microorganisms; also known as *bactericidal*

gestation—the period of development from conception to birth

government institution—a public health care facility that receives most of its funding from local, state, or federal sources

government plan—a health care plan funded by a government agency. Government plans are available for active military personnel and their dependents and for veterans. Medicaid and Medicare are also government-funded health care programs

group dynamics—the way in which individual group members relate to one another

H

health care cost containment—measures designed to lower health care costs that aim to create an affordable health care system for all Americans

health care team—a group of health care professionals who often have a variety of health-related backgrounds, education, and experiences

health informatics—a broad category of health data and related health care occupations that uses information technology to manage and share files containing medical records, test results, prescription history, billing details, and health insurance coverage; also known as *medical informatics*

Health Insurance Portability and Accountability Act (HIPAA)—a law that was enacted to protect a patient's right to privacy; it protects a patient's personal health information from being used or shared without the patient's written consent

health maintenance organization (HMO) plan—a health insurance plan that provides coverage only if the care is delivered by a member of the plan's hospital, physician, or pharmacy panel

health savings account (HSA)—a monetary account commonly paired with a high-deductible health insurance plan that allows individuals to pay for qualified medical care using tax-free HSA dollars until they meet their deductibles. Any funds remaining in an HSA at the end of each year are rolled over and can be saved for future use

hepatitis—a disease that causes inflammation of the liver

hereditary—inherited genetically; there is a greater likelihood that offspring may develop hereditary diseases or disorders if one or both parents have the disease or disorder

Hippocratic oath—was an oath written by Hippocrates of Cos that serves as the moral basis for many medical regulations and guidelines still in use today

histology—the study of the microscopic structure of tissue

holistic—treating both mind and body

Holter monitor—a portable EKG device worn by a patient

home health care—care provided in a patient's home through community health departments, visiting nurses' associations, hospital-based case managers, and home health agencies

homeopathy—a holistic system of healing that focuses on stimulating the body's ability to heal itself by giving very small doses of highly diluted substances

hospice—a care program focused on reducing pain, symptoms, and stress during the last stage of terminal illnesses

host—the person to whom a pathogen is transported after leaving the reservoir host

human dignity—the quality or state of acknowledging individuals' worthiness; to value human dignity is to respect the inherent worth and uniqueness of individuals

human immunodeficiency virus (HIV)—a virus that slowly wears down a person's immune system and, in most cases, causes the person to develop acquired immune deficiency syndrome (AIDS)

human rights—the fundamental rights of all people

I

immigrate—to settle in a new country

implied consent—when a patient gives permission for his or her care, but without a formal written agreement

incapacitated—being unable to make one's own medical decisions

incident report—a document completed by health care providers when a patient or a provider has been exposed to a biohazard; also known as an *exposure report*

independent-living facility—a group of apartments or houses for residents who can take care of themselves and are mobile, yet need some help with daily activities; it may offer meals and other social activities in a community setting

informed consent—when a patient is presented with information regarding his or her care and voluntarily consents to particular treatments or procedures

initiative—the ability to act and make decisions without the help or advice of others

in-network provider—a health care provider who has a contract with a managed care insurance plan

inpatient—a person who remains in an acute care facility, such as a hospital, for more than 24 hours

in-service education—on-site education and training provided by many hospitals and health care agencies for nurses and others employees

intentional torts—deliberate acts intended to cause harm

interdisciplinary team—a group of health care professionals with varied medical educations, backgrounds, and experiences who work together to deliver the best possible care for each patient

intervention—an active treatment process, such as an exercise to improve muscle extension

intuitive problem solving—a problem-solving method whereby a person instinctively, without logical thinking, identifies a solution to a problem based on its similarity or dissimilarity to other problems

invasion of privacy—when a provider intentionally and unreasonably exposes a patient's body or reveals personal information without the patient's consent

invasive—a medical procedure that requires entering the body by using a tube, needle, or other device

K

kinesics—body movement, including facial expressions, gestures, and eye movement

Korotkoff sounds—the sounds of the heart heard through a stethoscope

L

laissez-faire leadership—a leadership style whereby the leader hands power over to the group members, which encourages independent activity by group members; also known as *nondirective leadership*

leadership—the ability to influence others while working toward a vision or goal

legal guardian—someone appointed by a judge to act for another person, such as a minor or a mentally incompetent adult

libel—when incorrect or damaging information is written about a person

licensed practical nurse (LPN)—a health care professional who performs many of the routine tasks of nursing under the direction of a physician or RN

licensure—the granting of a license to a health care professional who has met the fundamental standards for performing a job, as required by a state

litigation—a legal proceeding in a court

living will—a legal document that indicates what steps, if any, are to be taken in order to save or prolong a person's life

M

malpractice—a failure or negligence of duties or responsibilities on the part of a health care professional that results in injury, loss, or damage

managed care—a type of health insurance plan that establishes predetermined rates for services with health care providers such as doctors and hospitals, and puts providers in the position of managing patients' use of health care

manual dexterity—skill at working with one's hands

Medicaid—a government program that offers health insurance to many low-income and disabled people

medical asepsis—measures taken to control and reduce the number of pathogens present in an area or on an object; commonly called *clean technique*

medical coding—the set of symbols and numbers used to communicate specific treatments and diagnoses between a care facility and payment provider

medical informatics—a broad category of health data and related health care occupations that uses information technology to manage and share files containing medical records, test results, prescription history, billing details, and health insurance coverage; also known as *health informatics*

Medicare—the federally-funded health care program for older Americans

medication administration record (MAR)—a common name in hospitals for a written log of the medications given to a patient

message—the information a sender or source conveys, which begins the communication process

microbiology—the branch of biology that studies microorganisms and their effects on humans

military time—a 24-hour time cycle that counts the hours of the day from 0000 (12:00 a.m.) to 2359 (11:59 p.m.); it is the time-keeping method used by most health care institutions

minority group—a group of people with some physical or cultural characteristics that identify the people within it as different from the dominant group, such as race, religion, beliefs, or customs and practices

modality—a treatment tool, such as a hot or cold pack, whirlpool, nerve stimulation, ultrasound, or traction

morbidity—the incidence of disease in a population

mortality—the incidence of death in a population

multidisciplinary team—a cooperative group that includes professionals with different qualifications, skills, and areas of expertise

mycology—the study of fungi and yeasts

N

narrative format—the oldest and least structured medical documentation style that consists of a paragraph indicating the contact with the patient, what was done for the patient, and what outcomes resulted

negligence—careless or senseless behavior by a practitioner that results in harm

nondirective leadership—a leadership style whereby the leader hands power over to the group members, which encourages independent activity by group members; also known as *laissez-faire leadership*

noninvasive—a medical procedure that doesn't involve entering the body or breaking the skin

non-language sounds—sounds that do not use language but still communicate meaning, such as sighs, sobs, laughs, grunts, and so on

nosocomial infection—a new infection acquired in a health-care facility that is not attributable to a patient's original condition

nuclear medicine—the use of radioactive materials inside the body to create diagnostic images or to treat cancer and other diseases

nurse practice acts—laws established in each state to regulate the practice of nursing

nursing—caring for people who are ill, injured, or unable in some other way to care for themselves

O

Occupational Safety and Health Administration (OSHA)—the main federal agency responsible for ensuring the safety of workers through the enforcement of safety and health legislation

oral—involving the mouth

oral hygiene—keeping one's mouth clean

out-of-network provider—a health care provider who is not in a particular managed care health insurance plan

outpatient—a patient who is discharged within 23 hours, but may require ongoing treatment, care, and education

P

pandemic—an infectious disease that affects entire continents or even the world

paraphrasing—using one's own words or phrases to repeat what one has heard; restating

parasitology—the study of parasitic protozoa and worms

pathogens—disease-causing microorganisms, such as bacteria or viruses

pathology—the study of diseases, particularly their causes and effects

pathophysiology—the study of functional changes in the body as the result of disease

patient monitoring systems—an electronic device that keeps a constant electronic watch over a patient's activities and vital signs

perception phase—a stage of receiving information in which a person gives meaning to the information

periodontal—refers to the gums and bones that support the teeth

pharmaceutical—refers to manufactured medicinal drugs

pharmacology—the study of how drugs act in the body

point-of-service (POS) plan—a physician-coordinated health insurance plan that combines characteristics of both HMO and PPO plans

polysomnography—the study and diagnosis of sleep disorders

preferred provider organization (PPO) plan—a health insurance plan that allows patients to receive care from a non-plan provider, but requires them to pay a higher out-of-pocket price if they do so

premium—the monthly amount paid to a private insurance company for health insurance coverage

private insurance—a health insurance system that allows individuals to obtain group health benefits through an organization, such as an employer, a union, or an association

problem-oriented organization—a method of organizing information in written communication whereby a problem is identified and explained, and then instructions are provided for correcting the problem

professionalism—the demonstration of courteous, conscientious behaviors and qualities by workers in the workplace

prognosis—a medical opinion about the likely outcome of a condition or disease

proprietary institution—a for-profit health care facility, usually owned by a corporation

prospective payment system—a health insurance system that pays the health care provider a fixed amount based on the medical diagnosis or specific procedure, rather than on the actual cost of hospitalization or care; if the actual cost for care is greater than the fixed amount, the provider must absorb the additional expense

proxemics—the study of the spatial separation that individuals naturally maintain; personal space

public law—a body of law that focuses on issues between a government and its citizens

public service—contributing to the good of society through one's work with others

Q

quality assurance (QA)—a program for ensuring high quality performance of all functions in a project or facility

quality control (QC)—a program that monitors each phase of a process to make sure that chemicals and other materials used for tests are of acceptable quality and that instruments are working accurately

R

race—a group of people unified by specific physical characteristics, such as skin pigmentation, body stature, facial features, and hair texture

radiation burn—a lesion that results when the skin is overexposed to ultraviolet light or to radiation; similar to a thermal burn

radionuclide (radioisotope)—an unstable atom of an element that gives off radiation

radiopharmaceutical—a drug used in nuclear medicine imaging that is formed by binding a radionuclide to a stable molecule or compound

reception phase—the first phase of receiving information whereby a person takes in information without yet knowing what it means

reflecting—the communication technique of using open-ended statements to repeat back what has been heard

registered nurse (RN)—a health care professional who has graduated from an accredited nursing program and has been licensed by public authority to practice nursing

registration—a professional designation indicating that a professional has graduated from an accredited school and passed a standardized national exam administered by a nongovernmental agency; the names of professionals who have achieved this status often appear in national registries that can be checked by potential employers

rehabilitation—the restoration, after a disease or injury, of the ability to function in a normal or near-normal manner

rehabilitation center—a health care facility that specializes in services for patients needing physical or emotional rehabilitation or treatment of chemical dependency

reporting systems—In health care, processes and procedures used to collect various types of data pertaining to patient care and supply the data to government agencies and other providers

resource utilization—making better use of health care resources to cut costs

respiratory therapy—the treatment of patients with breathing and other cardiopulmonary disorders

restitution—compensation for a wrongful act that results in harm

root canal—the pulp-filled cavity in the root of a tooth

s

sanitization—the lowest level of infection control, involving the use of soap or detergent to thoroughly clean a surface

scientific problem solving—a systematic, seven-step, problem-solving process that involves problem identification, data collection, hypothesis formulation, plan of action, hypothesis testing, interpretation of results, and evaluation

selection phase—the last phase in the process of receiving information where a person's brain recognizes information as important or unimportant, which affects which pieces of information are remembered

sharps container—a puncture-resistant, leakproof disposable container for sharp items, such as hypodermic needles and scalpels

slander—incorrect or damaging information that is spoken about a person

SOAP format—a documentation format made up of four parts; subjective data, objective data, assessment, and plan

sonography—the use of high-frequency sound waves to produce images of organs and other structures in the body

source—the person or group that begins the communication process by sending a message

sphygmomanometer—a device that is used to measure blood pressure; commonly referred to as a blood pressure cuff

spirometry—a medical test in which a patient breathes into a machine (spirometer) to test lung function

statutory law—laws enacted by federal, state, and local legislators and enforced by the court system

sterile field—the germ-free area around a surgical patient where the operation is performed

sterilization—an infection control method by which all forms of microorganisms, including spores, are destroyed on inanimate objects and surfaces; sterilization is the highest level of infection control

stethoscope—a device that allows health care professionals to listen to the internal sounds of a patient

stress—physical and emotional tension brought on by physical, chemical, or emotional factors

stress test—a medical test that measures the response of the heart muscle to increased demands for oxygen

subacute care facility—a health care facility that fills the gap between hospitalization and rehabilitation, by providing care to patients who are stable and don't need acute care, yet need more complex treatment than can be found in a nursing or rehabilitation facility

subculture—a group of people who are members of a larger cultural group, but whose attitudes and behaviors reflect different beliefs and values from those of the larger culture

support services— a category of health care occupations that provide care to patients either directly or indirectly or create a therapeutic environment for providing health care; examples of professionals in this category are biomedical engineers, biomedical/clinical technicians, and industrial hygienists

suture—materials used to close wounds

T

teamwork—cooperation among team members to accomplish the task at hand

telemedicine—patient home health monitoring that collects data on patients' health from their homes; also known as *tele-monitoring*

telemonitoring —patient home health monitoring that collects data on patients' health from their homes; also known as *telemedicine*

telesurgical monitoring—a branch of medicine that combines multimedia, telecommunications, and robotic technologies to provide surgical care from a distance

therapeutic services—health care services that provide treatment for patients or animals and may also help clients to maintain or improve their health over time

thermal burn—a lesion that results when skin comes in contact with a hot liquid, solid, superheated gas, or flame

time management—the ability to complete work in a timely fashion, while skillfully handling any tasks, concerns, or issues that arise

tort—a wrongful act that results in harm, for which restitution must be made

trial-and-error problem solving—a problem solving technique that involves testing any number of solutions until one is found that solves a particular problem

TRICARE—a government health insurance system that provides medical coverage for active and retired service personnel and their dependents

U

unintentional torts—accidents or mistakes that are not planned or intended that result in harm to another

utilization review—a process in which an insurer reviews decisions by physicians and other providers about how much care to provide

V

value—a belief about the worth or importance of something that acts as a standard to guide one's behavior

value system—a person's ranked personal principles, which often lead to a personal code of conduct

vascular—a medical terms that refers to blood vessels

vector—a vehicle for carrying infection, such as contaminated food or water, disease-carrying insects, or objects like soil, drinking glasses, and improperly disinfected medical instruments

venipuncture—the drawing blood from a vein

virology—the study of viruses

virus—the smallest of all microorganisms

voluntary nonprofit institution—a community facility that receives federal, state, and local tax exemptions in exchange for providing a community benefit, such as services to Medicaid patients and those who are unable to pay

W

ward—a person under the guardianship of another person or government agency

working memory—a concept that describes how the brain stores and retrieves information from short-term and long-term memory

Index

Note: Page numbers followed by *f* indicate figures; those followed by a *t* indicate tables and those followed by a *b* indicate a box.

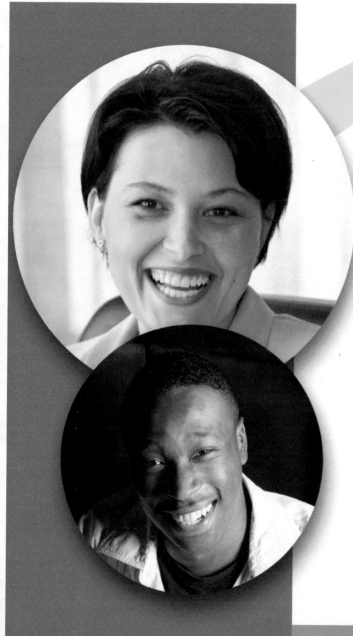
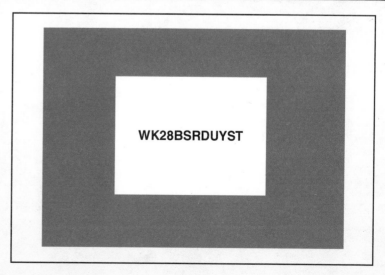